ALLE ZEIT WACH 1842

Cardiomyopathy and Myocardial Biopsy

Edited by
M. Kaltenbach F. Loogen E. G. J. Olsen

With the Collaboration of W.-D. Bussmann

Contributors

H.-J. Knieriem V. J. Ferrans and
H.-J. Becker W. Bircks W. Bleifeld H. Blömer
H.-D. Bolte G. Breithardt C. Brenner W.-D. Bussmann
W. Delius R. Guggenmoos P. Hanrath
D. Harmjanz F. Hehrlein E. H. Herman M. Hopf
R. Hopf M. Kaltenbach M. Keller G. Kober
A. Konrad W. Krelhaus H. Kuhn B. Kunkel
H. Lapp R. Lentz F. Loogen K. Loßnitzer P. Mathes
W. Mohr K. L. Neuhaus E. G. J. Olsen Y. Petersen
H. E. Riemann G. Sauer J. Schaper A. Schinz
W. Schmidt H. D. Schulte F. Schwarz H. Sebening
L. Seipel P. Spiller K.-U. Thiedemann A. Wirtzfeld

With 203 Figures

Springer-Verlag
Berlin Heidelberg New York 1978

Prof. Dr. med. M. KALTENBACH
Zentrum der Inneren Medizin,
Abteilung für Kardiologie,
Klinikum der Johann Wolfgang Goethe-Universität
Theodor-Stern-Kai 7
6000 Frankfurt/Main 70

Prof. Dr. med. F. LOOGEN
Direktor der I. Med. Klinik B der Universität Düsseldorf
Moorenstraße 5
4000 Düsseldorf 1

Dr. E.G.J. OLSEN, M.D., M.R.C.Path.
Consultant Pathologist
Department of Anatomy and Histology,
National Heart Hospital
Westmoreland Street
London W1M 8 BA

Priv.-Doz. Dr. med. W.-D. BUSSMANN
Zentrum der Inneren Medizin,
Abteilung für Kardiologie,
Klinikum der Johann Wolfgang Goethe-Universität
Theodor-Stern-Kai 7
6000 Frankfurt/Main 70

ISBN-13:978-3-642-66774-9 e-ISBN-13:978-3-642-66772-5
DOI: 10.1007/978-3-642-66772-5

Library of Congress Cataloging in Publication Data. Main entry under title: Cardiomyopathy and myocardial biopsy. Bibliography: p. Includes index. 1. Heart-Muscle-Diseases-Diagnosis. 2. Heart-Biopsy. I. Kaltenbach, Martin. II. Loogen, Franz, 1919. (DNLM: 1. Myocardial diseases, Primary-Diagnosis. 2. Biopsy-Methods. WG280 C268) RC685.M9C37 616.1'24'0758 77-13242.

Softcover reprint of the hardcover 1st edition 1978

Reproduction of the figures: Gustav Dreher GmbH, Stuttgart

2127-3130-543210

Foreword

The aim of this book is to give an up to date account of recent developments in the field of cardiomyopathy. Many authors, all experienced workers in their fields, – most from Germany – have contributed to this volume.

It would appear that the diagnosis of cardiomyopathy is now made more often than it was 10 years ago. The reason for this is probably not that the incidence of the disease has increased, but that it is better recognized. Where conventional clinical investigation may have failed to define the underlying disease process in a given patient, improved or more widely used diagnostic tools, such as selective coronary arteriography and endomyocardial biopsies, have contributed greatly to proper diagnosis. Furthermore, uniformity of terminology has also taken place during the last few years, permitting more accurate categorization of patients suffering from this entity. The difficult subject of terminology is discussed in a special section.

The first part of this volume, devoted to experimental cardiomyopathies, emphasizes the changes on the myocardium that may occur as the result of various agents. Next the technical aspects of obtaining fresh endomyocardial biopsies and the pathologic information that can be obtained, together with the prognostic significance of the biopsy material, is discussed in detail. The influence of hypertrophy and ischemia on human myocardium has also been highlighted in two chapters. Ventricular functional studies and angiography, noninvasive methods and other diagnostic procedures are also discussed in detail. The last section of the book deals with the natural history and the indications for surgical and medical treatment of hypertrophic obstructive cardiomyopathy.

We hope that this book will be of value to teachers, students and practitioners, not only those actively engaged in cardiology or the related specialities, but also those colleagues concerned with the clinical and pathologic diagnosis and treatment of cardiac disease with which they may occasionally come into contact.

M. Kaltenbach
F. Loogen
E. G. J. Olsen

Contents

Congestive Cardiomyopathy

Hypertrophic Obstructive Cardiomyopathy

List of Contributors

H.-J. BECKER, Priv.-Doz. Dr. med., Stadtkrankenhaus Hanau, Leimenstr. 20, 6450 Hanau

W. BIRCKS, Prof. Dr. med., Chirurgische Universitätsklinik Düsseldorf, Moorenstr. 5, 4000 Düsseldorf 1

W. BLEIFELD, Prof. Dr. med., II. Med. Klinik, Abt. Kardio/Angiologie, Universitätskrankenhaus Eppendorf, Martinistr. 52, 2000 Hamburg 20

H. BLÖMER, Prof. Dr. med., I. Med. Klinik rechts der Isar der Technischen Universität München, Ismaningerstr. 22, 8000 München 80

H.-D. BOLTE, Prof. Dr. med., Med. Klinik I, Klinikum Großhadern, Marchioninistr. 15, 8000 München

G. BREITHARDT, Dr. med., I. Med. Klinik B der Universität Düsseldorf, Moorenstr. 5, 4000 Düsseldorf 1

C. BRENNER, Dr. med., I. Med. Klinik B der Universität Düsseldorf, Moorenstr. 5, 4000 Düsseldorf 1

W.-D. BUSSMANN, Priv.-Doz. Dr. med., Zentrum der Inneren Medizin, Abteilung für Kardiologie, Klinikum der Johann Wolfgang Goethe-Universität, Theodor Stern-Kai 7, 6000 Frankfurt 70

W. DELIUS, Priv.-Doz. Dr. med., I. Med. Klinik rechts der Isar der Technischen Universität München, Ismaningerstr. 22, 8000 München 80

V. J. FERRANS, MD, Ph. D. Pathology Branch, National Heart and Lung Institute, National Institutes of Health, Bethesda, MD, 20014/USA

R. GUGGENMOOS, Dr. med., Kurotel 2002, Postfach 2002, 8730 Bad Kissingen

P. HANRATH, Priv.-Doz. Dr. med., II. Med. Klinik, Abt. Kardio/Angiologie, Universitätskrankenhaus Eppendorf, Martinistr. 52, 2000 Hamburg 20

D. HARMJANZ, Prof. Dr. med., Facharzt Innere Medizin, Chefarzt der Kardiologischen Abteilung des Allgemeinen Krankenhauses Celle, Siemensplatz 4, 3100 Celle

F. HEHRLEIN, Prof. Dr. med., Thoraxchirurgische Abteilung, Zentrum d. Chir. Klinikums der Universität, 6300 Gießen

E. H. HERMAN, Dr. med., Pathology Branch, National Heart and Lung Institute, National Institutes of Health, Bethesda, MD, 20014/USA

M. HOPF, Zentrum der Inneren Medizin, Abteilung für Kardiologie, Klinikum der Johann Wolfgang Goethe-Universität, Theodor Stern-Kai 7, 6000 Frankfurt 70

R. HOPF, Dr. med., Zentrum der Inneren Medizin, Abteilung für Kardiologie, Klinikum der Johann Wolfgang Goethe-Universität, Theodor Stern-Kai 7, 6000 Frankfurt 70

M. KALTENBACH, Prof. Dr. med., Zentrum der Inneren Medizin, Abteilung für Kardiologie, Klinikum der Johann Wolfgang Goethe-Universität, Theodor Stern-Kai 7, 6000 Frankfurt 70

M. KELLER, Zentrum der Inneren Medizin, Abteilung Kardiologie, Klinikum der Johann Wolfgang Goethe-Universität, Theodor Stern-Kai 7, 6000 Frankfurt 70

H.-J. KNIERIEM, Prof. Dr. med., Chefarzt des Institutes für Pathologie, Ev. Krankenhaus Bethesda, Heerstr. 219, 4100 Duisburg 1

G. KOBER, Prof. Dr. med., Zentrum der Inneren Medizin, Abteilung für Kardiologie, Klinikum der Johann Wolfgang Goethe-Universität, Theodor Stern-Kai 7, 6000 Frankfurt 70

A. KONRAD, Dr. med., Kurotel 2002, Postfach 2002, 8730 Bad Kissingen

W. KRELHAUS, Dr. med., I. Med. Klinik B der Universität Düsseldorf, Moorenstr. 5, 4000 Düsseldorf 1

H. KUHN, Priv.-Doz. Dr. med., I. Med. Klinik B der Universität Düsseldorf, Moorenstr. 5, 4000 Düsseldorf 1

B. KUNKEL, Dr. med., Zentrum der Inneren Medizin, Abteilung für Kardiologie, Klinikum der Johann Wolfgang Goethe-Universität, Theodor Stern-Kai 7, 6000 Frankfurt 70

H. LAPP, Prof. Dr. med., Abteilung II des Zentrums der Pathologie, Klinikum der Johann Wolfgang Goethe-Universität, Theodor Stern-Kai 7, 6000 Frankfurt 70

R. LENTZ, Dr. med., Zentrum der Inneren Medizin, Abteilung für Kardiologie, Klinikum der Johann Wolfgang Goethe-Universität, Theodor Stern-Kai 7, 6000 Frankfurt 70

F. LOOGEN, Prof. Dr. med., Direktor der I. Med. Klinik B der Universität Düsseldorf, Moorenstr. 5, 4000 Düsseldorf 1

K. LOSSNITZER, Priv.-Doz. Dr. med., Medizinische Klinik der Bundesknappschaft, 6603 Sulzbach

P. MATHES, Priv.-Doz. Dr. med., I. Med. Klinik rechts der Isar der Technischen Universität München, Ismaningerstr. 22, 8000 München 80

W. Mohr, Dr. med., Kurotel 2002, Postfach 2002, 8730 Bad Kissingen

K. L. Neuhaus, Dr. med., I. Med. Klinik B der Universität Düsseldorf, Moorenstr. 5, 4000 Düsseldorf 1

E. G. J. Olsen, MD, M.R.C. Path., Department of Anatomy and Histology, National Heart Hospital, Westmoreland Street, GB London WIM 8 BA

Y. Petersen, Zentrum der Inneren Medizin, Abteilung für Kardiologie, Klinikum der Johann Wolfgang Goethe-Universität, Theodor Stern-Kai 7, 6000 Frankfurt 70

H. E. Riemann, Prof. Dr. med., Abteilung für Allgemeine Röntgendiagnostik, Zentrum der Radiologie, Klinikum der Johann Wolfgang Goethe-Universität, Theodor Stern-Kai 7, 6000 Frankfurt 70

G. Sauer, Dr. med., I. Med. Klinik B der Universität Düsseldorf, Moorenstr. 5, 4000 Düsseldorf 1

Jutta Schaper, Dr. med., Max-Planck-Institut für Physiologische und Klinische Forschung, W. G. Kerckhoff-Institut, Abteilung für Experimentelle Kardiologie, Sprudelhof 11, 6350 Bad Nauheim

A. Schinz, Dr. med., I. Med. Klinik rechts der Isar der Technischen Universität München, Ismaningerstr. 22, 8000 München 80

W. Schmidt, Zentrum der Inneren Medizin, Abteilung für Kardiologie, Klinikum der Johann Wolfgang Goethe-Universität, Theodor Stern-Kai 7, 6000 Frankfurt 70

H. D. Schulte, Dr. med., I. Med. Klinik B der Universität Düsseldorf, Moorenstr. 5, 4000 Düsseldorf 1

F. Schwarz, Dr. med., Max-Planck-Institut für Physiologische und Klinische Forschung, W. G. Kerckhoff-Institut, Abteilung für Experimentelle Kardiologie, Sprudelhof 11, 6350 Bad Nauheim

H. Sebening, Priv.-Doz. Dr. med., I. Med. Klinik rechts der Isar der Technischen Universität München, Ismaningerstr. 22, 8000 München 80

L. Seipel, Priv.-Doz. Dr. med., I. Med. Klinik B der Universität Düsseldorf, Moorenstr. 5, 4000 Düsseldorf 1

P. Spiller, Dr. med., I. Med. Klinik B der Universität Düsseldorf, Moorenstr. 5, 4000 Düsseldorf 1

K.-U. Thiedemann, Dr. med., Max-Planck-Institut für Physiologische und Klinische Forschung, W. G. Kerckhoff-Institut, Abteilung für Experimentelle Kardiologie, Sprudelhof 11, 6350 Bad Nauheim

A. Wirtzfeld, Prof. Dr. med., I. Med. Klinik rechts der Isar der Technischen Universität München, Ismaningerstr. 22, 8000 München 80

Terminology

M. KALTENBACH

The terminology of cardiomyopathy, diseases not secondary to coronary heart disease, rheumatic or congenital heart disease, or arterial or pulmonary hypertension, is still rather confusing. Primarily because of the difficulty in defining this disease of which so little is known. Even the accuracy of the term *cardiomyopathy* is debatable and perhaps should be replaced more accurately by *myocardiopathy*. Furthermore, several names are often applied to the same type of cardiomyopathy. For example, muscular subaortic stenosis, idiopathic-hypertrophic subaortic stenosis, asymmetrical septal hypertrophy, and hypertrophic-obstructive cardiomyopathy apply to one disease entity and mean essentially the same thing. If it becomes clear that subaortic stenosis is only a more or less incidental finding, the term hypertrophic-obstructive cardiomyopathy would seem more appropriate. However, it may be necessary to change the name again since several authors have shown that the myocardium may only be one manifestation of a general disorder of the skeletal and cardiac muscles.

Based on clinical and hemodynamic findings, the classification of Goodwin and co-workers is that primarily used in Europe today. Three forms of cardiomyopathies are recognized:

Congestive, "dilated" cardiomyopathy (COCM)
Hypertrophic-obstructive cardiomyopathy (HOCM)
Restrictive-obliterative, constrictive cardiomyopathy (ROCM).

Alcohol-induced cardiomyopathy can be cited as a typical example of *congestive dilated cardiomyopathy*. Adriamycin-induced cardiomyopathy is another example of toxically induced damage to the myocardium, resulting in a dilated heart. Occasionally COCM may occur as a consequence of severe diffuse myocarditis, for example, as a final stage after diphtheric or virus myocarditis. In some patients a genetically determined origin is apparent (the familial form of COCM). In most patients, however, the etiology of the disease is unknown.

Apart from congestive heart failure, a manifestation of the late stage of the disease, the dilated left ventricle is the primary symptom. The left ventricular wall may be thickened as a consequence of hypertrophy, it may be normal, or it may even be thinner, in relation to the left ventricular diameter. However, left ventricular muscle mass is usually increased.

Therefore, the term congestive, dilated cardiomyopathy seems most appropriate.

Hypertrophic-obstructive cardiomyopathy can occur with or without subaortic stenosis, i.e., with or without an intraventricular systolic pressure gradient. Some patients, under resting conditions, do not show a gradient but on stimulation with substances such as catecholamines, show a marked or even very high gradient.

Some patients have significant mitral regurgitation, while others do not. Based on anatomic findings, forms with or without involvement of the free left ventricular wall – in addition to septal hypertrophy – have also been differentiated.

The left ventricle is approximately normal size with tendency to small enddiastolic and endsystolic volume. The thickness of the interventricular septum is almost always increased, and the free left ventricular wall is usually thicker than normal, with a ratio often exceeding 1.4 : 1.

The disease occurs frequently in several members of a family, according to some investigators, in over 50% of cases. Therefore a hereditary origin seems probable.

Restrictive-constrictive, obliterative cardiomyopathy is a heterogeneous group including primary and secondary myocardial diseases. Most are secondary, including sarcoidosis, lymphogranulomatosis, amyloidosis, and hemochromatosis. Inflammatory diseases such as myopericarditis and Löffler's disease are also included, as well as fibroelastosis of the endocardium.

This book is concerned with recent advances in congestive, dilated cardiomyopathy and the hypertrophic-obstructive form, while the restrictive/obliterative/constrictive type is only occasionally referred to.

Some differences in terminology occur in this book, an indication that the subject of cardiomyopathy is continually changing as our understanding increases. Of necessity, this will result in changes in terminology.

Forms of Cardiomyopathies

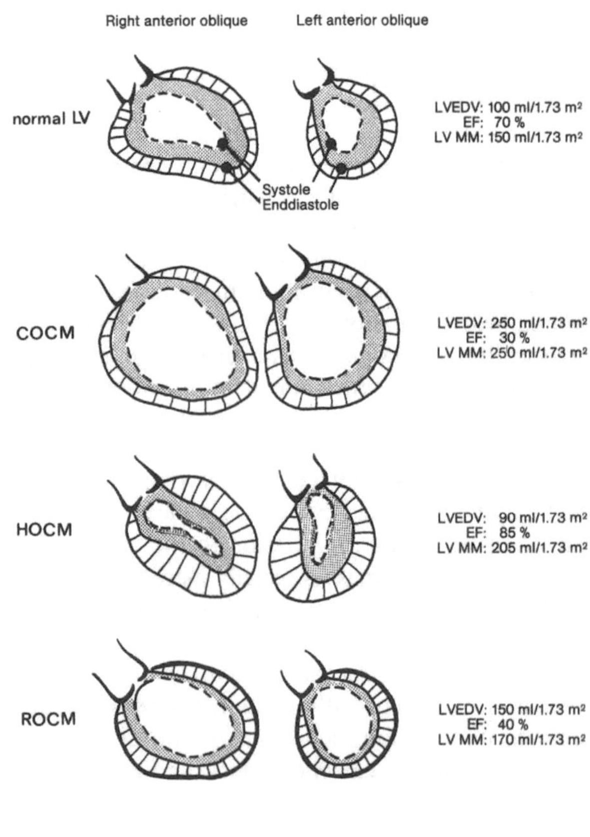

Classification of Cardiomyopathies

1. Idiopathic CM (> 50%)
2. Genetic CM, e.g., familial HOCM, familial COCM
3. Secondary CM

Infectious, infectious-toxic: Viral; Bacterial; Chagas'; Löffler's

Toxic: Alcohol, cobalt, narcotics, psycholeptics, adriamycin

Systemic disease: Sarcoidosis; Lymphogranulomatosis; Lupus erythematosus

Storage disease: Hemochromatosis; Amyloidosis

Neuromuscular: Progressive muscular dystrophy; HOCM?

Endocrine-metabolic: Hyperthyroidism; Acromegaly; Uremia

Reference

Goodwin, J. F.: Congestive and hypertrophic cardiomyopathies: A decade of study. Lancet *1970/I* 731

List of Abbreviations

The abbreviations are used herein both as the noun and adjective forms, e.g., CM stands for cardiomyopathy and cardiomyopathic

A–H	atrio-His interval
AS	aortic valve stenosis
ASH	asymmetric septal hypertrophy
CHD	coronary heart disease
CI	cardiac index
CM	cardiomyopathy, cardiomyopathic
COCM	congestive (dilated) cardiomyopathy
CT	cardiothoracic ratio
D/W	ratio of enddiastolic diameter to wall thickness
dp/dt_{max}	maximal rate of left ventricular pressure rise
ECG	electrocardiogram
EDP	enddiastolic pressure
EDV	enddiastolic volume
EDVI	endiastolic volume index
EF	ejection fraction
EMCB	endomyocardial catheter biopsy
ESV	endsystolic volume
ESVI	endsystolic volume index
HBE	His bundle electrogram
HNCM	hypertrophic nonobstructive cardiomyopathy
HOCM	hypertrophic-obstructive cardiomyopathy
IHSS	idiopathic hypertrophic subaortic stenosis
IP	instantaneous pressure
LAO	left anterior oblique
LBBB	left bundle branch block
LCM	latent cardiomyopathy
LV	left ventricle, left ventricular
LVEDP	left ventricular end-diastolic pressure
LVEDV	left ventricular end-diastolic volume
LVEDVI	left ventricular end-diastolic volume index
LVESVI	left ventricular endsystolic volume index
LVMM	left ventricular muscle mass
LVP	left ventricular systolic pressure
max dP/dt	maximal rate of left ventricular pressure rise
NYHA	New York Heart Association
RAO	right anterior oblique
RBBB	right bundle branch block
ROCM	restrictive obliterative (constrictive) cardiomyopathy
SAM	systolic anterior motion
SR	sarcoplasmic reticulum
SVI	stroke volume index
V_{cf}	velocity of circumferential fiber shortening
V_{pm}	peak measured velocity of contractile elements

Experimental Cardiomyopathies

1. Morphologic Changes of the Myocardium Induced by Different Toxic Agents

H.-J. Knieriem

Many poisons and toxic agents, such as arsenic, lead, and mercury, or drugs, such as chinidine, digitalis, and isoproterenol, can effect the myocardium either directly or indirectly by interfering with cell metabolism. Changes of the electrolyte content (e.g., potassium, sodium, calcium, and chloride) can decrease the efficiency of the myocardial cell. In addition, toxic agents may damage the endothelium of intramural vessels and consequently induce microcirculatory disturbances and ischemic lesions of the myocardium. As the result of the various morphologic effects, disseminated necroses, degenerative fatty degenerations, and hemorrhages can be found. Late sequelae or remnants of the toxic damage include dissiminated foci of fibrosis, small scars, and microcalcifications [18].

With regard to the differentiation of primary and secondary CMs the effects of ethanol are of particular importance. Alcoholic CM seems today the main differential diagnosis of COCM. In addition, primary toxic effect, of alcohol and also malnutrition (protein- and/or thiamine deficiency) must be considered. Furthermore, alcoholic CM can be complicated by additional toxic substances, such as cobalt, nickel, and arsenic.

The relationship between chronic alcoholism and heart disease was recognized as early as 1873 by Walshe and in 1884 by Bollinger and in 1929 by Aalsmer and Wenckebach. Historical descriptions make it obvious that quite different alcohol-induced alterations have been observed and described. In Munich beer heart (Bollinger) the tremendous volume load (up to 30 liters/day) in addition to the toxic effect of ethanol may be responsible for the cardiomegaly. Wenckebach recognized the relationship between alcoholic heart disease and the beri-beri heart disease, therefore explaining findings caused by thiamine deficiency. The observations of various Tubingian wine hearts (Münzinger) also showed side effects caused by chronic arsenic intoxication, similar to those seen in the 1930s in Scotland.

Today the spectrum of the disease "alcoholic CM" is still complex. New toxic agents such as cobalt and drugs are enhancing or masking the effect of ethanol.

Today, at least four groups of alcoholic CMs can be distinguished. 1. alcoholic CM caused by thiamine deficiency (substitution of thiamine is effective therapy); 2. alcoholic CM caused by thiamine deficiency *and* protein deficiency as observed in malnourished patients. Today these two groups of patients account for only about 10–15% of alcoholic CMs according to the social status and living conditions of these patients. But the disease can still be observed in chronic alcoholics who obtain almost their total calory requirements by alcohol. The largest group of patients today is the third group which is comprised of well-nourished alcoholics without protein or thiamine deficiency. In these patients the toxic effect of ethanol will be the primary cause of the CM, although not every alcoholic will suffer of alcoholic heart disease (only about 20%). With regard to alcoholic liver disease an average consumption of alcohol of about 100 g/day will be sufficient to produce liver disease. Restoration of the impaired ventricular function can be observed after withdrawal of alcohol. Also the electron-microscopic cell changes induced by alcohol are reversible [11, 16].

Electron-microscopic studies of human myocardial tissues of chronic alcoholics, particularly of persons who have consumed beverages, such as liquor or whiskey for many years, have shown an augmentation of large mitochondria [2, 9]. Some of these patients were not well-nourished, therefore additional protein or thiamine deficiency has to be taken into account. Almost the same increase and enlargement of mitochondria in the myocardium has been observed by us after observing experimental thiamine deficiency in rats (Fig. 1) [4]. The augmentation of mitochondria was confirmed by quantitative analyses. The ratio of mitochondria to myofibrils was increased. On the other hand biochemical studies demonstrated a marked decrease of pyruvate dehydrogenase activity in the myocardium as well as in the brain and liver. Even a single dose of thiamine given at the height of the thiamine deficiency caused regression of the morphologic changes and a normalization of the enzyme activity. Therefore, we presume that during thiamine deficiency there is an increase of insufficiently functioning mitochondria. The augmentation of such mitochondria may be interpreted as an adaptation of the myocardium according to the metabolic-energetic insufficiency caused by thiamine deficiency. In other cases foci of mycotolysis and degenerative changes of the myocardial cells have been described [2, 5, 9]. In myocardial biopsy specimen of chronic alcoholics intracellular fatty degeneration can also be observed. We have injected a 20% ethanol solution intravenously in rats for a period of 15 minutes [16]. Electron microscopically we found focal and mostly partial swelling of mitochondria within the myocardium of the left ventricle, septum and atria (Fig. 2). Fusion of their cristae, slight dilatation of sarcoplasmic reticulum, and edema of endothelial cells was also observed. These changes were reversible, as demonstrated in human subjects by Harmjanz and Klein. Therefore it seems unlikely that single acute alcoholic intoxications alone may induce progressive alcoholic CM.

New aspects of alcoholic CM were observed in 1965 and 1966 in the United States, Canada, and Belgium when many people died after the consumption of beer which contained cobalt chloride as an additive for foam stabilization. As in humans we could demonstrate within the myocardium of rats, treated with repeated injections of cobalt chloride, disseminated or even extensive necroses of the myocardium [14, 10]. Electron microscopy revealed severe swellings of mitochondria, dilatation of sarcoplasmic reticulum, disintegration of myofibrils as well as edema of endothelial cells. In addition electron-dense particles were found within the swollen mitochondria of those animals receiving 200–240 mg $CoCl_2$/kg for 10–15 days (Fig. 3). The content of cobalt within the myocardium and within the mitochondria was significantly increased, as was the cobalt/calcium ratio. The animals died because of heart failure induced by the withdrawal of calcium, causing an inhibited utilization of high-energy phosphates.

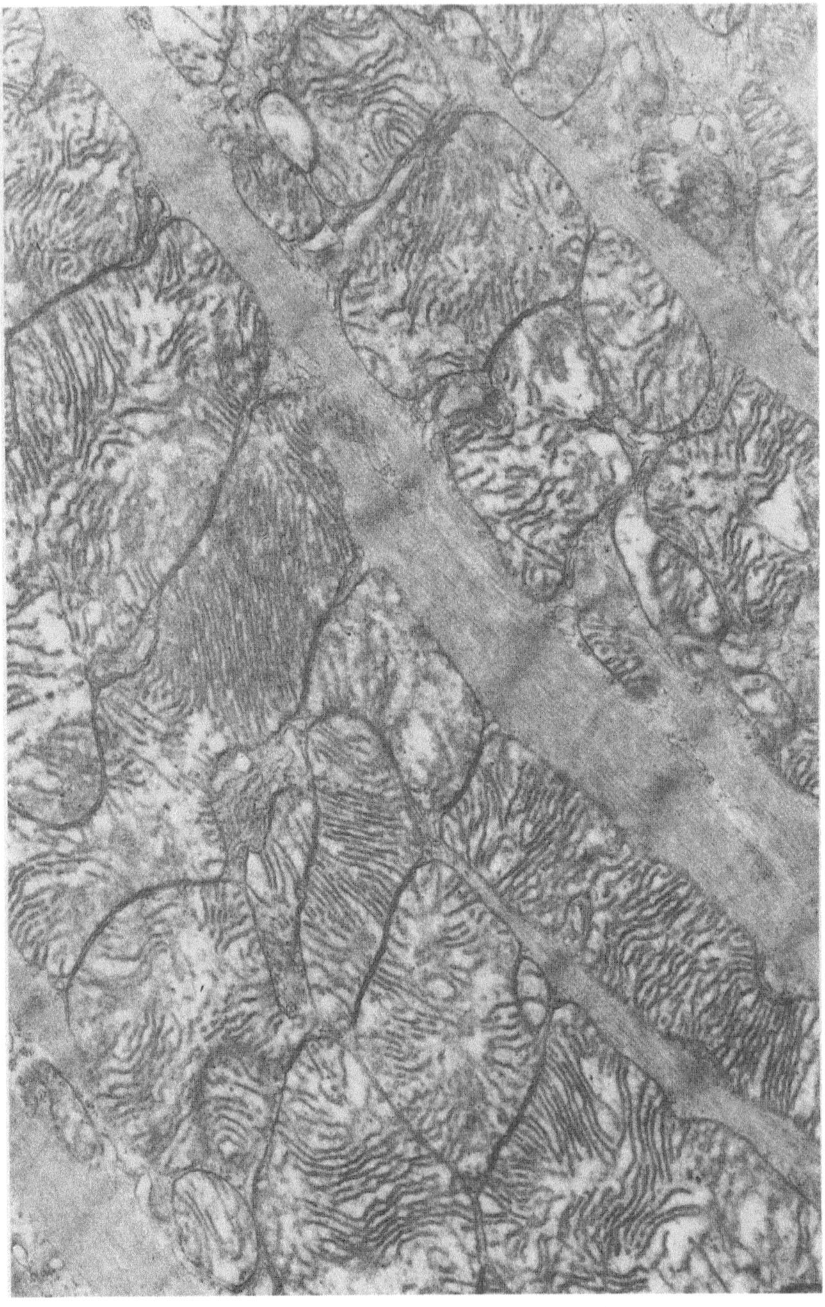

Fig. 1. Thiamine deficiency in the rat. Marked augmentation and enlargement of mitochondria between small myofibrils within myocardial cells. ×23000

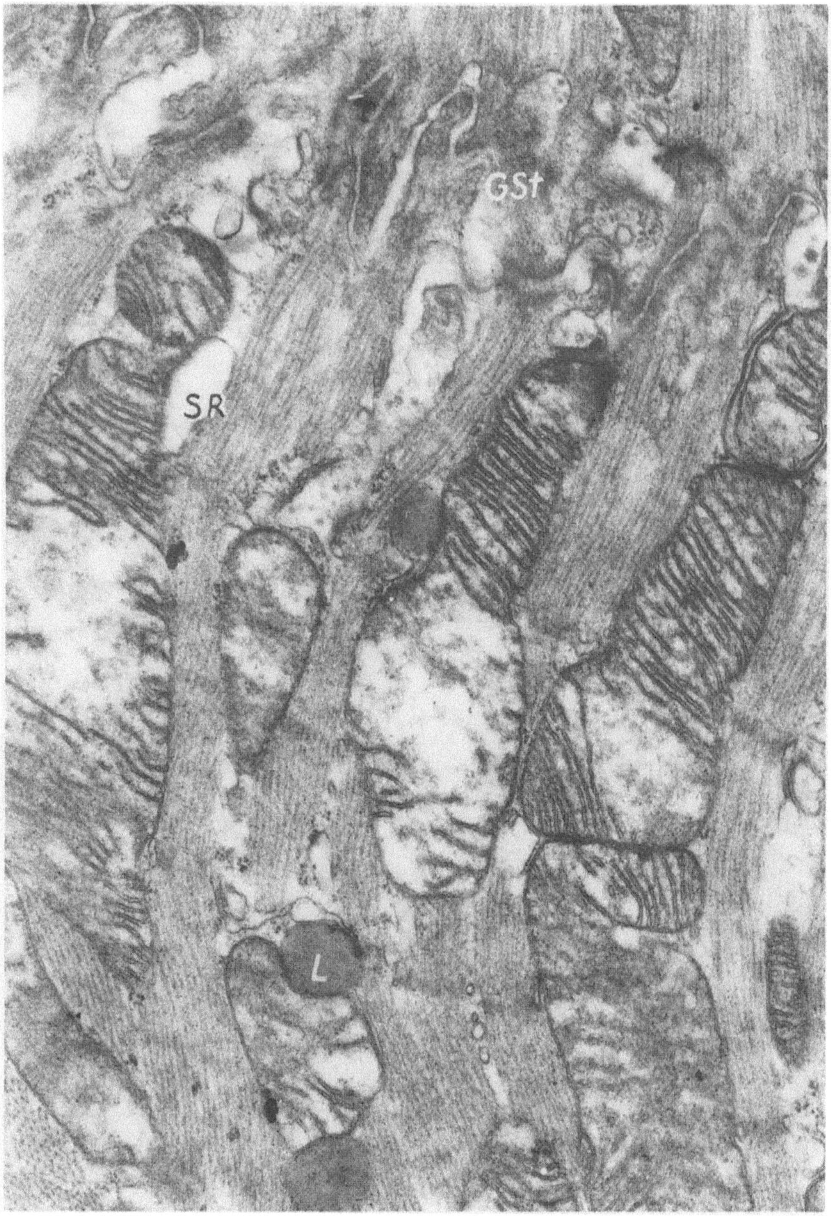

Fig. 2. Partial swelling of mitochondria in myocardial cells of the rat after infusion of 20% ethanol solution i.v. Slight dilatation of sarcoplasmic reticulum (*SR*) and intracellular lipid droplets (*L*). Intercalated disc (*GSt*). ×32000

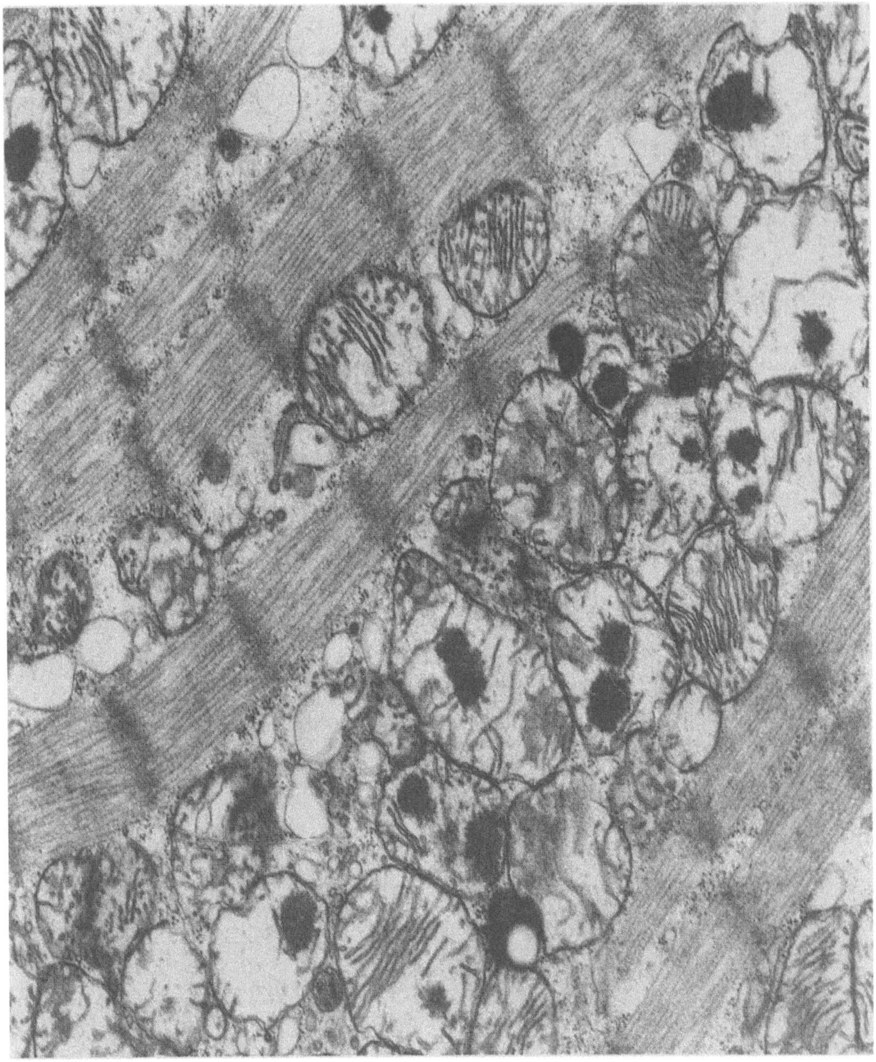

Fig. 3. Numerous osmiophilic particles (cobalt-calcium precipitations) within swollen and enlarged mitochondria of myocardial cells of the rat after repeated intraperitoneal injections of cobalt chloride solutions. × 22500

In myocardial biopsy specimens from human alcoholics we found either uncharacteristic morphologic changes, such as fatty degeneration of myocardial cells or other degenerative alterations of cell organelles similar to those found in CM (Fig. 4). As already mentioned, alcoholic CM can be further complicated by not only additives within the alcoholic beverages but by additional drugs abuse. We must be aware that in some individuals we not may be able to distinguish clearly all the different toxic agents affecting the myocardium.

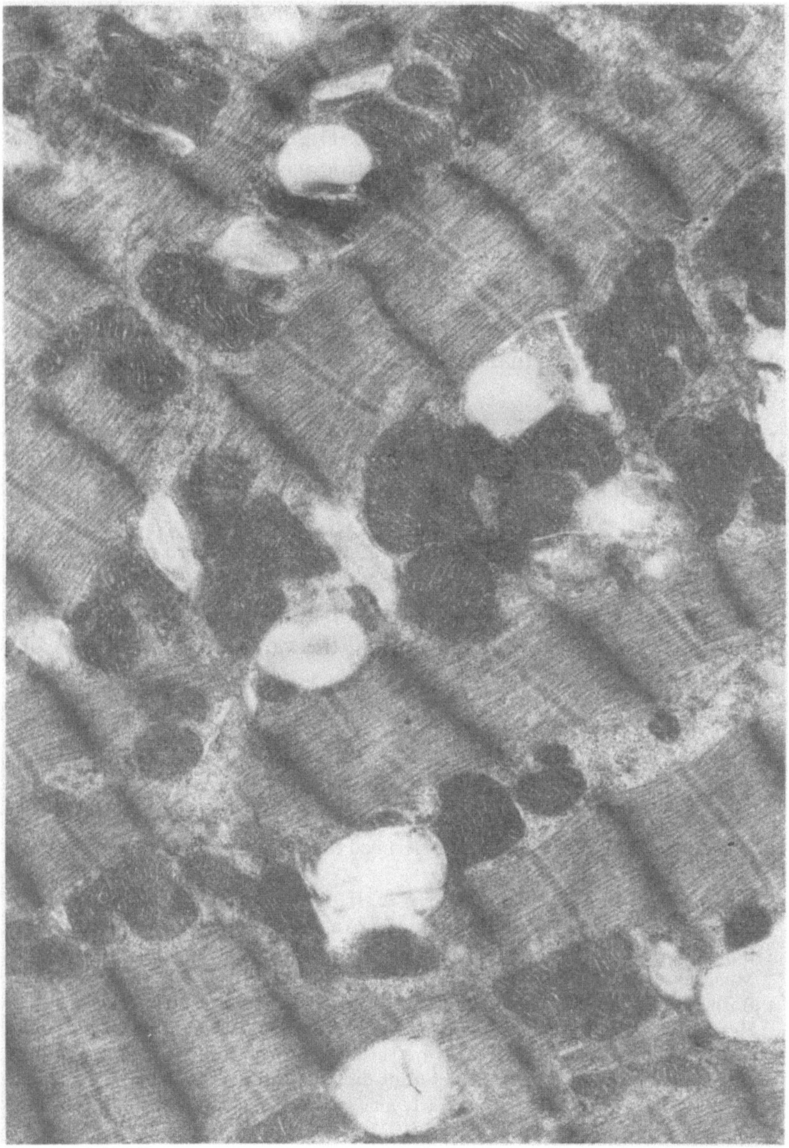

Fig. 4. Human myocardial biopsy specimen from right ventricle. Numerous intracellular lipid droplets within the cytoplasm in a case of presumed alcoholic COCM. ×14400

Changes of electrolyte concentrations may cause severe myocardial damage, depending on dosage and time of action. Myocardial necroses as a result of hyperkalaemia are well known. Increase in sodium and chloride may also lead to severe changes in the myocardium, especially a marked dilatation of the sarcoplasmic and tubular system of the myocardial cells. Such marked changes of the tubular system of the myocardium of dogs, treated by intravenous infusions of 30% sodium chloride solutions can be seen on Fig. 5. The animals died of ventricular flutter or energetic-hypodynamic heart failure.

Isoproterenol also can cause different myocardial changes according to the dosage and time of treatment [22, 7]. High doses of isoproterenol (Alupent, Aludrine, and epinephrine) will cause increased contractions of the myocardial cells. Electron microscopically, several, and often large herniations of sarcoplasmic bags protruding from one myocardial cell into the other are seen (Fig. 6) [20]. Such changes may sometimes also be present in biopsy specimen, if certain drugs are given prior to catheterization or if the biopsy procedure has taken place in a certain increased contractility stage. Higher doses of isoproterenol leads to disseminated necroses of the myocardium as well as to changes of the mitochondria.

Steroid CM has been extensively investigated by Selye. In our experiments we can confirm that corticosteroids alone may not produce myocardial damage, but necroses of the myocardium will occur if sodiumphosphate salts are also given [23, 21].

Morphologic findings of drug-induced CMs will be described in Chapter 2. The morphologic findings briefly described here should be taken as a short review of the multifactorial problems of "CM". Clinicians as well as morphologists must search intensively to reveal the various noxae which can complicate or obscure the disease picture.

References

1. Aalsmer, W.C., Wenckebach, K.R.: Herz und Kreislauf bei der Beri-Beri-Krankheit. Wien. Arch. inn. Med. *16*, 193 (1929)
2. Alexander, C.S.: Idiopathic heart disease. II. Electronmicroscopic examination of myocardial biopsy specimens in alcoholic heart disease. Amer. J. Med. *41*, 229 (1966)
3. Bollinger, O.: Über die Häufigkeit und Ursachen der idiopathischen Herzhypertrophie in München. Dtsch. med. Wschr. *12*, 180 (1884)
4. Bozner, A., Knieriem, H.-J., Meessen, H., Reinauer, H.: Die Ultrastruktur und Biochemie des Herzmuskels der Ratte im Thiaminmangel und nach einer Gabe von Thiamin. Virchows Arch. Abt. B Zellpath. *2*, 125 (1969)
5. Brigden, W., Robinson, J.: Alcohol heart disease. Brit. med. J. 1964 II 1283
6. Csapo, Z., Dusek, J., Rona, G.: Early alterations of the cardiac muscle cells in isoproterenol-induced necrosis. Arch. Path. *93*, 365 (1972)
7. Ferrans, V.J., Hibbs, R.G., Walsh, J.J.: Histochemical and electron microscopial studies on the cardiac necroses produced by sympathomimetic agents. Ann. N. Y. Acad. Sci. *156*, 309 (1969)
8. Hecht, A.: Einführung in experimentelle Grundlagen moderner Herzmuskelpathologie. Jena: VEB Fischer 1971
9. Hibbs, R.G., Ferrans, V.J., Black, W.C., Weilbacher, D.G., Walsh, J.J., Burch, G.E.: Alcoholic cardiomyopathy. An electronmicroscopic study. Amer. Heart J. *69*, 766 (1965)
10. Kasperek, K., Siller, V., Knieriem, H.-J.: Neutronenaktivierungsanalytische Bestimmung von Kobalt und Calcium bei der experimentellen Herzinsuffizienz durch Kobaltchlorid. Z. ges. exp. Med. *150*, 316 (1969)
11. Klein, H., Harmjanz, D.: Effect of ethanol infusion on the ultrastructure of human myocardium. Postgrad. med. J. *51*, 325 (1975)
12. Knieriem, H.-J.: Morphologische Grundlagen der Herzhypertrophie. Verh. dtsch. Ges. Kreisl.-Forsch. *38*, 1 (1972)

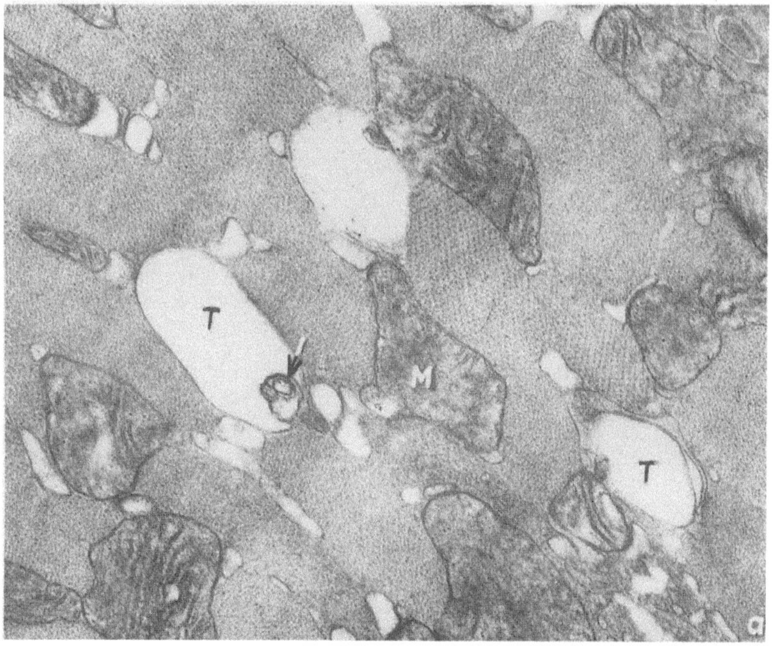

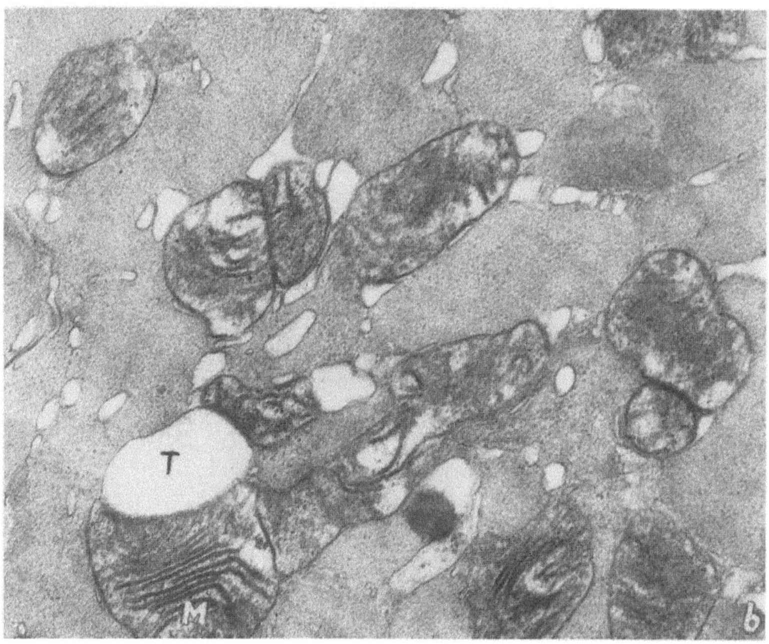

Fig. 5. Marked dilatation of the tubular system (I) within the myocardial cells of the dog after i.v. infusions of 30% sodium chloride solutions. Increased density of shrunken mitochondria. ×16500

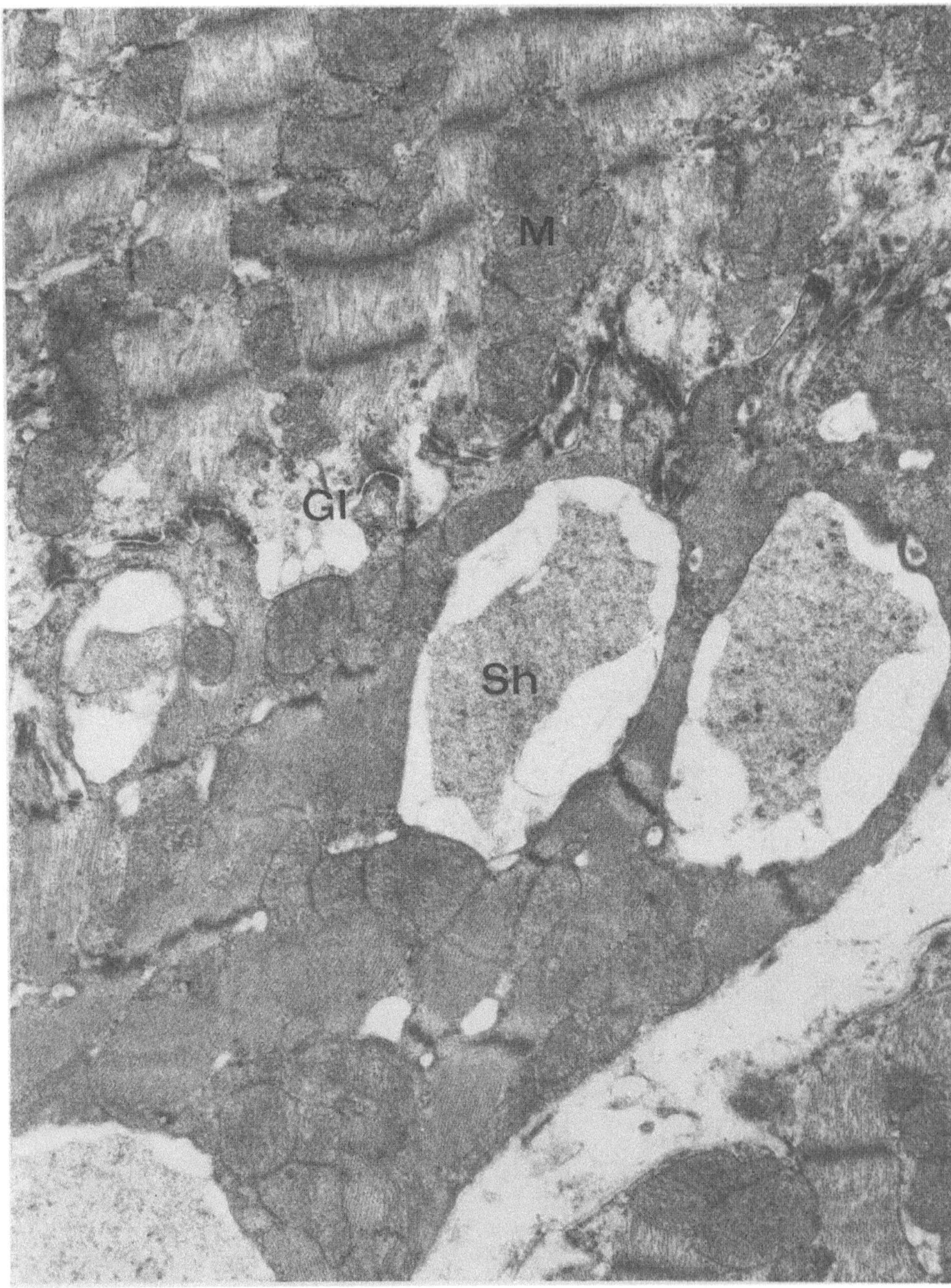

Fig. 6. Herniation of sarcoplasmic bags (*Sh*) and vacuoles in the immediate vicinity of the intercalated disc (*GL*) of the myocardial cells of the rat after 2 days of isoproterenol injections. Mitochondria (*M*). ×15600

13. Knieriem, H.-J.: Zur Differentialdiagnose zwischen Myokarditis und idiopathischer Kardiomyopathie aus pathologisch-anatomischer Sicht. Therapiewoche *24*, 1054 (1974)
14. Knieriem, H.-J., Herbertz, G.: Elektronenmikroskopische Befunde sowie photometrische und aktivierungsanalytische Ergebnisse bei experimenteller Herzinsuffizienz durch Kobaltchlorid. Virchows Arch. Abt. B *2*, 32 (1969)
15. Knieriem, H.-J., Krayenbühl, H.P., Meessen, H., Mehmel, H.: Die Ultrastruktur des Myokards bei experimenteller Herzinsuffizienz durch hypertone Kochsalzinfusionen. Z. Kreisl.-Forsch. *59*, 972 (1970)
16. Lacerda, P.R., Knieriem, H.-J., Bozner, A.: Die Ultrastruktur des Herzmuskels der Ratte nach akuter Alkoholintoxikation. Z. Kreisl.-Forsch. *58*, 97 (1969)
17. Meessen, H.: Morphologische Grundlagen der akuten und chronischen Myokardinsuffizienz. Verh. dtsch. Ges. Path. *51*, 31 (1967)
18. Meessen, H., Poche, R.: Pathomorphologie des Myokards. In: Das Herz des Menschen. Bargmann, W., Doerr, W. (eds.), Vol. II. Stuttgart: Thieme 1963
19. Münzinger, W.: Das Tübinger Herz. Arch. klin. Med. *19*, 449 (1887)
20. Pfitzer, P., Knieriem, H.-J., Dietrich, D., Herbertz, G.: Hypertrophie des Rattenherzens nach Isoproterenol. Virchows Arch. Abt. B Zellpath. *12*, 22 (1972)
21. Poche, R.: In: Herzkrankheiten. Reindell, H., Roskam, H. (eds.). Berlin–Heidelberg–New York: Springer-Verlag 1977
22. Rona, G., Kahn, D.S., Chappel, C.I.: Studies on infarctlike myocardial necrosis produced by isoproterenol: A review. Rev. Canad. Biol. *22*, 241 (1963)
23. Selye, H.: Experimental Cardiovascular Diseases. Part I. Berlin–Heidelberg–New York: Springer-Verlag 1970
24. Walshe, W.H.: Disease of the Heart and Great Vessels. London: Smith Elder 1873
25. Wenckebach, K.F.: Das Beriberiherz. Berlin and Vienna: Springer 1934

2. Cardiomyopathy Induced by Antineoplastic Drugs

V. J. Ferrans and E. H. Herman

Summary

Two types of CM are induced by drugs used in the treatment of cancer. The first, produced by anthracycline drugs (adriamycin and daunorubicin), is characterized by congestive heart failure, cardiac dilatation, and structural evidence of myocardial cellular degeneration. The second results from high doses of cyclophosphamide used in combination with other chemotherapeutic agents to ablate bone marrow in preparation for bone marrow transplantation. It is manifested by acute, fulminating cardiac failure, pericarditis, and myocardial microthrombosis. The pathogenesis of these CMs is discussed here.

Drug-induced CM may be defined as any type of heart muscle disease resulting either directly or indirectly from the administration of drugs or from exposure to chemical agents. Among the many drugs known to have cardiotoxic properties are sympathomimetic amines (isoproterenol, epinephrine and norepinephrine), cardiac glycosides, antihypertensives (hydralazine and minoxidil), vasoconstrictors, anticoagulants, hormones (thyroid hormone, insulin and corticosteroids), phenothiazines and other psychotherapeutic agents, antibiotics, antineoplastic agents (anthracyclines and cyclophosphamide), antimalarials (Plasmocid), emetine, histamine, anesthetics, vitamin D, ethanol, and a number of compounds of heavy metals [1]. Some of these agents, particularly when used in very large doses, have direct toxic or necrotizing effects on the myocardium; many others affect mainly the coronary circulation, with or without direct concomitant effects on the myocardium, and others act by precipitating unusual side effects or hypersensitivity reactions that involve the heart [1]. Regardless of the mechanism of action, most of these drugs exert acute rather than chronic effects manifested by the clinical picture of congestive or dilated type of cardiomyopathy. Anthracycline compounds constitute the main exception to this generalization. Until the introduction of daunorubicin and adriamycin, two anthracycline-type agents, the clinical use of a large number of powerful antimetabolites and antibiotics with antineoplastic properties had been associated with a remarkable paucity of clinically evident cardiac complications, perhaps because the main effects of most drugs used in the treatment of cancer are directed against rapidly growing and dividing cells, and because the effects on such cells overshadow any mild cardiac toxic effects of such drugs. In contrast to other clinically useful antineoplastic agents, both daunorubicin and adriamycin produce acute cardiac effects as well as a significant incidence of a unique syndrome of drug-induced chronic cardiomyopathy. This cardiomyopathy is characterized by congestive heart failure, cardiac dilatation, and structural evidence of severe myocardial cellular degeneration. More recently, a second syndrome of cardiomyopathy induced by antineoplastic drugs has been observed when high doses of cyclophosphamide are used in combination with other chemotherapeutic agents in patients undergoing ablation of bone marrow in preparation for bone marrow transplantation. This cardiomyopathy is manifested by acute, fulminating cardiac failure, pericarditis, and myocardial microthrombosis. The present communication reviews the clinical and pathologic features of these two types of cardiomyopathy produced by antineoplastic agents.

Anthracycline-Induced Cardiomyopathy

Daunorubicin, an antitumor antibiotic derived from *Streptomyces peucetius var caesius*, is structurally very similar to adriamycin (14-hydroxydaunomycin) [2–6]. Daunorubicin consists of a pigmented aglycone, daunomycinone, which is joined by a glycosidic linkage to the amino sugar, daunosamine. Both daunorubucin and adriamycin have a high degree of oncolytic activity against acute lymphocytic and acute myelocytic leukemias [7–9]. Adriamycin is especially effective in the therapy of solid tumors and is regarded as one of the most important new drugs in cancer therapy [5]. The clinical usefulness of adriamycin and daunorubicin has been limited by their cardiac toxicity rather than by myelosuppression, stomatitis, and gastrointestinal disturbances, which are the major toxic manifestations of therapy with both compounds [10–17].

Clinical Features

Two distinct types of cardiac effects have been observed after administration of daunorubicin and adriamycin. The first occurs during or immediately following intravenous infusion and consists of nonspecific electrocardiographic changes, such as sinus tachycardia, low QRS voltage, ST segment depression, T-wave alterations, and ventricular premature beats [16, 17]. Von Hoff *et al.* [17] reviewed the records of 5613 patients who had received daunorubicin therapy and found that the acute cardiac changes did not show a dose-dependent relationship in children or adults. Such changes did occur even at the lowest dosage levels and did not serve to predict the subsequent development of cardiomyopathy. The overall incidence of acute electrocardiographic changes in these daunorubicin-treated patients was only 0.8%, which may grossly underestimate the true incidence of these alterations since many of the patients did not undergo detailed cardiac studies while receiving the drug. Electrocardiographic changes have been reported in 11% of patients receiving adriamycin (see [12, 13, 16] for reviews). These abnormalities, as in the case of daunorubicin, are considered nonspecific and, in most instances, subside spontaneously during therapy or in the first few days after drug infusion. When given in high doses, both daunorubicin and adriamycin induce acute but reversible ECG changes, including ventricular arrhythmias, in a variety of experimental animals [15, 16, 18–20]. In addition, other cardiovascular alterations such as hypotension, increased coronary vascular resistance, and decreased ventricular function also have been reported [18].

The arrhythmias produced by both agents can be modified by a number of pharmacologic agents (see [19,20] for reviews) and appear to be unrelated to the future development of CM.

In contrast to the transient ECG changes, the second type of cardiac effect of anthracyclines is represented by a chronic CM that produces significant morbidity and mortality [10–17,21]. The cardiomyopathy is first manifested clinically by unexplained tachycardia, followed shortly thereafter by dyspnea, hepatomegaly, cyanosis, and finally by frank biventricular failure and cardiac dilatation. The failure is usually unresponsive to digitalis and diuretics. An important feature of this CM is that the onset of symptoms usually does not take place during the first few months of therapy. In fact, it may be delayed until several weeks or months after treatment is concluded. The average time from the last dose of daunorubicin to the onset of congestive heart failure was reported by Von Hoff *et al.* [17] to be 80 days (range, 2–280 days; median, 60 days). In that same series, 84% of the patients were in complete remission from their neoplasms at the time CM developed, and 79% of the patients with CM died as a result of that complication. Survival is brief, usually 1–10 days, averaging 2 days, once failure ensues [16]. The risk of developing CM increases markedly as the total cumulative doses of adriamycin or daunorubicin exceed 500 mg/m^2 body surface, although CM has been reported in patients receiving 55–220 mg/m^2 [21]. In a group of children receiving daunorubicin the incidence of CM was 9.9%, and the total dose in patients developing CM varied from 360 to 1260 mg/m^2 [14]. Radiation to the heart [22,23] and treatment with cyclophosphamide [21] enhance the severity of cardiac changes produced by adriamycin.

Cardiovascular Pathologic Findings

Gross cardiac pathologic findings in patients with anthracycline-induced cardiomyopathy consist of generalized cardiac dilatation, which may be accompanied by mural thrombosis, and congestion of the lungs and visceral organs [11,12,14]. These changes are indistinguishable from those in dilated CM of other causes. Microscopic findings include vacuolization, edema, lysis of myofibrils and atrophy of the cardiac muscle cells, and interstitial fibrosis. Inflammatory reaction is usually minimal or absent, even in areas of muscle cell necrosis. Vascular lesions are absent. Myocardial ultrastructural changes have been observed in the nuclei, myofibrils, mitochondria, sarcoplasmic reticulum, and T tubules. Nuclear alterations, found by Buja *et al.* [11,24] in 10% or less of nuclei of cardiac muscle cells of daunorubicin treated patients, consisted of the transformation of variable amounts of chromatin into thick fibers (160–200 Å in diameter), intermediate-sized fibers (70–100 Å in diameter) and thin filaments (30–40 Å in diameter [Fig. 1]). These alterations, which were reproduced *in vitro* by incubation of fragments of cardiac muscle from monkeys in tissue culture medium containing daunorubicin, were interpreted as representing various stages of uncoiling and unraveling of chromatin and were considered to be related to the phenomenon of intercalation of daunorubicin into DNA. Such nuclear lesions have not been found in animals given anthracyclines *in vivo* (as opposed to the *in vitro* incubation experiments of Buja *et al.* [11]); however, this has not been studied in

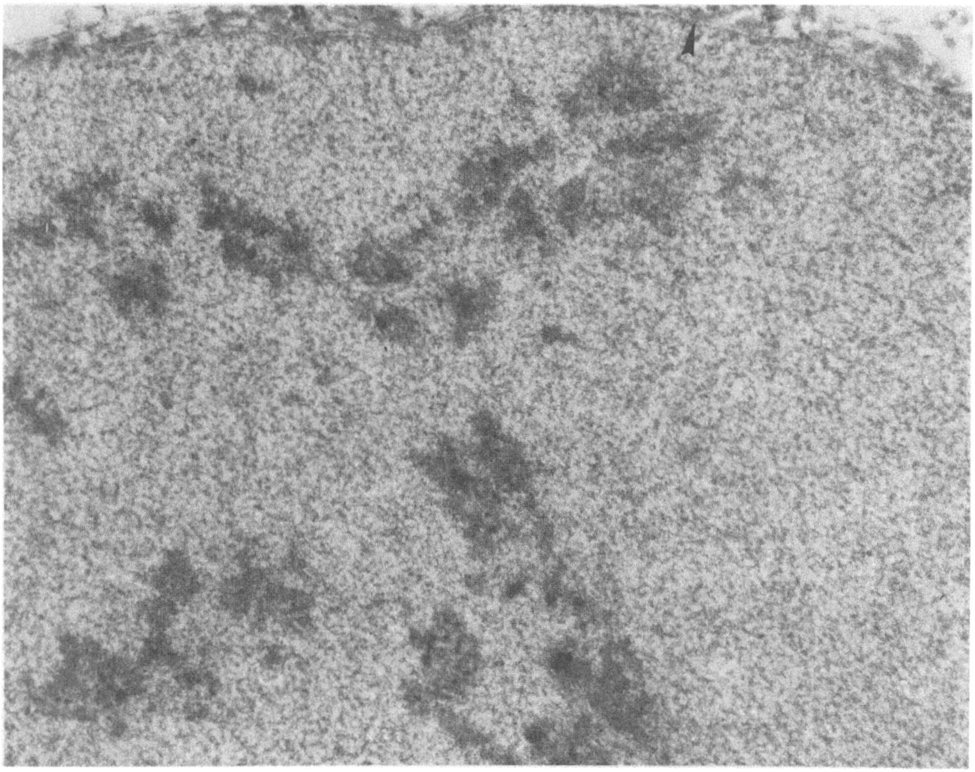

Fig. 1. Electron micrograph of part of nucleus of cardiac muscle cell from 5-year-old patient with acute lymphocytic leukemia who received 500 mg daunorubicin/m^2 body surface. The patient developed fatal cardiomyopathy. The chromatin shows severe changes characterized by unraveling into fine filaments that fill the nucleoplasm. Nuclear membrane is indicated by arrowheads. ×50000

sufficient detail. The myofibrils showed various degrees of lysis of the myofilaments, especially of the thick (myosin) filaments, and accumulations of Z-band material (Fig. 2). The mitochondria also showed lysis and frequently were associated with concentric lamellae (myelin figures). The sarcoplasmic reticulum showed variable degrees of swelling and fragmentation. The intercellular junctions showed a variety of changes related to dissociation of the cells, especially in areas of fibrosis. Changes similar to those just described have been observed in cardiac biopsies of patients receiving adriamycin [25].

Although a number of pathologic changes have been produced by the acute administration of large amounts of daunorubicin and adriamycin to experimental animals, including the mouse, rat, monkey, hamster, rabbit, and pig [15, 16, 23, 26–29], only the rabbit, monkey, and pig have been shown to develop a chronic dose-related CM with congestive heart failure comparable to that seen in the human. The dog has proven peculiarly resistant to anthracycline toxicity. The reasons for these species variations in drug response have not been established. In the rabbit, the species that has been most extensively studied [27, 28], the chronic

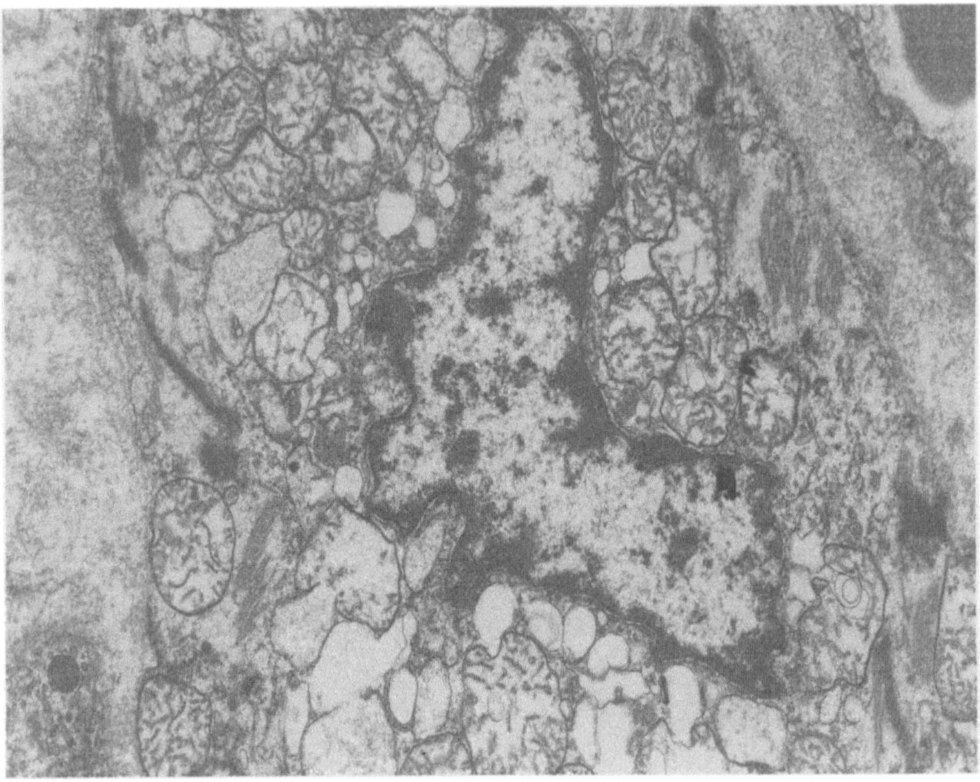

Fig. 2. Part of cardiac muscle cell from 7-year-old patient with acute lymphocytic leukemia who died of cardiomyopathy after receiving a total dose of 455 mg daunoribicin/m^2 body surface. Note interstitial edema, lysis of myofibrils, accumulation of small masses of Z-band material, and dilatation of sarcoplasmic reticulum. Most of the nuclear chromatin is peripherally aggregated, but some is in the form of fine strands. ×15000

cardiac clinical and morphologic changes have a reasonably close resemblance to those in humans; however, in the rabbit the vacuolization (Fig. 3 and 4) of muscle cells ("adria" cells), which is caused by dilatation of the sarcoplasmic reticulum and T tubules, is much more extensive than in man and the cardiac lesions have a preferential distribution around blood vessels. In addition, the rabbit exhibits two extracardiac complications which are impairment of chondro-osteogenesis and severe renal toxicity [15]. The latter is characterized by proteinuria, loss of glomerular foot processes and vacuolar destruction of glomeruli; tubular degeneration with associated protein casts; thickening of the basement membranes of Bowman's capsule; and a peculiar type of enlargement of tubular epithelial cells, with mosaic-like aggregates of chromatin in the central areas of the nuclei. The bone lesions are of particular interest because anthracyclines are avidly bound (as are tetracyclines) by bone, from which they may be released over a long period of time. Both adriamycin and daunorubicin induce genital, renal, and mammary neoplasms in rats [15]. Tumor induction by these drugs has not been reported in other species.

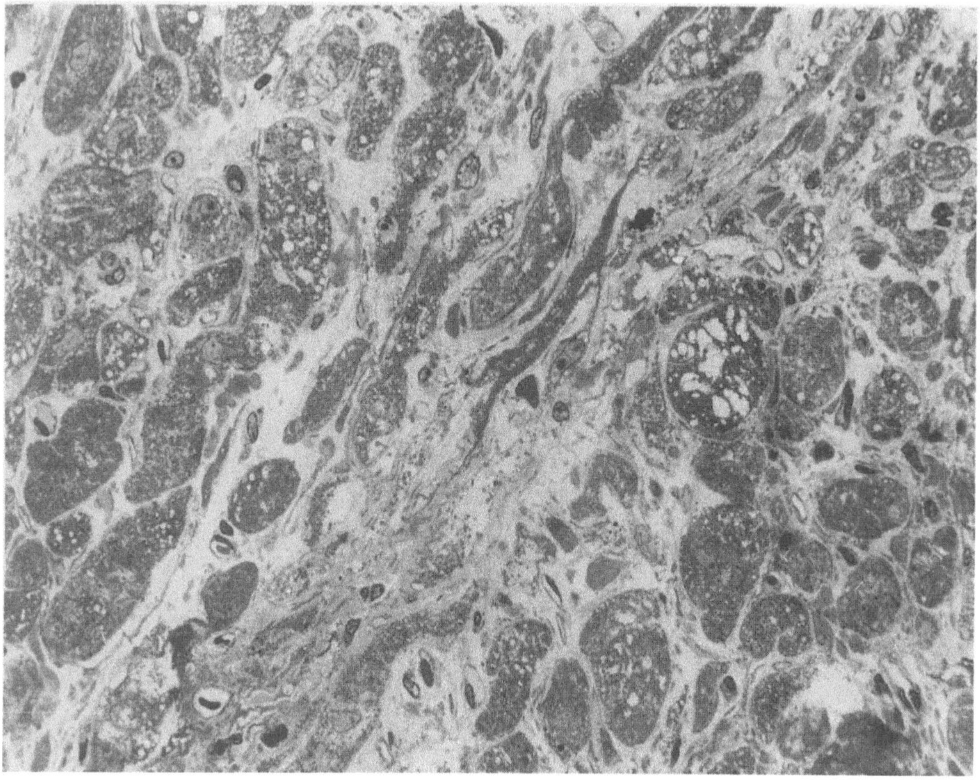

Fig. 3. Light micrograph of $\frac{1}{2}$-μ-thick section of plastic-embedded myocardium of rabbit with adriamycin-induced cardiomyopathy (total dose = 20 mg/kg body wt.); showing interstitial edema and fibrosis and marked vacuolization of the muscle cells. Compare with Fig. 4. Alkaline toluidine blue stain. ×400

Pathogenesis

The pathogenetic mechanisms of anthracycline-induced CM have been of great interest, not only from the standpoint of therapy but also from the standpoint of utilizing these drugs for developing animal model systems for the study of COCM. The exact mechanism by which the delayed, chronic cardiotoxicity of anthracyclines is mediated has not been elucidated. It remains to be determined whether the chronic and acute toxicities are qualitatively different phenomena, or whether the chronic toxicity simply results from the additive effect of small amounts of acute damage occurring each time the drugs are given. Several complex biochemical alterations are known to be produced by adriamycin and daunorubicin, and it seems likely that each of these changes plays a contributory role in the pathogenesis of the CM. These alterations (see [15, 16] for review) include: 1. binding of the drugs to nuclear and mitochondrial DNA (i.e., intercalation or insertion of the drug molecules into both strands of the DNA helix), with damage to the DNA structure and inhibition of the synthesis of DNA and

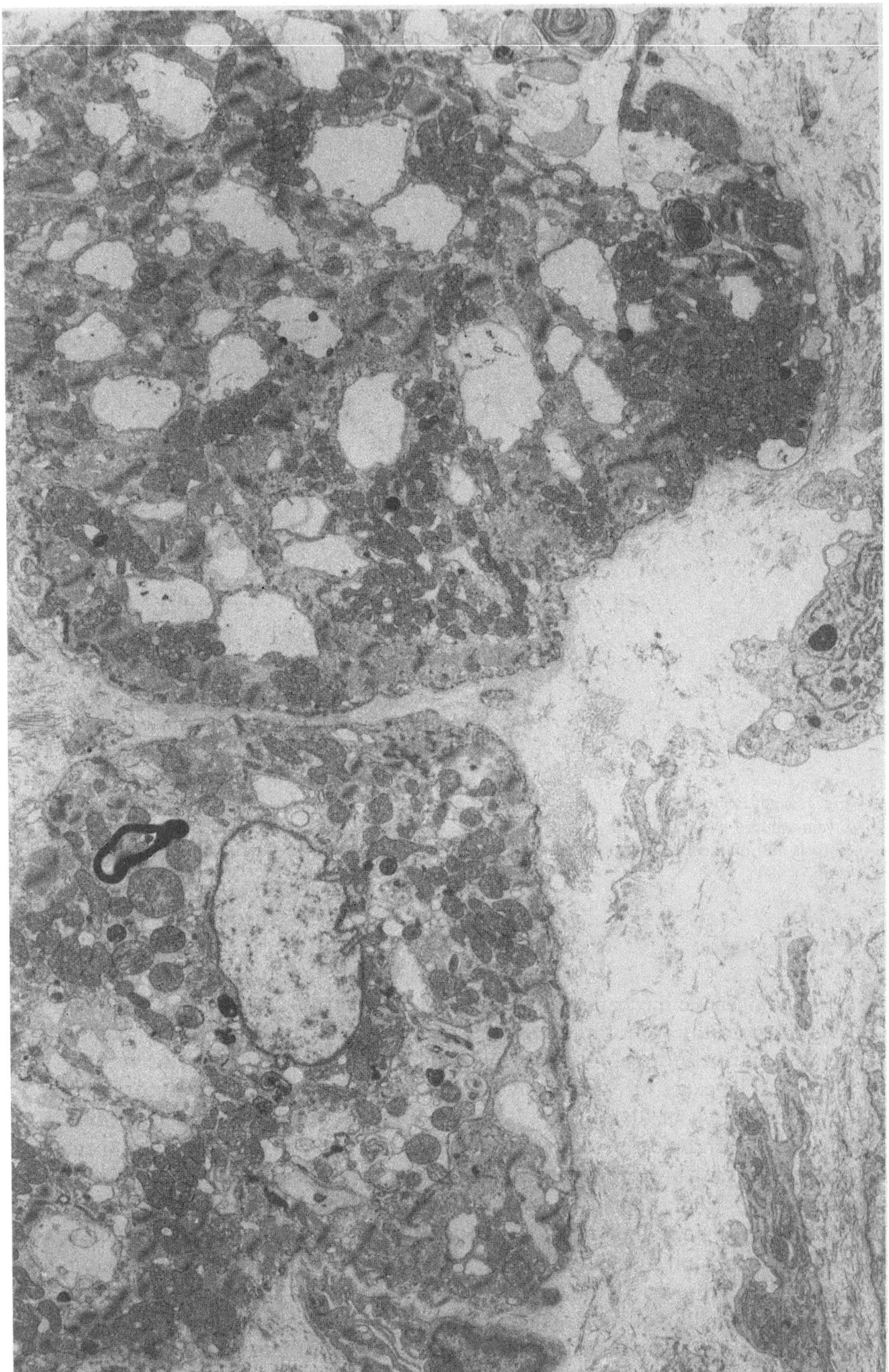

RNA; 2. inhibition of Na- and K-dependent ATPase; 3. other membrane effects leading to marked elevations in the intracellular concentration of Na, Ca, and water; 4. disturbances of mitochondrial function caused by the inhibition by anthracyclines of coenzyme Q_{10}-containing enzyme systems in the mitochondrial electron transport chain; 5. reactions that are mediated by free radical groups and lead to peroxidation of membrane lipids, and 6. endothelial cell damage (such as occurs with radiation therapy). Daunorubicin and adriamycin are known to bind to nuclear DNA in cardiac muscle, as shown by fluorescence microscopy and biochemical studies, and it is thought that the ability of these drugs to bind the DNA is responsible for their antitumor effect. Buja *et al.* [11,24] postulated that the binding of these drugs to the DNA of a cell type, such as cardiac muscle, that does not reproduce itself leads to long-term damage that cannot be repaired and that eventually will result in cardiac dysfunction as the renewal of proteins becomes progressively more inadequate to meet the needs of protein turnover. Incorporation of precursors into heart DNA of adult animals is believed to occur mainly in nuclei of endothelial and connective tissue cells and in mitochondria of muscle cells [30]. Mild to moderate endothelial damage has been found in acute experiments [30, 31], but it seems unlikely to account for the profound degenerative changes that anthracyclines cause in the muscle cells.

Daunorubicin and adriamycin have some similarities to the digitalis cardiac glycosides. These similarities might provide a basis for some of the membrane and ionic changes reported, such as the increased concentrations of myocardial calcium in rabbits treated chronically with adriamycin [28]. Intracellular overloading with calcium is a well-recognized mechanism for cardiac cellular damage and could be related to the pathogenesis of anthracycline-induced CM; however, elevated calcium levels were noted in rabbits at a time when CM was not apparent [28]. Intracellular myocardial calcium concentrations have been found to increase when membrane Na-K ATPase is inhibited by digitalis compounds, and adriamycin decreases the activity of this enzyme system isolated from rabbit heart (Gonsalvez, M. and Blanco, M., unpublished data). It is not known whether these effects occur *in vivo* since inhibition *in vitro* occurs only in the absence of calcium. Both daunorubicin and adriamycin are potential chelating agents and could alter the intracellular concentrations not only of calcium but also of other divalent cations such as Mg, Zn, and Cu. Dietary imbalances of these agents are known to lead to a variety of cardiovascular alterations [32]. It should be noted that ICRF 159, an antineoplastic derivative of EDTA, has been found to reduce the formation of aglycone metabolites and certain toxic effects of adriamycin and daunorubicin [20]. The role of changes in intracellular ionic concentration in the pathogenesis of anthracycline-induced CM remains to be established.

Bertazzoli *et al.* showed that ubiquinone, given simultaneously with adriamycin, prevented to a very significant extent the chronic cardiac toxicity of the

---

◁ Fig. 4. Electron micrograph of same tissue as shown in Figure 3. Two adjacent cardiac muscle cells (upper and lower left) in area of edema and fibrosis (center and lower right) show marked vacuolization, nuclear alterations (chromatin disruption), myelin figures, myofibrillar loss and intracellular edema. The vacuolization is due to severe dilatation of the sarcoplasmic reticulum. ×6000

latter drug in the rabbit [33, 34]. It should be pointed out, however, that ubiquinone also is capable, as is α-tocopherol, of counteracting the peroxidation of membrane lipids. As reviewed by Myers *et al.* [35, 36], drugs such as adriamycin and daunorubicin can initiate lipid peroxidation by facilitating the transfer of electrons from endogenous compounds such as NADPH to oxygen, resulting in the formation of superoxides that can decompose to hydroxy radicals, peroxy radicals, and hydrogen peroxide. These in turn can oxidize unsaturated fatty acids in membranes to lipid peroxides. Two observations [35, 36] indicate that lipid peroxides may have some role in the pathogenesis of anthracycline toxicity: First, the administration of very large doses of α-tocopherol reduces significantly the acute toxicity and mortality of adriamycin in the mouse; secondly, malondialdehyde, a product of the peroxidation and subsequent decomposition of unsaturated fatty acids, is readily detected in the hearts of mice for 2–6 days after the administration of adriamycin, but not in the hearts of control animals or of animals treated with both adriamycin and α-tocopherol. Preliminary data [36] obtained on the P388 ascites tumor suggest that the binding of adriamycin to tumor cell nuclei and the antineoplastic effect of the drug are not affected by α-tocopherol. Nevertheless, the exact relationship between lipid peroxidation and anthracycline CM in the human remains unclear. The cardiac lesions induced by adriamycin and daunorubicin in the rabbit and mouse are morphologically different in several respects [37, 38] from those in deficiency of selenium and α-tocopherol, the only other types of CM in which lipid peroxidation is known to play a pathogenetic role. (It is possible, however, that such differences are due to differences in sites of release of the offending free radicals.) Perhaps more importantly, the lipid peroxidation theory does not provide a satisfactory explanation for the long delay between administration of the drug and the onset of cardiac failure. Thus, the evidence just reviewed shows that anthracyclines produce a multiplicity of biochemical effects that can lead to cardiac muscle damage. The relative importance of these effects remains to be assessed critically, particularly from the standpoint of the selective blocking of the CM potential of these drugs without interfering with their antineoplastic properties.

Cardiomyopathy Induced by Cyclophosphamide-Based High-Dose Combination Chemotherapy

High-dose chemotherapy utilizing primarily cyclophosphamide has been used in varying doses and combinations as a preparatory regimen before bone marrow transplantation. Initial studies at the National Cancer Institute suggested that a total dose of 180 mg cyclophosphamide/kg body wt., given over 4 days, provided inadequate immunosuppression and antileukemic effect in patients with refractory leukemia. In an effort to gain more immunosuppressive and antineoplastic effects, Graw and associates developed a combination chemotherapy protocol (BACT) utilizing bischlorethyl nitrosourea, cytosine arabinoside, cyclophosphamide, and 6-thioguanine [39]. Of 15 patients treated on this protocol, four died of an acute lethal myopericarditis, which appears to be a unique clinical and pathological entity.

Clinical Features

Three of the four patients in this report were given the 4-day BACT regimen consisting of cyclophosphamide, 45 mg/kg/day (total dose, 180 mg/kg); 6-thioguanine, 100 mg/m^2 q. 12 h for $3^1/_2$ days (total dose 700 mg/m^2); cytosine arabinoside, 100 mg/m^2 q. 12 h for $3^1/_2$ days (total dose 700 mg/m^2); and bis-chlorethyl nitrosourea, given as a single dose of 200 mg/m^2 on day 3. The fourth patient received the 6-day BACT regimen, a modification of the above with cyclophosphamide given for 6 days (total dose 270 mg/kg body wt.), cytosine arabinoside and 6-thioguanine given for $5^1/_2$ days each (total dose of 1100 mg/m^2), and the nitrosourea as a single dose of 200 mg/m^2 on day 3. Twenty-four hours after the last dose of chemotherapy, all four patients received an infusion of either allogenic or autologous bone marrow.

The four patients had similar clinical courses [40] which differed from those of patients dying of cardiac failure produced by daunorubicin or adriamycin [11, 41, 42]. From 5–9 days after the initiation of the BACT regimen, cardiac toxicity became manifest by dyspnea, orthostatic hypotension, fluid retention, tachycardia, decreased voltage on ECG, and pericardial effusion. In all 4 patients, the effusion was initially a nonhemorrhagic, nonmalignant exudate, and the myopericarditis progressed rapidly for 2–6 days to a fatal low-output state despite treatment with digitalis, diuretics, catecholamines, dopamine, and repeated pericardiocentesis. No patient had significant preexisting cardiac, hepatic, or renal dysfunction. During therapy no patient developed severe renal, hepatic, or coagulation dysfunction, although all had moderate elevations of partial thromboplastin time, and three of four developed moderate elevations of creatinine. None of the four had raised creatine-phosphokinase level or laboratory or clinical evidence of disseminated intravascular coagulation.

Cardiovascular Pathologic Findings

The hearts of all three patients studied at necropsy were increased in weight. Fibrinous pericarditis, severe interstitial edema, intramyocardial extravasation of blood, fibrin-platelet microthrombi in cardiac capillaries, and fibrin strands in the interstitium, were present in all three hearts (Figs. 5–7). Ultrastructural study of the lungs of one patient revealed the presence of rare fibrin thrombi within capillaries. Multifocal cardiac necroses, found in two patients, were characterized by severe hypercontraction bands, myofibrillar damage and lysis, intramitochondrial electron-dense inclusions, and fibrin strands within the cytoplasm of the muscle cells. The other patient showed less severe changes, which consisted of small focal areas of myofibrillar lysis and occasional intramitochondrial inclusions and were interpreted as representing early cellular damage. In all three patients a few nuclei of cardiac muscle cells showed alterations similar to those produced by anthracyclines.

Pathogenesis

The lesions involving the cardiac muscle cells of the subjects of this report are nonspecific and occur in other forms of myocardial injury. In contrast, the

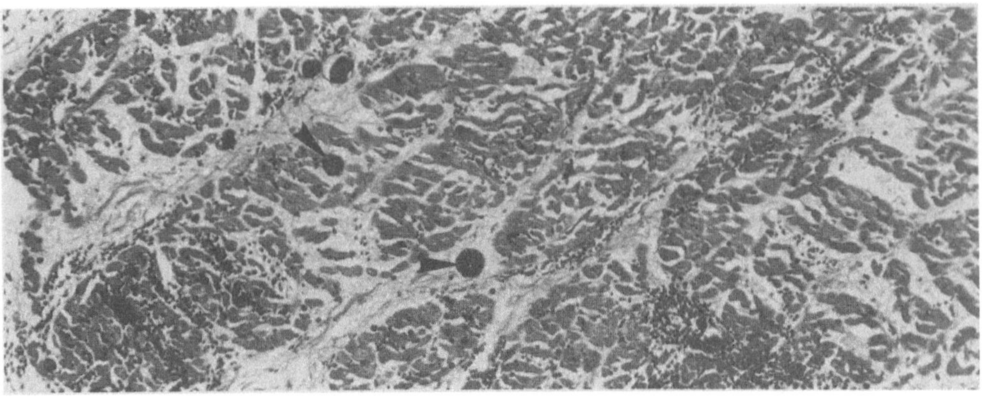

Fig. 5. Light micrograph of left ventricular myocardium of 15-year-old patient who developed acute, fatal cardiomyopathy after receiving cyclophosphamide-based combination chemotherapy (see text) in preparation for bone marrow transplantation for the therapy of acute lymphocytic leukemia. Severe edema, hemorrhage, and several microthrombi (*arrowheads*) are present. H&E, ×100

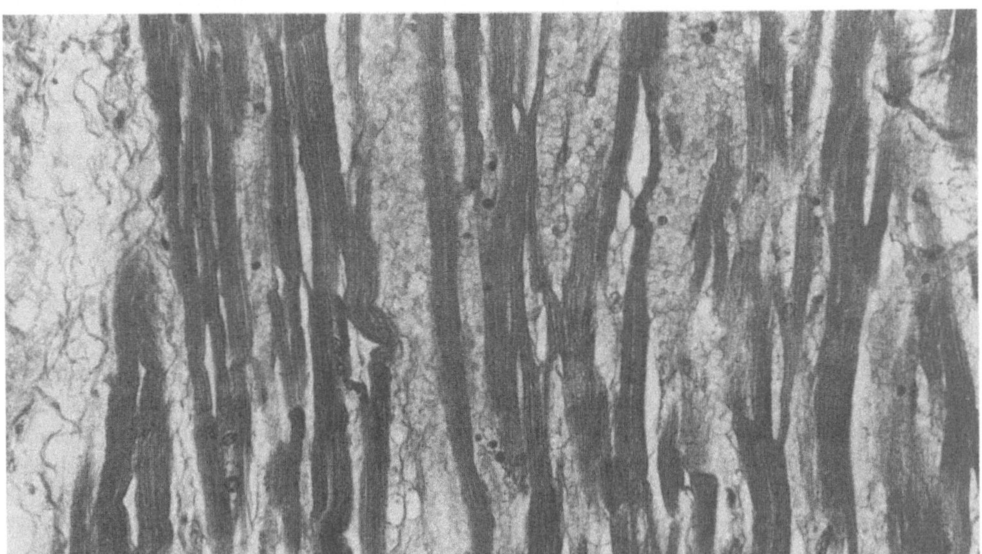

Fig. 6. Same tissue as in Figure 5, showing hemorrhage and interstitial edema. H & E, ×250

Fig. 7. Electron micrograph of fibrin thrombus that has occluded a capillary in myocardium of same patient as in Figures 5 and 6. Adjacent cardiac muscle cells appear damaged, and myofilaments appear indistinct, presumably because of adsorption of plasma proteins. ×35000 ▷

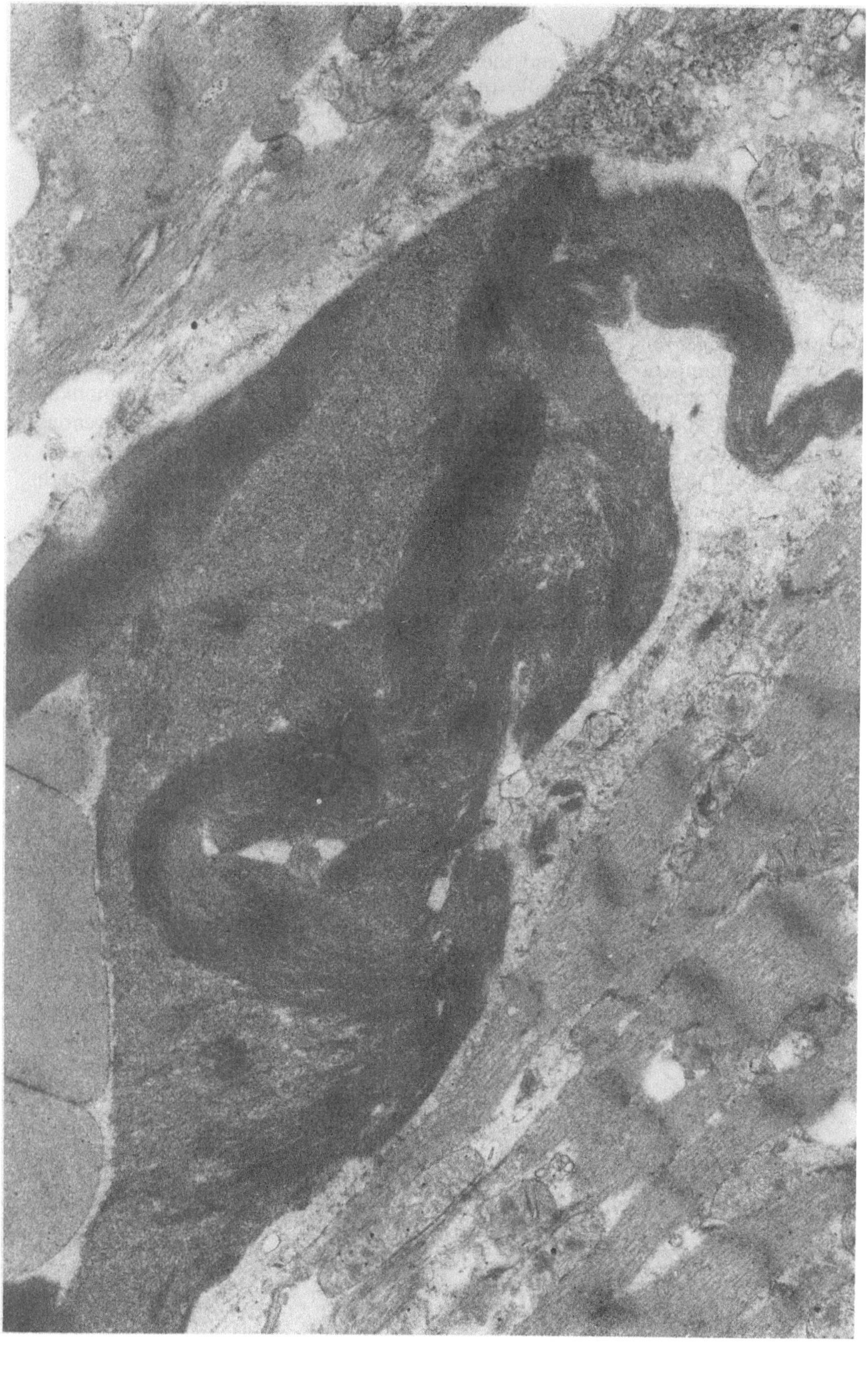

capillary microthrombosis and the strands of fibrin in myocardial interstitium and within cardiac muscle cells are highly unusual features. Fibrin deposition within cardiac muscle cells has been described only in rats with experimentally induced hypertension [43]. Cardiac microthrombi have been reported in patients with disseminated intravascular coagulation [42]. Microthrombosis in myocardium also is found in pigs with deficiency of selenium and vitamin E, in which endothelial damage also occurs [37, 38]. In the human, the combination of pericarditis and acute cardiac microthrombi with fibrin deposits in the interstitium and muscle cells has been observed only in the clinical setting of cyclophosphamide-based high-dose chemotherapy with associated acute cardiotoxicity.

The administration of large doses of cyclophosphamide induces edema and hemorrhage in suckling-rat brains, in the lungs and hearts of dogs, in monkey hearts, and in the urinary bladder of rats, dogs, and humans. The intravenous administration, to dogs of 500 mg cyclophosphamide/kg body wt. results in a marked fall in the voltage of the QRS complex after 2 or 3 hours and in death from pulmonary edema and intractable cardiac failure in another 30–90 min. In monkeys, 200 mg cyclophosphamide/kg body wt. given over 4 days are tolerated, but 240 mg/kg given over 4 days results in a diffuse hemorrhagic diathesis most prominent in the myocardium (see [40] and [41] for reviews). In man, 180 mg cyclophosphamide/kg body wt. given over 4 days without other accompanying chemotherapy has not resulted in cardiac toxicity [39]. One case of cardiac toxicity has been reported at 200 mg cyclophosphamide/kg body wt. given over 4 days [44], and at higher doses (240 and 270 mg/kg) two cases have been reported [45–48].

The light and electron microscopic findings in these three patients suggest that large doses of cyclophosphamide-based chemotherapy induce cardiac failure basically through direct endothelial damage. This damage would lead to capillary microthrombosis and increased permeability of endothelium, with leakage of plasma proteins and erythrocytes into the myocardial interstitium and into the myocardial muscle cells. Similarly, it appeared that exudation of large amounts of protein-rich fluid into the pericardial cavity was responsible for the pericardial effusions in our patients. The exact nature of the cardiac endothelial damage produced by the chemotherapy could not be determined in the present study because the endothelium in the tissue samples that we examined showed postmortem autolytic changes.

References

1. Buja, L.M., Ferrans, V.J., Roberts, W.C.: Drug-induced cardiomyopathies. Adv. Cardiol. *13*, 330–348 (1974)
2. Grein, A., Spalla, C., DiMarco, A., Canevazzi, G.: Descrizione e classificazione di un attinomicete (Streptomyces peucetius sp. Nova). Produttore di una sostanza ad attività antitumorale: la daunomicina. G. Microbiol. *11*, 109–118 (1963)
3. DiMarco, A., Gaetani, M., Dorigotti, L., Soldati, M., Bellini, O.: Daunomycin: A new antibiotic with antitumor activity. Cancer Chemother. Rep. *38*, 31–38 (1964)
4. DiMarco, A., Gaetani, M., Scarpinato, B.: Adriamycin (NSC-123, 127): New antibiotic with antitumor activity. Cancer Chemother. Rep. *53*, 33–37 (1969)
5. Blum, R.H., Carter, S.K.: Adriamycin. A new anticancer drug with significant clinical activity. Ann. intern. Med. *80*, 249–259 (1974)
6. Maral, R., Bourat, G., Ducrot, R., Fournal, J., Ganter, P., Julou, L., Koenig, F., Myon, J., Pascal, S., Pasquet, J., Populaire, P., DeRatuld, Y., Werner, G.H.: Etude toxicologique et activité antitumorale experimentale de la rubidomycine (13,057 RP). Pathol. Biol. *15*, 903–908 (1967)
7. Jones, B., Holland, J.F., Morrison, A.R.: Daunorubicin (NSC-82151) in the treatment of advanced childhood lymphoblastic leukemia. Cancer Res. *31*, 84–90 (1971)
8. Malpas, J., Scott, R.: Daunorubicin in acute myelocytic leukemia. Lancet *1969/I*, 465–470
9. Holton, C.P., Lonsdale, D., Nora, A.H., Thurman, W.G., Vietti, T.J.: Clinical study of daunomycin (NSC-82151) in children with acute leukemia. Cancer *22*, 1014–1017 (1968)
10. Bonadonna, G., Monfardini, S.: Cardiac toxicity of daunorubicin. Lancet *1969/I*, 837
11. Buja, L.M., Ferrans, V.J., Mayer, R.J., Roberts, W.C., Henderson, E.S.: Cardiac ultrastructural changes induced by daunorubicin therapy. Cancer *32*, 771–778 (1973)
12. Lefrak, E.A., Pitha, J., Rosenheim, S., Gottlieb, J.A.: A clinicopathologic analysis of adriamycin cardiotoxicity. Cancer *32*, 302–314 (1973)
13. Rinehart, J.G., Lewis, R.P., Balcerzak, S.P.: Adriamycin cardiotoxicity in man. Ann. intern. Med. *81*, 475–478 (1974)
14. Halazun, J.F., Wanger, H.R., Gaeta, J.F., Sinks, L.F.: Daunorubicin cardiac toxicity in children with acute lymphocytic leukemia. Cancer *33*, 545–554 (1974)
15. Young, D.M.: Pathologic effects of adriamycin (NSC-123, 127) in experimental systems. Cancer Chemother. Rep. *6*, Part 3, 159–175 (1975)
16. Lenaz, L., Page, J.A.: Cardiotoxicity of adriamycin and related anthracyclines. Cancer Treat. Rev. *3*, 111–120 (1976)
17. Von Hoff, D.D., Rozencweig, M., Layard, M., Slavik, M., Muggia, F.M.: Daunomycin-induced cardiotoxicity in children and adults. A review of 110 cases. Amer. J. Med. *62*, 200–208 (1977)
18. Herman, E.H., Mhatre, R.M., Lee, I.P., Vick, J., Waravdekar, V.S.: A comparison of the cardiovascular actions of daunomycin, adriamycin and N-acetyldaunomycin in hamsters and monkeys. Pharmacology (Basle) *6*, 229–241 (1971)
19. Herman, E.H., Mhatre, R.M., Lee, I.P., Waravdekar, V.S.: Prevention of the cardiotoxic effects of adriamycin (NSC-123, 127) and daunomycin (NSC-82151) in the isolated dog heart. Proc. Soc. exp. Biol. *140*, 234–239 (1972)
20. Herman, E.H., Mhatre, R.M., Chadwick, D.P.: Modification of some toxicological effects of daunomycin by ICRF 159. Toxicol. Appl. Pharmacol. *27*, 517–526 (1974)
21. Minow, R.A., Benjamin, R.S., Gottlieb, J.A.: Adriamycin cardiomyopathy—an overview with determination of risk factors. Cancer Chemother. Rep. *6*, Part 3, 195–201 (1975)
22. Billingham, M.E., Bristow, M.R., Mason, J.W., Daniels, J.R.: Endomyocardial biopsy evidence of radiation enhancement of adriamycin cardiotoxicity. Circulation *53*, *54*, Suppl. II, II–23 (1976)
23. Eltringham, J.R., Fajardo, L.F., Stewart, J.R.: Adriamycin cardiomyopathy: enhanced cardiac damage in rabbits with combined drug and cardiac irradiation. Radiology *115*, 471–472 (1975)
24. Buja, L.M., Ferrans, V.J., Rabson, A.S.: Letter: Unusual nuclear alterations. Lancet *1974/I*, 402–403
25. Bristow, M.R., Mason, J.W., Billingham, M.E., Daniels, J.R.: Endomyocardial biopsy and systolic time intervals in detection of adriamycin cardiotoxicity. Circulation *53*, *54*, Suppl. II, II–80 (1976)
26. Chalcroft, S.C.W., Gavin, J.B., Herdson, P.B.: Fine structural changes in rat myocardium induced by daunorubucin. Pathology *5*, 99–105 (1973)

27. Jaenke, R.S.: An anthracycline antibiotic-induced cardiomyopathy in rabbits. Lab. Invest. *30*, 292–304 (1974)
28. Olson, H.M., Young, D.M., Prieur, D.J., Leroy, A.F., Reagan, R.L.: Electrolyte and morphologic alterations of myocardium in adriamycin-treated rabbits. Amer. J. Pathol. *77*, 439–454 (1974)
29. Rosenoff, S.H., Olson, H.M., Young, D.M., Bostick, F., Young, R.C.: Adriamycin-induced cardiac damage in the mouse. J. nat. Cancer Inst. *55*, 191–194 (1975)
30. Gross, N.J., Getz, G.S., Rabinovitz, M.: Apparent turnover of mitochondrial deoxyribonucleic acid and mitochondrial phospholipids in the tissues of the rat. J. Biol. Chem. *244*, 1552–1562 (1969)
31. Stewart, J.R., Fajardo, L.F.: Radiation-induced heart disease. Clinical and experimental aspects. Radiol. Clin. North Am. *9*, 511–531 (1971)
32. Underwood, E.J.: Trace Elements in Human and Animal Nutrition. New York: Academic Press 1971.
33. Bertazzoli, C., Sala, L., Tosana, M.G.: Antagonistic action of ubiquinone on the experimental cardiotoxicity of adriamycin in the isolated rabbit heart. IRCS Med. Sci. *3*, 367 (1975)
34. Bertazzoli, C., Sala, L., Solcia, E., Ghione, M.: Experimental adriamycin cardiotoxicity prevented by ubiquinone *in vivo* in rabbits. IRCS Med. Sci. *3*, 468 (1975)
35. Myers, C.E., McGuire, W., Young, R.: Adriamycin: amelioration of toxicity by α-tocopherol. Cancer Treat. Rep. *60*, 961–962 (1976)
36. Myers, C.E., McGuire, W., Liss, R.H., Ifrim, I., Grotzinger, K., Young, R.C.: Adriamycin: the role of lipid peroxidation in cardiac toxicity and tumor response. Science *197*, 165–167 (1977)
37. Van Vleet, J.F., Ferrans, V.J., Ruth, G.R.: Ultrastructural alterations in nutritional cardiomyopathy of selenium-vitamin E deficient swine. I. Fiber lesions. Lab. Invest. *37*, 188–200 (1977)
38. Van Vleet, J.F., Ferrans, V.J., Ruth, G.R.: Ultrastructural alterations in nutritional cardiomyopathy of selenium-vitamin E deficient swine. II. Vascular lesions. Lab. Invest. *37*, 201–211 (1977)
39. Graw, Jr., R.G., Lohrmann, H.-P., Bull, M.I., Decter, J., Herzig, G.P., Bull, J.M., Leventhal, B.G., Yankee, R.A., Herzig, R.H., Krueger, G.R.F., Bleyer, W.A., Buja, L.M., McGinniss, M.H., Alter, H.J., Whang-Peng, J., Gralnick, H.R., Kirkpatrick, C.H., Henderson, E.S.: Bone-marrow transplantation following combination chemotherapy immunosuppression (B.A.C.T.) in patients with acute leukemia. Transplant. Proc. *6*, 349–354 (1974)
40. Applebaum, F.R., Strauchen, J.A., Graw, R.G., Savage, D.D., Kent, K.M., Ferrans, V.J., Herzig, G.P.: Acute lethal carditis caused by high-dose combination chemotherapy. A unique clinical and pathologic entity. Lancet *1976/I*, 58–62
41. Buja, L.M., Ferrans, V.J.: Myocardial injury produced by antineoplastic drugs. In: Recent Advances in Studies on Cardiac Structure and Metabolism, Vol. 6, Pathophysiology and Morphology of Myocardial Cell Alteration, Fleckenstein, H., Rona, G. (eds.). Baltimore: University Park Press 1975, pp. 487–497
42. Buja, L.M., Ferrans, V.J., Graw, Jr., R.G.: Cardiac pathologic findings in patients treated with bone marrow transplantation. Hum. Pathol. *7*, 17–45 (1976)
43. Hüttner, I., Rona, G., More, R.H.: Fibrin deposition within cardiac muscle cells in malignant hypertension: an electron microscopic study. Arch. Pathol. *91*, 19–28 (1971)
44. Buckner, C.D., Clift, R.A., Fefer, A., Funk, D.D., Glucksberg, H., Ramberg, R.E., Storb, R., Thomas, E.D.: Aplastic anemia treated by marrow transplantation. Transplant. Proc. *5*, 913–916 (1973)
45. Santos, G.W., Sensenbrenner, L.L., Burke, P.J., Colvin, O.M., Owens, A.H., Bias, W., Slavin, R.: Marrow transplants in man utilizing cyclophosphamide: summary of Baltimore experience. Exp. Hematol. *20*, 78–81 (1970)
46. Santos, G.W., Sensenbrenner, L.L., Burke, P.J., Colvin, O.M., Owens, A.H., Bias, W., Slavin, R.E.: Marrow transplantation in man following cyclophosphamide. Transplant. Proc. *3*, 400–404 (1971)
47. Santos, G.W., Sensenbrenner, L.L., Burke, P.J., Mullins, G.M., Bias, W., Tutschia, P.J., Slavin, R.E.: The use of cyclophosphamide for clinical marrow transplantation. Transplant. Proc. *4*, 559–564 (1972)
48. Buckner, C.D., Rudolph, R.H., Fefer, A., Clift, R.A., Epstein, R.B., Funk, D.D., Neiman, P.E., Slichter, S.J., Storb, R., Thomas, E.D.: High-dose cyclophosphamide therapy for malignant disease. Toxicity, tumor response, and the effects of stored autologous marrow. Cancer *29*, 357–365 (1972)

3. Hereditary Cardiomyopathy in the Syrian Golden Hamster:

Influence of Verapamil as Calcium Antagonist

K. Lossnitzer, W. Mohr, A. Konrad, and R. Guggenmoos

Introduction

Coronary sclerosis, arterial and pulmonary hypertension, valvular or septal abnormalities, bacteria, and viruses have been regarded as primary causes of myocardial disease. During the past 20 years, great interest has been focused on other factors, especially hormones and toxins that may produce myocardial cell damage. In addition, we became aware that pathology of heart muscle may also be of familial nature, thus suggesting genetic origin.

In order to denote diseases of the heart muscle of unknown and unusual etiology and pathogenesis the clinical term CM was introduced by Brigden [1]. It must be emphasized that this term covers not only myocardial degeneration but also cardiac hypertrophy and several myocardial dysfunctions leading to cardiac insufficiency.

Very often it seems impossible to evaluate the extracardiac etiology and pathogenesis of the CMs. Moreover, the interrelationships between distinct clinical, morphologic, functional, and biochemical phenomena are not yet fully understood. Therefore, it appears as a promising way to search at least for a more general pathogenetic basis of cardiac cell damage. Büchner [2] established cellular hypoxydosis as a clue to myocardial degeneration, whereas Fleckenstein [4] more specifically favors deficiency or blockage of utilization of high-energy phosphates in cardiac cells. Using the isoproterenol-treated rat as a pharmacologic model, he established the chalenging hypothesis that flooding of the myocardial cytosol with calcium ions – interfering with the excitation-contraction process – is a crucial factor in whether or not myocardial cells will undergo degeneration.

This concept would become a general principle if *any* noxious stimulus attacking the cardiac cell caused at least this stereotypic or nonspecific reaction. However, from the molecular-biologic level, discrimination between specific etiologies of the different CMs is impossible. Therefore the question arises whether knowledge of etiology is helpful in order to prevent myocardial degeneration. The answer seems to be no if one could beneficially manipulate the nonspecific, molecular myocardial reactions. If, for instance, calcium overloading of myocardial cells played a general and determinant pathogenetic role in myocardial degeneration and could be counteracted successfully by pharmacologic agents, investigation of specific etiology doesn't appear to be of great importance. Furthermore, should functional myocardial changes or hypertrophy regress with an antidegenerative therapy, their interrelationship with myocardial degeneration would become evident.

Previous studies in genetically CM hamsters demonstrated myocardial calcium overload with the onset of myocardial degeneration [10]. For the reasons given above, it seems particularly important to evaluate the pathogenetic role of disturbed myocardial calcium metabolism in these animals and to determine whether it can be influenced by a so-called calcium antagonistic substance. Until now five pharmacologic agents are known to have calcium antagonistic properties, i.e., to interfere with the excitation-contraction coupling process of the musculature by reducing the transmembrane calcium conductivity: Diltiazeme, Fendiline, Nifedipine, Prenylamine, and Verapamil. Prevention of myocardial degeneration in the spontaneous CM hamsters by application of one of these drugs would favor the hypothesis of Fleckenstein [4] and possibly encourage clinicians to use these drugs in the treatment of human CM.

Materials and Methods

Genetically CM hamsters of both sexes from the BIO 8262 inbred strain and healthy control hamsters of inbred strain CLAC were used. The CM animals are afflicted with a degenerative myocardial disease and with muscular dystrophy. Detailed description of the genetic background of the animals as well as of the morphologic appearance of heart and skeletal musculature and of some biochemical and functional features is given elsewhere [8–12, 14]. The hereditary disease can be labeled as secondary CM since the heart muscle is involved within a disorder of the striated musculature. Clinical, electrocardiographic, morphologic, chemical, and cytophotometric investigations could not reveal striking cardiac hypertrophy in the myopathic animals [13, 15]. Therefore, the CM of the hamsters seems to be of the dilative type since hemodynamic studies [18] revealed a decrease in cardiac performance with no indication for restrictive cardiomyopathy.

The CM hamsters of strain BIO 8262 and the healthy control hamsters of strain CLAC were housed under identical conditions in air-conditioned rooms with artificial light in a 12-h day and night cycle. Normal laboratory diet (Ssniff-H hamster chow) and tap water were offered ad libitum.

1 a) Myocardial Calcium Content as a Function of Dose of Isoproterenol

Thirty-day-old CM hamsters do not show any histopathologic signs of the CM thus being in the prenecrotic phase of the disease [14]. Earlier experiments showed that isoproterenol will provoke an increased uptake of radiocalcium as well as elevation of total myocardial calcium content in these animals 6 hours after subcutaneous injection [9].

A total of 178 healthy (strain CLAC) as well as CM (strain BIO 8262) hamsters at age 30 days was used for the experiments. Of each strain, 10 animals were untreated. Eight groups of 9 or 10 animals of each strain were injected s.c. with increasing doses of isoproterenol (0.03, 0.1, 0.3, 1.0, 3.0, 10.0, 30.0, 100.0 mg/kg body wt.). Six hours after administration of isoproterenol the treated and the untreated animals were anesthetised with ether and killed. Their hearts were excised. The left ventricular wall with septum was prepared for calcium analysis by atomic absorption spectrophotometry as described elsewhere [7,10].

1b) Myocardial Calcium Content as a Function of Time after Isoproterenol

For these experiments 268 healthy (strain CLAC) as well as CM (strain BIO 8262) hamsters of age 30 days were used. Of each strain, 10–15 animals were untreated. Ten groups consisting of 9–15 animals of each strain were injected s.c. with 1 mg isoproterenol/kg body wt. At 7.5, 15, and 30 min and, 1, 2, 4, 8, 16, 32, and 64 h after the administration of isoproterenol, the treated as well as the untreated animals were sacrificed after anesthesia with ether. Their hearts were excised and prepared for calcium analysis as already described.

2. Action of Verapamil on Isoproterenol-Induced Myocardial Calcium Uptake

A total of 53 CM hamsters (strain BIO 8262) at age 30 days were used in this study. Ten animals were untreated, ten animals received 1 mg isoproterenol s.c./kg body wt., and 4 groups of 7–11 animals each were injected s.c. with increasing doses of Verapamil (1, 3, 5, and 10 mg/kg body wt.) and simultaneously with 1 mg isoproterenol s.c./kg body wt. Six hours after the administration of isoproterenol the treated and the untreated hamsters were anesthetised with ether and sacrificed. Their hearts were excised and prepared for calcium analysis.

3. Action of Verapamil on Spontaneous Myocardial Calcium Uptake

For this series 38 CM hamsters (strain BIO 8262) were used. Twenty-eight animals (age 30 days) were divided into 3 groups and injected s.c. with 1, 5, and 10 mg Verapamil/kg body wt. twice daily for 30 days. Ten hamsters were untreated. On the 60th day of life the animals were anesthetised with ether and killed. Their hearts were excised and prepared for calcium determination.

4. Action of Verapamil on Spontaneous Myocardial Degeneration

For this histologic study 27 CM hamsters (strain BIO 8262) were used. Seventeen 30-day-old animals were injected s.c. with 10 mg Verapamil/kg body wt. twice daily for 30 days. Ten hamsters served as controls and were untreated. On the 60th day of live the animals were anesthetised with ether, killed, and their hearts excised. From the formaline-fixed tissue paraffin sections (7 μm) were performed and stained with hematoxylin-eosin.

Since the treatment of the hamsters with Verapamil was carried out at different times between 1973 and 1976, the hearts were not cut uniformly. For histologic evaluation we differentiated between fresh necroses and resorptive changes. The quantity of the pathologic changes was estimated by an approximative counting of the foci per section. In cases of more than one section of a heart, the foci found were given in percent of the total of the sections examined.

In our earliest experiments only one section was made through the middle of both ventricles in a plane horizontal to the heart axis. In the second series three planes were studied. The hearts were cut as in the first series; however, from the apical part, two additional sections parallel to the heart axis were taken. In our recent experiments four planes of the hearts were evaluated for pathologic changes. Two sections were cut in horizontal plane projection, and from the apical part two sections were cut parallel to the heart axis, as described above.

Results

1 a) Myocardial Calcium Content as a Function of Dose of Isoproterenol

In Figure 1 the behavior of the myocardial calcium content in healthy and CM 30-day-old hamsters is demonstrated as a function of dose of isoproterenol. The detailed values are enlisted in Table 1. The myocardial calcium content of untreated hamsters (of both strains) is 7.6 mEq/kg dry wt. Comparing the dose-effect curves (Fig. 1) it is obvious that myocardial calcium accumulation becomes increasingly augmented with increasing doses of isoproterenol in the CM hearts. The dose of 0.1 mg isoproterenol/kg body wt. is already effective in slightly elevating myocardial calcium content in both strains of hamsters; however, beyond the dose of 0.3 mg/kg, calcium accumulation in CM hearts significantly exceeds that in controls. At the dose of 100 mg isoproterenol/kg body wt., the myocardial calcium content amounts 30.9 ± 7.75 mEq/kg dry wt. in the CM hamsters, whereas it reached only 20.0 ± 2.07 mEq/kg dry wt. in the control animals.

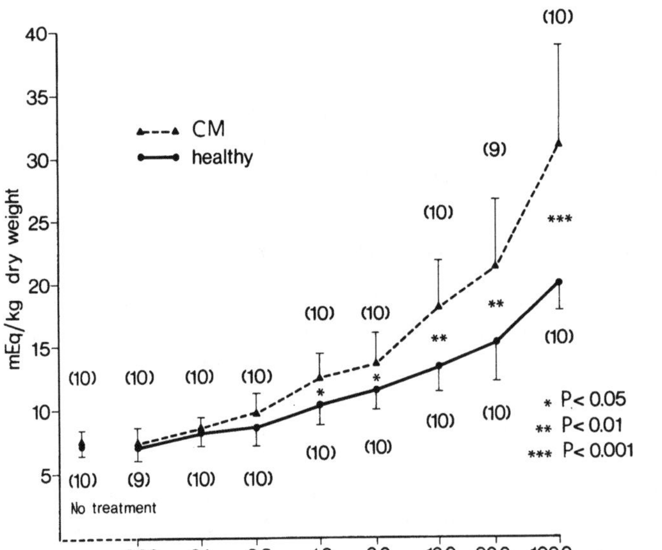

Fig. 1. Myocardial calcium content (mean ± s.d.) in 30-day-old healthy (strain CLAC) and CM (strain BIO 8262) hamsters as a function of dose of isoproterenol. The measurements were carried out 6 h after s.c. isoproterenol administration. Numbers in parentheses represent the number of animals studied

Table 1. Myocardial calcium content in 30-day-old healthy (strain CLAC) and CM (strain BIO 8262) hamsters 6 h after s.c. injection of various doses of isoproterenol. The values represent the mean ± s.d. Numbers in parentheses are the number of hearts analysed.

	Myocardial calcium content (mEq/kg dry wt.)	
	Strain CLAC	Strain BIO 8262
Untreated	7.6 ±0.98 (10)	7.6 ±1.03 (10)
Isoproterenol treated		
0.03 mg/kg	7.1 ±1.00 (9)	7.2 ±0.96 (10)
0.1 mg/kg	8.7 ±0.70 (10)	8.6 ±0.80 (10)
0.3 mg/kg	8.6 ±0.86 (10)	9.7 ±1.76 (10)
1.0 mg/kg	10.4 ±1.55 (10)	12.4 ±1.97 (10)[a])
3.0 mg/kg	11.5 ±1.53 (10)	13.6 ±2.40 (10)[a])
10.0 mg/kg	13.3 ±1.95 (10)	17.9 ±3.83 (10)[b])
30.0 mg/kg	15.2 ±3.06 (10)	21.1 ±5.50 (9)[b])
100.0 mg/kg	20.2 ±2.07 (10)	30.9 ±7.75 (10)[c])

[a]) $P < 0.05$
[b]) $P < 0.01$
[c]) $P < 0.001$

1b) Myocardial Calcium Content as a Function of Time after Isoproterenol

In Figure 2 the behavior of the myocardial calcium content in healthy and CM 30-day-old hamsters is shown as a function of time after 1 mg isoproterenol s.c./kg

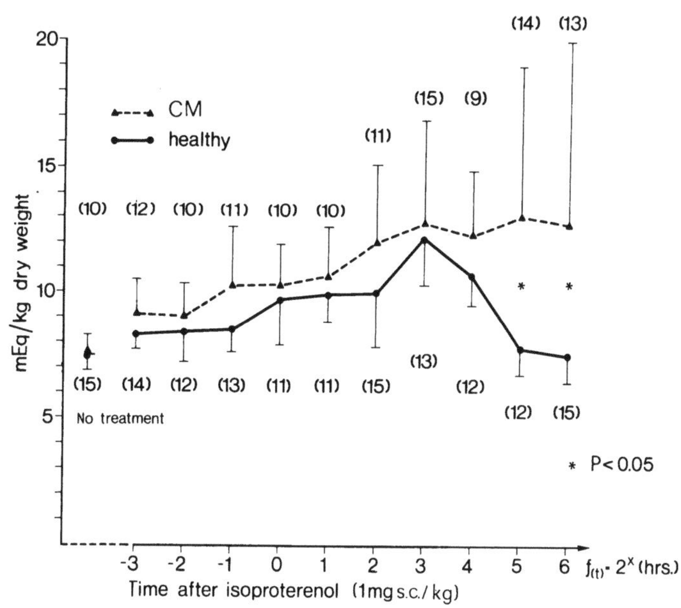

Fig. 2. Myocardial calcium content (mean ± s.d.) in 30–33-day-old healthy (strain CLAC) and CM (strain BIO 8262) hamsters as a function of time after isoproterenol administration. The measurements were carried out 7.5 min to 64 h after the s.c. injection of 1 mg isoproterenol/kg body wt. Numbers in parentheses represent the number of animals studied

body wt. The detailed values are given in Table 2. The myocardial calcium content of untreated CM animals is 7.5 ±0.76 mEq/kg dry wt., and does not differ from that of untreated healthy controls, which is 7.6 ±0.59 mEq/kg. Amazingly, only $7^1/_2$ min after the s.c. isoproterenol injection myocardial calcium content begins to increase and continues for the next 8 h. During this period myocardial calcium accumulation runs parallel to CM and healthy hearts, although the calcium content of the CM hearts is constantly higher. Eight hours after isoproterenol injection, a climax is reached. Myocardial calcium content is 12.8 ±3.96 mEq/kg dry wt. in the CM hearts and 12.2 ±1.86 mEq/kg dry wt. in the healthy control hearts. Later, myocardial calcium content declines in the controls, approaching basic values again 32 h after isoproterenol injection, whereas that of the CM hamsters remains elevated during the rest of the observation period up to 64 h.

Table 2. Myocardial calcium content in 30–33-day-old healthy (strain CLAC) and CM (strain BIO 8262) hamsters at various intervals after s.c. injection of 1 mg isoproterenol/kg body wt. The values represent the mean ± s.d. Numbers in parentheses are the number of hearts analysed.

	Myocardial calcium content (mEq/kg body wt.)	
	Strain CLAC	Strain BIO 8262
Untreated	7.6 ±0.59 (15)	7.5 ±0.76 (10)
After isoproterenol		
7.5 min	8.3 ±1.16 (14)	9.1 ±1.36 (12)
15 min	8.4 ±0.95 (12)	9.0 ±1.26 (10)
30 min	8.5 ±1.76 (13)	10.3 ±2.33 (11)
1 h	9.7 ±1.87 (11)	10.3 ±1.60 (10)
2 h	9.9 ±1.11 (11)	10.6 ±2.04 (10)
4 h	10.0 ±2.16 (15)	12.0 ±3.11 (11)
8 h	12.2 ±1.86 (13)	12.8 ±3.96 (15)
16 h	10.7 ±1.23 (12)	12.3 ±2.56 (9)
32 h	7.8 ±1.13 (12)	13.0 ±6.03 (14)[a])
64 h	7.5 ±1.11 (15)	12.7 ±7.31 (13)[a])

[a]) $P < 0.05$

2. Action of Verapamil on Isoproterenol-Induced Myocardial Calcium Uptake

Table 3 shows the myocardial calcium contents of 30-day-old CM hamsters in the prenecrotic stage of their CM with and without treatment. Here, the calcium content of untreated animals is 7.9 ±1.84 mEq/kg dry wt. Six hours after administration of 1 mg isoproterenol s.c./kg body wt. it rises up to 10.8 ±2.02 mEq/kg dry wt., which is about 37% above base level. When calcium antagonistic Verapamil is administered in increasing doses simultaneously with the standard dose of 1 mg isoproterenol/kg body wt., a dose-dependent decrease of the isoproterenol-induced calcium accumulation can be observed. While 1 mg Verapamil s.c./kg body wt. is nearly ineffective in this respect (10.3 ±1.36 mEq/kg dry wt.), 3 and 5 mg s.c./kg can considerably restrict myocardial calcium overload (8.9 ±1.17 and 8.3 ±0.65 mEq/kg dry wt., respectively). Doses of 10 mg

Verapamil s.c./kg body wt. do completely counteract 1 mg isoproterenol/kg body wt. (8.0 ±1.11 mEq/kg dry wt.).

Table 3. Myocardial calcium content in 30-day-old CM hamsters (strain BIO 8262) after s.c. administration of isoproterenol and Verapamil. The values represent the mean ± s.d. Numbers in parentheses are the number of hearts analysed.

	Myocardial calcium content (mEq/kg dry wt.)
Untreated	7.9 ±1.84 (13)
Isoproterenol (1 mg/kg)	10.8 ±2.02 (10)
Verapamil (1 mg/kg) plus isoproterenol (1 mg/kg)	10.3 ±1.36 (7)
Verapamil (3 mg/kg) plus isoproterenol (1 mg/kg)	8.9 ±1.17 (7)
Verapamil (5 mg/kg) plus isoproterenol (1 mg/kg)	8.3 ±0.65 (11)
Verapamil (10 mg/kg) plus isoproterenol (1 mg/kg)	8.0 ±1.11 (8)

3. Action of Verapamil on Spontaneous Myocardial Calcium Uptake

Table 4 displays the myocardial calcium contents of 60-day-old CM hamsters with and without chronic treatment with Verapamil. In the untreated group the average calcium content is 269.9 ±295.4 mEq/kg dry wt. It declines with increasing doses of Verapamil. Already the chronical application of 1 mg Verapamil s.c./kg body wt. twice daily considerably counteracts myocardial calcification. The average calcium content is reduced to 85.8 ±136.6 mEq/kg dry wt. The dose of 10 mg Verapamil s.c./kg body wt. twice daily is fully effective in suppressing the spontaneous myocardial calcification. The myocardial calcium content under this treatment is 9.9 ±2.15 mEq/kg dry wt. and does not differ from that value, which was gained in previous studies from 61–82-day-old healthy hamsters and amounted to 8.85 ±1.10 mEq/kg dry wt. [10].

Table 4. Myocardial calcium content in 60-day-old CM hamsters (strain BIO 8262) after chronic treatment with Verapamil. The values represent the mean ± s.d. Numbers in parentheses are the number of hearts analysed.

	Myocardial calcium content (mEq/kg dry wt.)
Untreated	269.9 ±295.40 (13)
Verapamil 2 × 1 mg/kg	85.8 ±136.56 (5)
Verapamil 2 × 5 mg/kg	33.5 ± 32.63 (10)
Verapamil 2 × 10 mg/kg	9.9 ± 2.15 (13)

4. Action of Verapamil on Spontaneous Myocardial Degeneration

Figure 3 depicts the results of the histologic studies. In the first series with only one myocardial section evaluated (dots) none of the five Verapamil-treated

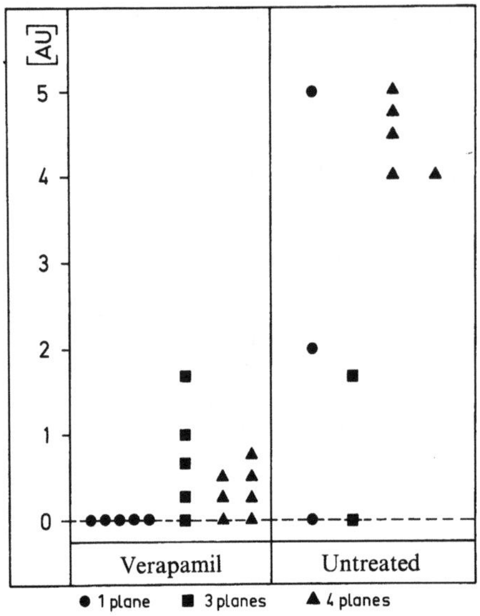

Fig. 3. Morphologic changes of the myocardium in chronically Verapamil-treated and untreated 60-day-old CM hamsters (strain BIO 8262). The animals received 10 mg Verapamil/kg body wt. twice daily for 30 days. The treatment started on the 30th day of life. The results are plotted on an arbitrary scale (*AU*). The different symbols represent different experimental series studied at different times with different numbers of sections through the heart

hamsters exhibited morphologic abnormalities, whereas severe structural changes could be detected in the myocardium of two out of three untreated animals. The changes consisted of necroses with resorption and of calcification partially located in giant cells. In the second series (squares), in which three different myocardial planes were cut, the results were not as distinct as in the first series. The treated hamsters revealed to some extent older necroses with resorptive changes and calcification. In one out of two untreated animals morphologic abnormalities were not detected. In the last experimental series with four planes studied (triangles) only a few structural alterations of minor degree could be seen in seven treated hamsters. Not quite fresh necroses with cellular infiltration, calcification, and fibrosis were seen in untreated animals. In addition, the heart of one animal showed evidence of very fresh necroses without resorptive changes.

Discussion

Earlier experiments revealed that myocardial degeneration in the CM hamsters is accompanied by myocardial calcium accumulation [10]. Histologic investigations suggested that after the 40th day of life, a rapid cardiac cell decay with coagulation necrosis occurs, as well as a slow degeneration process with calcification, which induces formation of myocardial giant cells [14]. In 30-day-old hamsters, which do not yet exhibit histologic signs of myocardial degeneration, the myocardial calcium content does not differ from that of healthy controls. However, 6 h after the fairly low dose of 1 mg isoproterenol s.c./kg body wt. radiocalcium uptake was strikingly higher in the prospective CM hearts than that in hearts of equally treated healthy control animals [9]. Thus, a latent disturbance on the myocardial calcium metabolism can be assumed. In order to get further insight into the possibly disturbed myocardial calcium metabolism, total myocardial calcium content was measured in 30-day-old CM and healthy hamsters as a function of dose and as a function of time after administration of isoproterenol. The results of these experiments, described here, fully agree with our earlier findings with radiocalcium. Latent disturbance of myocardial calcium metabolism seems to exist unequivocally in the prospective cardiomyopathic hamsters. Morphologic-functional correlative experiments in rats revealed increased permeability of the sarcolemma as an early and significant event during the evolution of isoproterenol-induced cardiac muscle cell lesions [16]. It appears as if the CM heart muscle cells are impaired to counterbalance isoproterenol-induced flooding with calcium. A very similar behavior is reported when transient ischemic myocardium is reperfused [17].

As Verapamil – a calcium antagonistic drug known to blockade specifically transmembrane calcium conductivity of the sarcolemma [6] – was effective in preventing isoproterenol-induced myocardial calcium overload in our experiments, the question arose as to whether this substance might also be able to counterbalance spontaneous calcium accumulation in the CM hamster hearts. Chronic treatment of the cardiomyopathic hamsters with Verapamil was successful in suppressing not only the spontaneous myocardial calcification but also the occurrence of most of the degenerative lesions in the CM animals. Therefore, it seems reasonable that spontaneous manifestation of disturbed myocardial calcium metabolism is represented by the histologically detectable changes of the hamster CM. Disturbance of myocardial calcium metabolism turned out to be the determinant factor for the development of degenerative cardiac lesions in an inherited spontaneous CM of the hamster as well as in the pharmacologic disease model of a isoproterenol-treated rat [4]. Thus, the chalenging hypothesis of Fleckenstein, who considers myocardial calcium overload to play a key role in the pathogenesis of myocardial necroses, seems to become a more general principle for the evolution of degenerative myocardial processes. The successful results of Ciplea and Bock [3], who induced cardioprotection by oral application of another calcium antagonistic substance (fendiline), further support this principle.

Recently, Kaltenbach *et al.* [5] began treating with oral doses of Verapamil humans suffering from HOCM, who were previously treated with beta blockers. There was an impressive improvement in clinical symptoms, in the ECG signs of left ventricular hypertrophy, and of radiologically measured heart volume. Although it has not yet been clarified whether the calcium antagonistic drug acted beneficially by interfering directly with the CM heart muscle cells of the patients, the therapeutical advantage by application of a calcium antagonistic drug is apparent. Since the correlation between distinct clinical, morphologic, functional, and biochemical phenomena of CM has not yet been established, considerable research is required to disclose the certainly intriguing problems of this disease and its therapy.

Summary and Conclusions

In Syrian golden hamsters of the CM inbred strain BIO 8262, latent disturbance of the myocardial calcium metabolism was demonstrated by different degrees of calcium accumulation after isoproterenol administration. Dose-effect and time-course studies were made on 30-day-old prospective CM hamsters in the pre-necrotic stage of their disease and in healthy control animals. By acute and chronic application of the calcium antagonistic substance Verapamil, isoproterenol-induced and spontaneous myocardial calcium accumulation, which accompanies myocardial degeneration in these hamsters, was prevented. Furthermore, the histologic manifestation of the CM, coagulation necrosis and giant cell formation, could also be suppressed by chronic application of Verapamil. Hence, disturbed myocardial calcium metabolism and histologic manifestation of the CM seem to be closely interlinked.

The successful treatment of human HOCM by application of Verapamil and the beneficial therapeutic effect of this drug in the hamster CM support the hypothesis of Fleckenstein [4], who considers myocardial calcium overload as a determining factor for myocardial degeneration. However, distinct clinical, morphologic, functional, and biochemical phenomena require intense study of the variety of degenerative myocardial diseases before this hypothesis can find general acceptance.

References

1. Brigden, W.: Uncommon myocardial diseases. Lancet *1957/II*, 1179–1184, 1234–1249
2. Büchner, F.: Die Pathologie der zellulären und geweblichen Oxydationen. Die Hypoxydosen. In: Handbuch der allgemeinen Pathologie. Springer-Verlag: Berlin-Heidelberg-New York 1957
3. Ciplea, A.G., Bock, P.R.: Kardioprotektion durch perorale Anwendung des Calcium-Antagonisten Sensit. Verhütung isoproterenol-bedingter Myokardnekrosen bei Ratten. Arzneimittel-Forsch. *26*, 1819–1826 (1976)
4. Fleckenstein, A.: Specific inhibitors and promoters of calcium action in the excitation-contraction coupling of heart muscle and their role in the promotion or production of myocardial lesions. In: Calcium and the Heart. London-New York: Academic Press 1971
5. Kaltenbach, M., Hopf, R., Keller, M.: Calciumantagonistische Therapie bei hypertroph-obstruktiver Kardiomyopathie. Dtsch. med. Wschr. *101*, 1284–1287 (1976)
6. Kohlhardt, M., Bauer, B., Krause, H., Fleckenstein, A.: Differentiation of the transmembrane Na and Ca channels in mammalian cardiac fibers by the use of specific inhibitors. Pflügers Arch. ges. Physiol. *335*, 309–322 (1972)
7. Lossnitzer, K., Bajusz, E.: Water and electrolyte alterations during the life course of the BIO 14.6 Syrian golden hamster. A disease model of a hereditary cardiomyopathy. J. mol. cell. Cardiol. *6*, 163–177 (1974)
8. Lossnitzer, K.: Genetic induction of a cardiomyopathy. In: Handbuch der experimentellen Pharmakologie. Berlin-Heidelberg-New York: Springer-Verlag 1975
9. Lossnitzer, K., Janke, J., Hein, B., Stauch, M., Fleckenstein, A.: Disturbed myocardial calcium metabolism – A possible pathogenetic factor in the hereditary cardiomyopathy of the Syrian hamster. In: Recent Advances in Studies on Cardiac Structure and Metabolism, Vol. V, Myocardial Call Damage. Baltimore-London-Tokyo: University Park Press 1975a
10. Lossnitzer, K., Steinhardt, B., Grewe, N., Stauch, M.: Charakteristische Elektrolytveränderungen bei der erblichen Kardiomyopathie des Syrischen Goldhamsters (Stamm BIO 8262). Basic Res. Cardiol. *70*, 508–520 (1975b)

11. Lossnitzer, K., Stauch, M., Mohr, W., Burkhardt, H.: Die Kardiomyopathie des syrischen Goldhamsters. Krankheitsmodell einer sekundären Kardiomyopathie. Therapiewoche *26*, 1730–1743 (1976)
12. Lossnitzer, K., Grewe, N., Konrad, A., Stauch, M.: Elektrokardiographische Veränderungen bei der erblichen Kardiomyopathie des syrischen Goldhamsters. Verh. dtsch. Ges. inn. Med. *82*, 1057–1060 (1977a)
13. Lossnitzer, K., Grewe, N., Konrad, A., Adler, J.: Electrocardiographic changes in cardiomyopathic Syrian hamsters (strain BIO 8262). Basic Res. Cardiol. *72*, 421–435 (1977b)
14. Mohr, W., Lossnitzer, K.: Morphologische Untersuchungen an Hamstern des Stammes BIO 8262 mit erblicher Myopathie und Kardiomyopathie. Beitr. Path. *153*, 178–193 (1974)
15. Mohr, W., Lossnitzer, K., Schwarz, J.: The cardiomyopathy of the Syrian hamster. Hypertrophic or dystrophic? (1977) (Submitted for publication)
16. Rona, G., Boutet, M., Hüttner, I., Peters, H.: Pathogenesis of isoproterenol-induced myocardial alterations: Functional and morphological correlates. In: Recent Advances in Studies on Cardiac Structure and Metabolism, Vol. III, Myocardial Metabolism. Baltimore-London-Tokyo: University Park Press 1973
17. Shen, A.C., Jennings, R.B.: Kinetics of calcium accumulation in acute myocardial ischemic injury. Amer. J. Path. *67*, 441–452 (1972)
18. Stauch, M., Lossnitzer, K.: Left ventricular function in Syrian hamsters of different ages with hereditary cardiomyopathy. In: Recent Advances in Studies on Cardiac Structure and Metabolism, Vol. VI, Pathophysiology and Morphology of Myocardial Cell Alteration. Baltimore-London-Tokyo: University Park Press 1975

Myocardial Biopsy: Technical Aspects, Problems

4. Technical Aspects, Experiences, and Complications of Right and Left Ventricular Endomyocardial Biopsy

G. KOBER, B. KUNKEL, H.-J. BECKER, W.-D. BUSSMANN, and M. KALTENBACH

Surgical procedures [5,25] include access to the heart by thoracotomy or from the epigastrium. Today direct transcutaneous puncture of the left ventricle [3,20], and more recently endomyocardial biopsy procedures from right and left ventricles are preferred. When considering a biopsy, benefit to the patient must be weighed against possible complications.

Patients

Since 1971, we investigated 143 patients in order to verify the diagnosis of suspected COCM. Prior to biopsy clinical investigations, right and left heart catheterization, angiocardiography, and selective coronary arteriography were done in all patients. The number of patient biopsies during recent years has increased eightfold due to refinement of the technique and decrease in the rate of complications. All specimens were obtained under fluoroscopic control. Right ventricular biopsies were taken from the septal wall and left ventricular samples from the diaphragmatic wall or occasionally from apical or distal septal areas.

Methods

The right ventricle was reached transvenously through the punctured or opened femoral vein. In the first studies a relatively rigid and curved endomyocardial bioptome, developed by Konno and Sakakibara[1], was introduced through Seldinger's technique or by an incision in the femoral vein. In the advanced stages of study, a thinner and more flexible forceps[2] was introduced via a pilot catheter[3] which was advanced through the opened saphenous vein up to the right ventricle. Its position was confirmed by pressure measurements and injection of contrast media. Left ventricular biopsies were performed by introducing either Olympus[4] or Machida[5] forceps through the right brachial artery. Left ventricular hemodynamic and angiographic evaluation as well as selective coronary arteriography were performed prior to the biopsy. The same arterial access could

[1] USCI, catalogue no. 9400
[2] R. Wolf, 7134 Knittlingen, PE type of forceps 197z
[3] Lutz & Co., 5 Köln 60, tubing material
[4] Olympus, type BF5 B_2
[5] Machida, type FFC-BR-10W

be used for both procedures. Before biopsy, the pilot catheter was retracted into the ascending aorta to avoid splinting and stiffening of the forceps. For routine examination the Olympus forceps was used. The thinner Machida instrument was reserved for patients with delicate or narrow brachial arteries (Table 1).

Table 1. Techniques of right and left ventricular biopsy.

	Right ventricle		Left ventricle	
Type of forceps	Konno/USCI 9400	Wolf 197z	Olympus BF_5 B_2	Machida FFC-BR-10W
Diameter (mm)				
Tip	2.5	2.3	1.8	1.3
Shaft	2.0	2.0	1.6	1.2
Access to vascular System	Puncture of the femoral vein	Opening of the great saphenous vein	Opening of brachial artery	
Insertion method	Puncture set Vygon 1129.09	Pilot catheter Messrs. Lutz u. Co.	Pilot catheter UMI 1308–3888 (tip was cut)	Pilot catheter USCI 5435 (tip was cut)
Outer diameter				
(mm)	3.0	3.2	8	
(F)	10			7

Transvenous Biopsy of the Right Ventricle (Konno's Method)

In 25 patients the Konno bioptome [12], used by many groups [8,9,11,12,14, 19,23], was introduced transcutaneously into the femoral vein. This bioptome is relatively rigid and curved at the tip to facilitate access to the right ventricle. The curve of the instrument, however, often causes difficulties; when advancing through the inferior vena cava, it may become entangled in other veins, e.g., the hepatic veins. The procedure may sometimes require considerable time and effort and make it impossible to obtain several specimens without great discomfort to the patient.

Transvenous Biopsy of the Right Ventricle ("Wolf" Forceps Via a Pilot Catheter)

In contrast to the Konno method, several biopsies can be obtained without difficulties and in a relatively short time if a pilot catheter is employed. Additional advantages are that pressure can be measured and small injections of contrast media can verify the position of the catheter and forceps. Great saphenous vein cutdown was necessary for introduction of the larger diameter forceps. A disadvantage is the stiffening of the straight forceps in the pilot catheter during removal of the specimens. On the other hand, when the catheter is withdrawn before sampling, the forceps may turn into the outflow tract of the right ventricle.

Retrograde Transarterial Biopsy of the Left Ventricle

The "Olympus" forceps has a flexible shaft which decreases the risk of perforation of the cardiac wall. This forceps is essentially the same as the King's-endomyocardial bioptome used by Richardson [18], Brooksby *et al.* [6], and Ali [2]. Despite the use of thin-walled pilot catheters with very smooth surfaces, it is sometimes impossible to insert the forceps into delicate brachial arteries. In these cases the thinner forceps of Machida via a 7F pilot catheter are used. This instrument is delicate but is prone to malfunction especially in patients with rigid endocardia. Despite this disadvantage the forceps is a good alternative in cases with narrow brachial arteries. Both methods allow excision of several specimens from the left ventricle in a short period of time without significantly prolonging cardiac catheterization.

Cardiac muscle biopsies were performed in 143 patients using the various methods, already described (Table 1). If possible, two specimens were taken from different areas of the ventricle for microscopic evaluation and a third for electron-microscopic analysis. In the left ventricle triple biopsies could be performed.

Results

The patients examined with the different methods are listed in Table 2. All techniques produced specimens large enough for analysis, i.e., between 1.0 and 2.0 mm^2. The lower success rate in obtaining biopsies of the right ventricle was 85%, partly due to the technical difficulties initially encountered. Irrespective of the method, some patients complained of chest pain during sampling which coincided with ventricular extrasystoles. In some patients the turning of the Konno instrument caused an unpleasant, painful sensation. The patients' discomfort and the stiffness of the instrument made retrograde probing of the left

Table 2. Data from patients examined from techniques listed in Table 1.

	Biopsies 6/71–9/77	Number of patients	Sufficient specimens	Complaints	Complications	
right ventricle	Konno biotome	25	85%	Chest pain during turning of biotome, premature beats	Hemopericardium Puncture Thoracotomy	2 1 1
	Pilot catheter Wolf-forceps	19		Chest pain (premature beats) during excision of specimen	Hemopericardium Puncture Thoracotomy	2 1 1
left ventricle	Olympus	88	100%	Heart pain	Transient perception Discorder 22 h after biopsy AV Block 3° transitory Tamponade (puncture)	1 1 1
	Machida	11				

ventricle extremely difficult. This is probably the reason why left ventricular biopsies with the Konno bioptome have seldom been described.

Complications

As indicated in Table 2, myocardial biopsies are not without risk to the patient. In four patients, hemopericardia occurred during right ventricular biopsy. Hemodynamic signs of cardiac tamponade developed within 30 min and could be controlled initially by paracentesis of the pericardium and by insertion of an indwelling catheter. In two patients bleeding stopped following aspiration, and two patients required a thoracotomy. In both patients operated on the punctured area was located in the anterior wall of the right ventricle about 1 cm from the septal wall area chosen as the site for biopsy. In both cases the patients suffered from severe COCM and had severely damaged ventricles and thin ventricular walls. Biopsying resulted in puncture of the ventricular wall. Following closure of the iatrogenic defect, both patients recovered without further complications.

In one case tamponade occurred during left ventricular biopsy. This could be controlled by pericardial aspiration. Another patient with severe cardiomegaly due to COCM and atrial fibrillation developed a transitory unilateral perception disorder, two hours before the planned discharge from hospital and 22 hours after the biopsy. This was considered to be related to the biopsy, even though the primary disease as well as the atrial fibrillation could be the cause of the disturbance. In a third patient a transient 3° a-V block was observed.

There were no serious embolic complications which can particularly occur after left ventricular biopsy. Combinations of heparin and salicylates are always given in these cases, which possibly explains the low incidence of embolic complications. On the other hand, bleeding complications, e.g., hemopericardia, may be provoked partially by this therapy.

Discussion

At various hospitals myocardial biopsies were performed routinely for evaluation of CMs, particularly if the diagnosis were somewhat doubtful. The technique provides valuable information on morphology of the myocardium even in the early stages of the disease. Postmortem investigations yield less information because disease processes of any etiology are usually at their end stage.

Microscopic, electron-microscopic, and fluorescence microscopic evaluations of the material verified the diagnosis in some cases while in other cases suspected COCM initially was confirmed. These findings also correlated with clinical severity and prognosis. Some cases involved discrepancies between morphology, clinical, and angiographic data. A follow-up of these patients revealed a clear correlation between the morphology and the course of the disease. Only a few authors consider a preoperative morphologic examination of cardiac muscle necessary in patients with valve disease [4]. A specific indication for the procedure exists for patients with cardiac transplantation because morphologic evaluation permits early recognition of rejection phenomenon before the appearance of other signs, such as ECG [7].

In the future, more detailed analyses of biopsy material may reveal important information regarding etiology and therapy of myocardial diseases of unknown etiology. Examinations such as hemodynamic and angiographic investigations including selective coronary arteriography and elaborate serologic tests have not contributed to the solution of most of the problems in CMs.

Biopsies can only be carried out in a sufficient number of cases if a technically good, quick, and low risk method is available. The bioptome, particularly the King's instrument [18], fulfills these criteria. Samples must be obtained from several sites, because the disease process may be localized and one specimen may not be representative. Several samples also supply sufficient material to analyse other parameters, e.g., biochemistry.

Surgical methods [5, 17, 22, 25], such as thoracotomy using various approaches, have largely been abandoned because they constitute a major undertaking. Samples can also be obtained through direct transthoracic puncture of the apical area of the heart by means of a Vim-Silverman or Menghini needle, but this has been undertaken by only a few groups [3, 17, 20, 21, 23]. Injuries of the coronary arteries, perforations of the ventricle, pneumothoraces, or hemothoraces [17, 20] are a constant serious potential risk.

The catheter biopsy technique is the most widely accepted method permitting a transvenous recovery of endomyocardial tissue, especially from the right ventricle. Many groups [8, 9, 11, 12, 14, 19, 23] employ primarily the instrument developed by Konno and Sakakibara [12]. Due to the special design of the instrument, insertion into the right ventricle is often complicated and does not allow multiple biopsies or left ventricular biopsies. These difficulties can be overcome by using a pilot catheter in combination with a different type of forceps.

Our experience as well that of others [6a and personal communications] indicate that even carefully performed ventricular biopsies carry a potentially high risk of complications. This applies especially to severely ill patients in advanced stages of CMs. This risk is minimized if the specimens are definitely obtained from the septal wall and the thin anterior right ventricular wall is avoided. Specimens sometimes include all wall structures, even the pericardium [6a].

Retrograde biopsy of the left ventricle via the brachial artery is a time-saving procedure compared to other methods. The pilot catheter is exchanged with the Sones catheter used for coronary arteriography and ventriculography by means of a guide wire. Thus, hemodynamic and angiographic evaluations as well as the biopsy can be performed together without causing additional discomfort for the patient. The risk of ventricular perforations with subsequent hemopericardia is lower than in right ventricular biopsies, because of the considerable thickness of the left ventricular wall. Comparative studies on biopsy material from the left and right ventricle of the same patient revealed more severe changes in the left ventricular muscle; this included patients with aortic and mitral valve disease [6]. Our own angiographic findings suggest pronounced disturbances of both right and left ventricular function in patients with CMs [8].

In left ventricular biopsies systemic and especially cerebral emboly have been reported in the literature [6a]. So far we have not encountered this problem, possibly because of our choice of routinely administered premedication (heparin and salicylates). The risk of bleeding complications is, however, increased.

Considering the relatively small number of patients examined with this technique, particularly in view of the complications of right ventricular biopsies, the procedure should not be undertaken without serious consideration. It carries potentially a greater risk than other catheter techniques, including selective coronary arteriography [11]. Hemopericardium is a serious complication and may require immediate surgical intervention. Therefore the procedure can only be undertaken in institutes where a thoracic surgeon is available at all times.

Indications for biopsy include all stages of suspected CMs. Biopsies can now be carried out with relative ease. Clarification at an early stage of the disease seems important in view of possible therapeutic consequences which may influence the progression of the disease. Moreover, ventricular biopsies are potentially dangerous and may cause complications when performed during final stages of disease. This applies mainly to right ventricular biopsies in cases of severely enlarged and thin walled chambers.

Summary

Experiences with different catheter biopsy techniques in 143 patients with CMs are reported. Between 1971 and 1977, 44 patients had right and 99 patients left ventricular biopsies. In every case two or more specimens were taken. The complication rate in right ventricular biopsy was much higher (four times tamponade) than after left ventricular biopsy. The amount of tissue taken from the myocardium was sufficient for analysis in each case of left, but not in all right ventricular biopsies.

Due to a higher complication rate and lower effectiveness, transvenous right ventricular biopsies were given up in favor of left ventricular biopsies. The use of a thin-walled pilot catheter simplifies the introduction of the bioptome via the brachial artery. With this technique multiple biopsies can be obtained in a short time without much discomfort to the patient.

Appendix

Tables 3 and 4 list unpublished investigations of endomyocardial biopsies performed by seven West German groups. We would like to express our thanks to these investigators for kindly making their data available to us and for permission to publish these.

It should be noted that the administration of premedication was not uniform and that different techniques, including transthoracic puncture have been used.

Table 3. Data from endomyocardial biopsies.

Clinic	Biopsy methods[a]	Premedication	Patients[b]	Specimens per patient	Ventricular biopsy Left	Ventricular biopsy Right
Deeg, Schneider Würzburg	Konno (Olympus)	None	110 (100)	1–3	2	108
Harmjanz Celle	Konno (Olympus)	None	85	2–3	–	85
Kober, Kaltenbach Frankfurt	Konno Wolf-Biotom Olympus Machida	Heparin Salicylates 1.5 g/d	143 (136)	2–3	 59 10	25 19
Kuhn, Loogen Düsseldorf	Konno (73) Olympus (109)	None	182	1–3	16	166
Schlepper Bad Nauheim	Transthoracic puncture	Anesthesia Intubation Xylocain Intensive care unit	40	1	40	
Zebe, Kübler Heidelberg	Konno (RV) Olympus (RV + LV)	None	109	2	99 (left + right = 5)	10

[a] Methods in parentheses were rarely used. [b] Numbers in parentheses are the numbers of patients where adequate biopsy material was obtained.

Table 4. Data from endomyocardial biopsies.

Clinic	Complications[a]	Therapy	Consequence	Complaints[a]
Deeg, Schneider Würzburg	Cardiac tamponade (RV) (1)	Surgery	–	Occasional dyspnea and chest pain
Harmjanz Celle	–	–	–	In ~10% chest pain often > 12 h
Kober, Kaltenbach Frankfurt	Cardiac tamponades (RV) (4) Tamponade (LV) (1) AVB III° transitory (1) transitory sensation disorder (1)	Puncture 2 × Thoracotomy 2 × Puncture Pacemaker	– –	Transitory chest pain Chest pain for 2 h (1)
Kuhn, Loogen[b] Düsseldor	RSB (RV) (1) LSB (LV) (1) AV Block II° (1) AV Block III° in LSB (1)	Conservative	–	Seldom transitory chest pain
Schlepper Bad Nauheim	Transitory premature beats	Xylocain, routinely	–	–
Zebe, Kübler Heidelberg	Sepsis (1) Transitory cerebrale ischemia during atrial fibrillation (1)	Conservative		Transitory chest pain (1)

[a] Number of patients indicated in parentheses [b] All complications were transitory

References

1. Alexander, C.S., Gobel, F.L.: Diagnosis of idiopathic hypertrophic subaortic stenosis by right ventricular septal biopsy. Amer. J. Cardiol. *34*, 142–151 (1974)
2. Ali, N.: Transvenous endomyocardial biopsy using the gastrointestinal biopsy (Olympus GFB) catheter. Amer. Heart J. *87*, 294–297 (1974)
3. Bercu, B., Heinz, J., Choudhry, A.S., Cabrera, P.: Myocardial biopsy. A new technic utilizing the ventricular septum. Amer. J. Cardiol. *14*, 675–678 (1964)
4. Björk, V.O., Hultquist, G.: Ultrastructural, enzyme, histochemical and light microscopic investigation of the myocardium in cases undergoing open heart surgery. Scand. J. Thorac. Cardiovasc. Surg. *1*, 27–41 (1967)
5. Brainbridge, W.V., Niles, N.R.: Left ventricular drill biopsy. J. Thorac. Cardiovasc. Surg. *47*, 685–686 (1964)
6. Brooksby, A.B., Jenkins, B.S., Coltart, D.J., Webb-Peploe, M.M.: Left-ventricular endomyocardial biopsy. Lancet *1974/II*, 1222–1225

6a. Brooksby, I.A.B., Swanton, R.H., Jenkins, B.S., Webb-Peploe, M.M.: Long sheat technique for introduction of catheter tip manometer or endomyocardial bioptome into left or right heart. Brit. Heart J. *36*, 908–912 (1974)

7. Caves, P.K., Schulz, W.P., Dong, E., Stinson, E.B., Shumway, N.E.: New instrument for transvenous cardiac biopsy. Amer. J. Cardiol. *33*, 264–267 (1974)
8. Guldner, N., Kober, G., Schäfer, G., Bussmann, W.-D., Hopf, R., Kaltenbach, M.: Volumenparameter des linken und rechten Ventrikels bei Kardiomyopathien. Z. Kardiol., Suppl. *2*, 7 (1975) (Abstr 7)
9. Harmjanz, D.: Problems of myocardial biopsy. Postgrad. med. J. *51*, 291–292 (1975)
10. Harmjanz, D., Reale, E., Luciano, L., Ostertag, P.: Die Endomyokard-Biopsie als Hilfsmittel in der Diagnostik von Myokarderkrankungen. Verh. dtsch. Ges. inn. Med. *77*, 1263–1266(1971)
11. Kaltenbach, M., Becker, H.-J., Kober, G., Martin, K.-L., Bussmann, W.-D., Petersen, P., Lutz, E., Bartelt, K.-M.: Erfahrungen mit der Sones-Technik bei 1000 selektiven Koronarangiographien. Verh. dtsch. Ges. Kreisl.-Forsch. *40*, 426–429 (1974)
12. Konno, S., Sakakibara, S.: Endo-myocardial biopsy. Dis. Chest *44*, 345–350 (1963)
13. Kuhn, H., Breithardt, G., Knieriem, H.-J., Loogen, F., Both, A., Schmidt, W.A.K., Stroobandt, R., Gleichmann, U.: Die Bedeutung der endomyokardialen Katheterbiopsie für die Diagnostik und die Beurteilung der Prognose der kongestiven Kardiomyopathie. Dtsch. med. Wschr. *100*, 717–723 (1975)
14. Kunkel, B., Kober, G., Lapp, H., Leuschner, U., Kaltenbach, M.: Vergleich klinischer, licht- und elektronenmikroskopischer Befunde bei Kardiomyopathien. Z. Kardiol., Suppl. *2*, 27 (1975)
15. Mösslacher, H., Slany, J.: Myokardbiopsie. Z. Kreisl.-Forsch. *60*, 289–291 (1971)
16. Müller, S., Müller, P., Richter, G.: Transvenöse und transarterielle Endomyokardbiopsie mit einem Katheter-Bioptom. Z. Kreisl.-Forsch. *60*, 291–303 (1971)
17. Raffensberger, J., Driscoll, J.F., Sutton, G.C., Weinberg, M.: Myocardial biopsy. Arch. Surg. *89*, 1021–1028 (1964)
18. Richardson, P.J.: King's endomyocardial bioptome. Lancet *1974/I*, 660–661
19. Richardson, P.J.: Catheter technique for endomyocardial biopsy. J. Cardiovasc. Technology *16*, 31–37 (1974)
20. Shirey, E.K., Hawk, W.A., Mukerji, D., Effler, D.B.: Percutaneous myocardial biopsy of the left ventricle. Experience in 198 Patients. Circulation *46*, 112–122 (1972)
21. Sutton, D.C., Sutton, G.C.: Needle biopsy of the human ventricular myocardium: review of 54 consecutive cases. Amer. Heart J. *60*, 364–370 (1960)
22. Sutton, G.C., Driscoll, J.F., Gunnar, R.M., Tobin, J.R.: Exploratory mediastinotomy in primary myocardial disease. Prog. cardiovasc. Dis. *7*, 83–97 (1964)
23. Timmis, C.G., Gordon, S., Baron, R.H., Brough, A.J.: Percutaneous myocardial biopsy. Amer. Heart J. *70*, 499–504 (1965)
24. Torp, A.: Endomyocardial biopsy. Scand. J. Thorac. Cardiovasc. Surg. *7*, 253–261 (1973)
25. Weinberg, M., Egbert, H.F., Lynfield, J.: Diagnostic biopsy of the pericardium and myocardium. Arch. Surg. *76*, 825–829 (1958)

5. Myocardial Biopsies

D. Harmjanz

Problems of Myocardial Biopsy

The various techniques for obtaining myocardial biopsies are potentially harmful, and one must select very carefully the candidates for this procedure. These patients must be those in whom the myocardial disease can be determined by no other methods – due to the cause, the extent, or the stage of the disorder. Thus the selection of patients is the task of the clinical cardiologists, not the catheterization team. Moreover, whether or not this procedure is undertaken depends on the availability of histologic back-up facilities. The cardiologists and histologists should discuss individual cases in advance of the biopsy. The fixation method and the extent of examination of the specimens should be determined in order to help reduce unnecessary and uninformative examinations.

The site of the proposed biopsy should also be selected in advance, because several myocardial diseases are more likely to be found in the left ventricle. For example, IHSS commonly occurs in the left ventricular septum. Thus, knowledge of the topographic distribution of the disease improves the outcome of the examination.

The optimal time for biopsy depends on the stage of the underlying disease. We should remember that little is known of the morphologic course of myocardial diseases in humans. For example, an inflammation may have already healed, so the histologic examination will show only scars, and the etiology cannot be determined at this time. Other signs, such as swelling of the mitochondria, may be transitory, as we have demonstrated in a case of alcoholic CM. On the other hand, timing cannot be accurately determined until more is known about the natural course of the various myocardial diseases. Thus a vicious circle is set up.

Standardizing the data taken for patients undergoing myocardial biopsy may be a solution to the problem. In collaboration with Dr. Olsen, National Heart Hospital, and Dr. Richardson, King's College Hospital, London, a questionnaire has been formulated. In this way we hope to get more information concerning these unsolved problems.

Hospital: Date: **Cardiac Biopsy**

Name: Catheterization no:
male/female: Unit no:
Age: Race: Biopsy no:

Clinical Diagnosis: cardiac
systemic

Indication for Biopsy:

History (general):

History (special): duration of the cardiac disease
date of onset of the patient's symptoms
cardinal symptoms

present class of the N. Y. Heart Association
drugs prescribed

drug response alcohol intake

Clinical Findings: dyspnoea at rest: on exertion: cyanosis:
oedema: neck veins: liver:
blood pressure: pulmonary congestion:
heart rate at rest: rhythm:
signs of ventricular hypertrophy right: left:
signs of ventricular scar: valvar disease:

Chest X-ray: cardio-thoracic ratio:

Ecg:

Catheterization data: RA LA RV LV LVEDP
PA aorta

cardiac output:

Angiography: RV LV
ejection fraction of LV: coronaries:

Site of Biopsy: RV LV
no. of samples: fixation solution:

Biopsy Diagnosis:

Myocardial Biopsy and Pathology in Cardiomyopathies

6. Postmortem Findings and Histologic, Histochemical, and Electron Microscopic Findings of Myocardial Biopsies

E. G. J. Olsen

Introduction

The clinical classification of CMs [3, 4, 9], defined as a heart muscle disease of unknown cause or association [10], is used here. COCM, the type most commonly encountered, is of world-wide distribution. It is known by a variety of names which were reviewed by Cockshott *et al.* as early as 1967.

The age at which patients present is usually over 35 years [2], but the age range in those cases personally examined has varied from 16–84 years. At autopsy

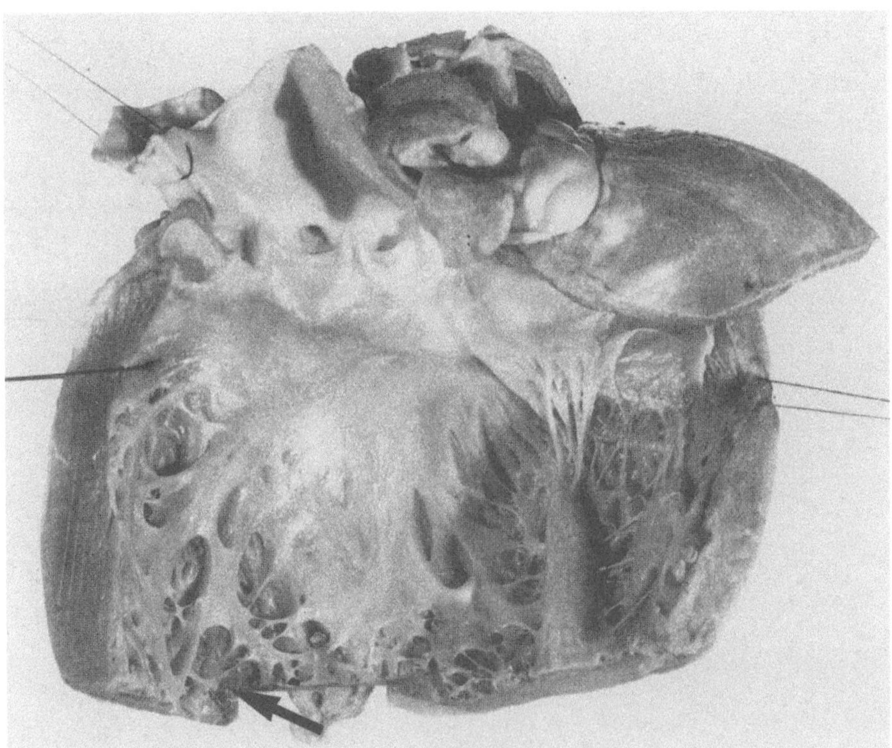

Fig. 1. Part of the opened left ventricle is displayed, showing severe dilatation of the chamber and endocardial thickening. Despite hypertrophy, the myocardial wall thickness is normal (due to dilatation). Note the thrombus at the lower margin of the photograph (*arrow*)

the hearts are usually overweight, between 400 and 750 g [11]. In three instances weights greater than 1000 g have been registered (personal observation).

The striking feature at autopsy is that all cardiac chambers are often severely dilated and the muscle is extremely soft, flabby (Fig. 1), and frequently pale. Despite hypertrophy, the ventricular walls may be of normal thickness, 2–3 mm at the conus and 15 mm at the left ventricular wall, due to the severe degree of dilatation masking the hypertrophy [12]. The endocardium is frequently thickened and thrombus is superimposed in over 60% of cases [16], located particularly in the apical region. Transverse sections of the ventricles show not infrequently fine fibrous replacement, particularly in long-standing cases, usually limited to the inner layers of the myocardium. This contrasts with the distribution in cases of proven viral etiology where foci of fibrosis are scattered throughout the entire thickness of the myocardial wall. The coronary arteries are usually completely unobstructed and free from atheroma, although this depends on the age at death. Occasionally in elderly patients, some flecks of arteriosclerosis may be found narrowing the arterial lumina, but the severe changes observed in the myocardium are out of all proportion to the mild degree of atherosclerosis which may be encountered. By definition, there are no other lesions in the heart and no other associated conditions elsewhere in the body which could result in myocardiac failure.

Histologically, the appearances are characteristically nonspecific. The myocardial fibers are regularly arranged and severely attenuated (Fig. 2). Nuclear

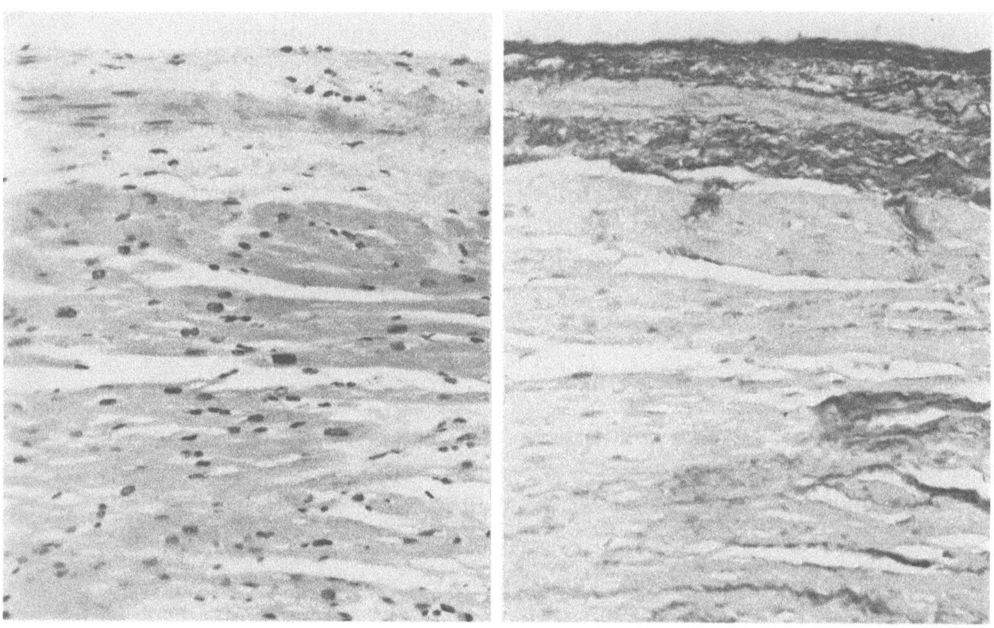

Fig. 2. Photomicrograph from a patient who died as the result of COCM. The myocardial fibers are regularly arranged and nuclear changes of hypertrophy are seen, but the diameter of the fibers is normal, due to attenuation. The endocardium is thick. Note the severe hypertrophy of the smooth muscle component. Left, H & E. Right, Weigert's elastic Van Gieson. Both, ×200

changes of hypertrophy such as blunting of the nuclear poles, pyknosis, or vesicular changes are clearly seen, but due to the attenuation of the fibers, their diameters may fall within the normal range, that is, 5–12 μ. Occasionally small necrotic foci which have incited an inflammatory reaction are found [15]. The small vessels are usually absolutely normal. Interstitial fibrous tissue may have increased and areas of fibrous replacement may be present. These, as already mentioned, are confined to the inner layers of the myocardium. The endocardium is thickened and the smooth muscle component is often prominent, denoting that dilatation has been present for some time (see Fig. 2).

Material and Methods

The criteria established from the study of postmortem material have been strictly applied to fresh endomyocardial biopsies obtained from 199 patients in whom the principal suspected diagnosis was COCM. The tissue was recovered either by the Konno instrument [22, 5] or the King's College Hospital instrument [20]. There were 131 males and 68 females, aged 7–65 years, averaging 44.3 years. The average number of biopsies per patient was 3.2, and right ventricular biopsies alone were performed in 191 patients. In the remaining eight patients, only the left ventricle was sampled. Thirteen patients underwent simultaneous right and left biopsies.

During the last five years, tissue has been received from 11 London centers and from four in the Federal Republic of Germany. Morphologic evaluation was carried out without prior knowledge of the suspected clinical diagnosis.

The techniques and methods employed for morphologic and electron-microscopic examination have previously been summarized [14]. Histologic examination was carried out on every biopsy and electron-microscopic evaluation on all those where sufficient material existed after tissue for histologic examination had been selected. Histochemical analysis was restricted to the material submitted from the London centers.

Results

Histology

The characteristic histologic appearances were those of a dilated ventricular chamber consisting of regularly arranged, hypertrophied, attenuated myocardial fibers and smooth muscle hypertrophy in the overlying thickened endocardium.

Histochemical Analysis

When biopsy material was first analysed (1972) a wide spectrum of histochemical and cytochemical analyses were carried out, including ATPase (calcium activated) and alkaline phosphotase. Subsequent experience gave consistent results, and it became evident that many of the changes observed were secondary to heart failure. At the present time the material is analysed for succinic dehydrogenase, which reflects the activity of other similar types of enzymes, glycogen, acid, and alkaline phosphotase. The changes observed with light microscopy varied with the clinical stage. In the majority of cases, though heart failure had been present, apparent increase in succinic dehydrogenase and phosphotases was obtained. Glycogen was also frequently slightly increased (Fig. 3), but a decrease was observed in some biopsies, corresponding to the third stage of hypertrophy [8].

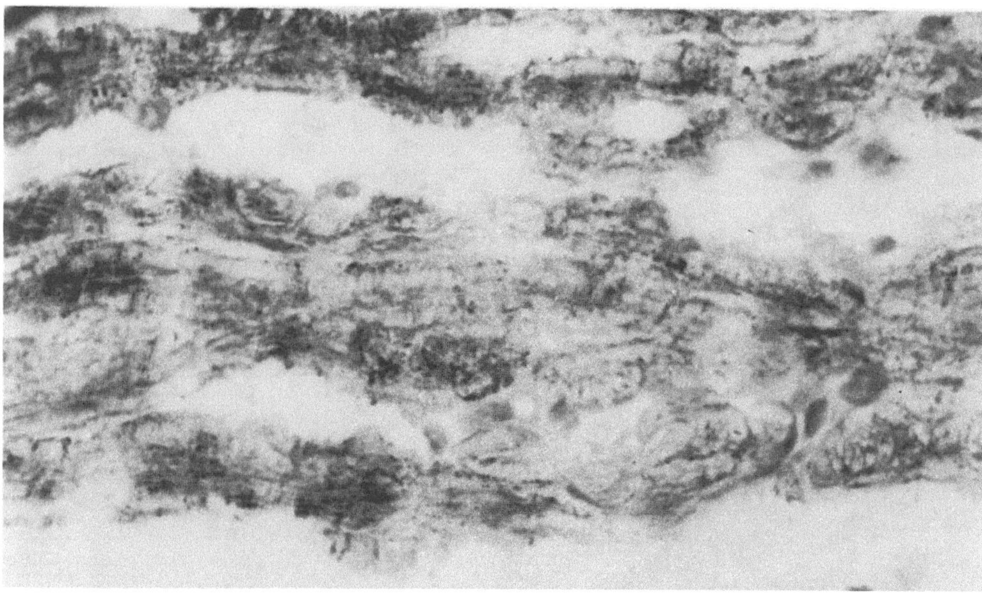

Fig. 3. Photomicrograph of right ventricular biopsy obtained by bioptome, stained for glycogen. In some cells a mild increase is noted. Periodic acid Schiff, ×800

Electron-Microscopic Examination

Changes of hypertrophy, i.e., an increase in mitochondria showing variability in size and shape, an increased number of ribosomes, an enlarged Golgi apparatus, increased convolutions of nuclear membranes, and irregular, dilated T tubules, were found, in short, the changes of hypertrophy previously described by Olsen [13] and Maron *et al.* [7].

Changes similar to those seen in mild hypoxia, consisting of swelling and cristolysis (Fig. 4) and foci of dissolution of the protein elements of myofibrils, were occasionally encountered. Necrotic foci with disruption of the sarcolemma were occasionally found. Not infrequently some irregular arrangement of myofibrils was seen (Fig. 5), including those of frequent cross-over between myocardial fibrils, but these findings were never as severe or as extensive as those encountered in typical cases of hypertrophic CM (with or without obstruction).

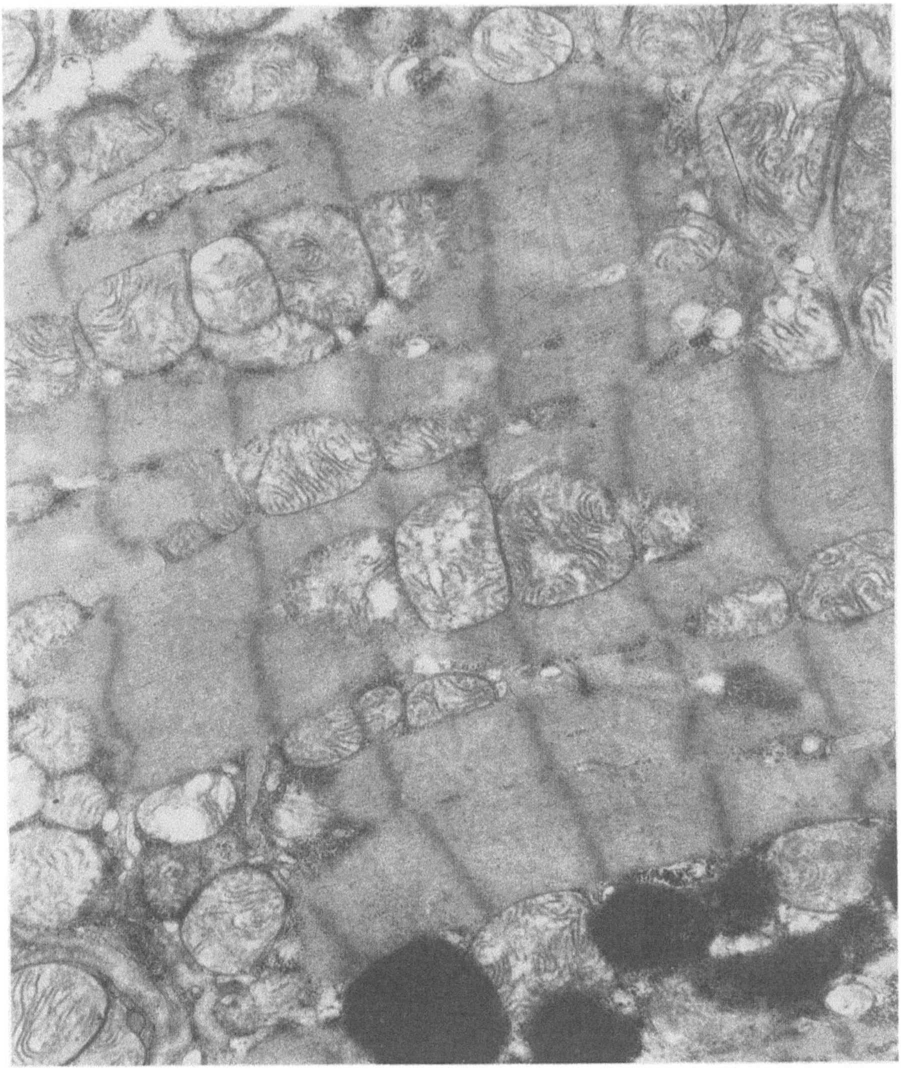

Fig. 4. Electronmicrograph showing regularly arranged myocardial fibrils. There is an increase in mitochondria, showing variation in size and shape. Some of the mitochondria are swollen and also show evidence of cristolysis. The electron-dense particles near the lower border of the photograph are lipofuscin granules. Uranyl acetate and lead citrate, ×12600

The results were summarized, after discussion with the referring physician, into the following categories:

Suspected clinical diagnosis confirmed: Material was categorized into this group if all the criteria enumerated above were present. 101 patients fell into this category.

No pathological evidence (other findings): This included those patients where either no abnormality whatever was found, severe hypertrophy without dila-

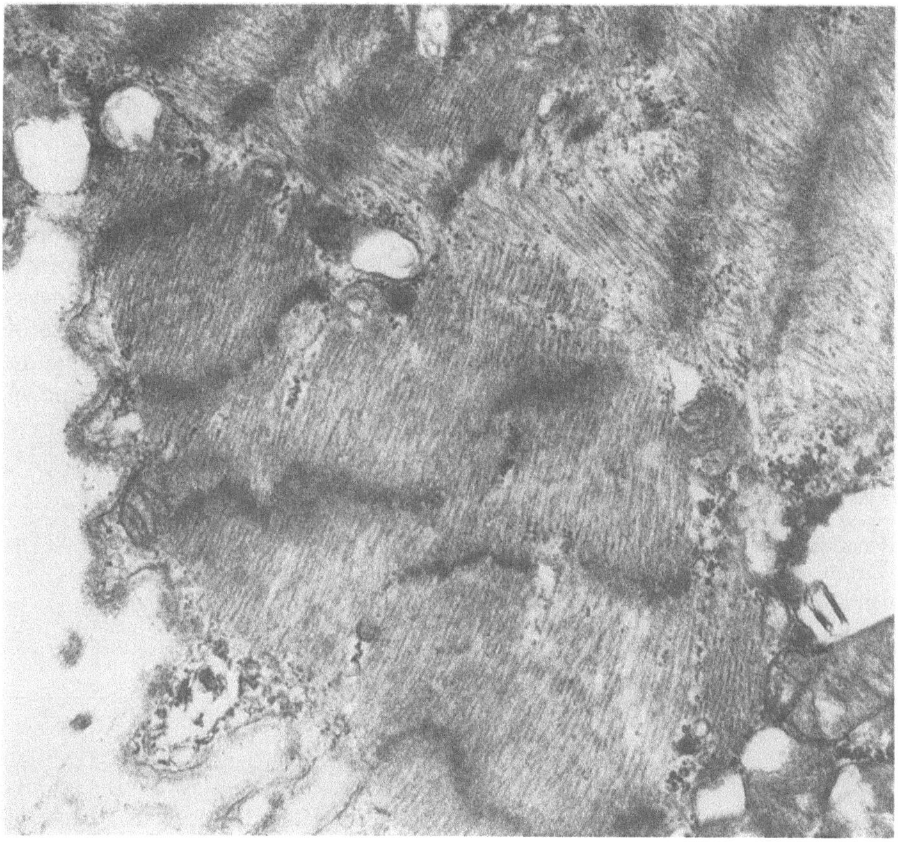

Fig. 5. Electron micrograph from a patient suffering from COCM, showing irregular arrangement of myocardial fibrils. Uranyl acetate and lead citrate, ×32000

tation was evident, or other conditions such as myocarditis were found. Forty-six patients belonged to this group.

Unhelpful results: Under this heading material was grouped if either myocardium or endocardium only was received, or where there was insufficient material to interpret the results meaningfully.

Failed biopsy: This group consisted of 18 patients where no material was recovered.

The results are summarized in Table 1.

Table 1. Results of biopsy material obtained from patients suspected of COCM.

Total number	Confirmed	No pathologic evidence (Other Findings)	Unhelpful results	Failed biopsy
199	101 (51%)	46 (23%)	34 (17%)	18 (9%)

Confirmation of the suspect clinical diagnosis and no pathologic evidence (other findings) were considered to be of help by the referring physicians, that is, in 74% of the patients analysed.

The group of 46 patients are detailed in Table 2. In eight cases clinically unsuspected myocarditis was found to be present, and in two cases, hypertrophic CM. Similar findings were reported by Kuhn *et al.* [6], who in six out of 25 patients found different pathology from that clinically suspected. The most interesting patients in this group were those where either myocardial hypertrophy without dilatation or no abnormalities were found. In some of these patients only minor unexplained abnormalities, such as LBBB or immunologic idiosyncracy, were found, and these patients may well belong to the latent phase of COCM. Regular clinical follow-up and possible sequential biopsy examination may shed light on the natural history of COCM, of which so very little is known at present.

Table 2. Material in which no pathologic evidence was found (other findings)[a]

Myocardial hypertrophy, no evidence of dilatation	18
Normal	14
Myocarditis	8
Severe hypertrophy; no dilatation; (hypertension)	3
Hypertrophic CM	2
Small vessel disease	1

[a] Total Number: 46

An entirely separate group, so far not discussed, consisted of 61 patients (Table 3). In 39 of these patients the principal suspected diagnosis as a cause of heart failure, was myocarditis. In 26 of these, no pathologic evidence of present or past infection was evident, and the nonspecific changes compatable with a clinical diagnosis of COCM were found.

Included in this group are 33 patients who complained of angina, but in whom coronary arteriograms were absolutely normal. Studies of lactate estimations have also been undertaken in a small number of cases [21]. It has been suggested by some that this may be one of the presenting symptoms which later might develop into the COCM, while other authorities believe that this is an entirely different group of patients.

Table 3. Endomyocardial biopsies

From 61 patients in whom the principal suspected diagnosis was:	
Myocarditis	26
"Puerperal" CM	1
Hypertrophic CM	1
Small vessel disease? (Normal coronary angiogram)	33

In all patients, changes consistent with a diagnosis of COCM was made.

M: 37 F: 24 Age range: 10–54 Average age: 36.8 yr

Discussion

The recovery of fresh endomyocardial tissue by means of the bioptome has become increasingly popular, and reports on this procedure have been published from many countries. This subject has been reviewed by Olsen [18].

From time to time doubt has been expressed as to whether morphologic examination is of value. This particularly applies to those patients suspected of COCM, and it can reasonably be argued that one makes a positive "diagnosis" on negative findings. Clinically, the diagnosis is achieved by excluding cardiac or extracardiac conditions which could result in a dilated heart. Morphologically the clinical suspicion can be confirmed by excluding entities such as myocarditis, small vessel disease, and degenerative or infiltrative diseases of the myocardium. This has been achieved on material from 101 patients of the 199 examined. Although the number of cases in which unexpected pathology has been found is small (for example, myocarditis in eight and hypertrophic CM in two), this alone justifies the procedure and is helpful to the physician. Furthermore, of the 39 cases of suspected myocarditis, 26 showed no evidence other than that of a dilated heart, which also adds to the useful information that can be gained.

Persuasive evidence has been reported by Kuhn and co-workers [6] that prognosis of patients can be assessed by applying a point system to the biopsy material at electron microscopic level. My own experience with 25 patients has not yielded consistent results, and this should be explored further. Bouhour [1] also sounded a note of caution regarding prognosis.

From Table 1 it is clear that in 74% of patients, helpful information can be obtained. The question then arises whether or not the small ventricular samples reflect accurately the state of the rest of the myocardium. The ultimate confirmation can be obtained by examining the cases at postmortem. The number of reported instances is small. Sekiguchi and Konno [23] reported good correlation in 15 patients, and Olsen [19] found good correlation in seven out of nine cases. If the underlying disease process is widespread, or if the lesion can be accurately located, representative biopsies are likely to be obtained by multiple sampling [17].

Morphologic examination is also of great value as a base line for interpretation of other investigations being undertaken at an ever increasing rate, such as detailed biochemical analysis, virologic and immunologic studies.

Summary

The characteristic macroscopic and microscopic findings at autopsies have been detailed. The histologic criteria have been applied to fresh endomyocardial tissue obtained by means of a bioptome. 199 patients in whom the principal suspected diagnosis was COCM have been analyzed histologically, histochemically, and ultrastructurally. In 101 patients confirmation of the suspected clinical diagnosis was possible, but in 46 cases uncharacteristic or different pathology was found. It was considered that both these categories have yielded useful information (74% of the patients analysed).

A separate group of 61 patients in whom the principal diagnosis was not COCM has also been included. In 26 patients suspected of myocarditis, no evidence other than that of a dilated heart was found. In 33 patients, the presenting symptom was angina, but these patients showed no abnormalities in the arteries on coronary arteriography. At all levels of morphologic investigation no abnormalities of the small vessels were found.

It is concluded that multiple ventricular samples are likely to yield helpful information if the disease process is widespread, or where site of the lesion can be accurately defined. Furthermore, morphologic evaluation is extremely valuable, not only diagnostically, but also as an important adjunct to other types of investigation, such as biochemical, virologic, or immunologic analyses.

The support of the British Heart Foundation is gratefully acknowledged.

References

1. Bouhour, J.B., Petitier, H., De Lajartre, A.Y., Almazor, M., Nicolas, G., Horeau, J.: La biopsie myocardique dans les myocardiopathies congestives en apparence primitives. Arch. Mal. Cœur *69*, 485 (1976)
2. Cockshott, W.P., Thorpe, G.J., Ikeme, A.C.: Radiological aspects of heart muscle disease in Nigerian adults. Circulation *36*, 460 (1967)
3. Goodwin, J.F.: Congestive and hypertrophic cardiomyopathy: A decade of study. Lancet *1970/I*, 731
4. Goodwin, J.F.: Primary myocardial disease. Spectrum of cardiomyopathy and current classification. Singapore med. J. *14*, 358 (1973)
5. Konno, S., Sakakibara, S.: Endomyocardial biopsy. Dis. Chest *44*, 345 (1963)
6. Kuhn, H., Breithardt, G., Knieriem, H.-J., Loogen, F., Both, A., Schmidt, W.A.K., Stroobandt, R., Gleichmann, U.: Die Bedeutung der endomyokardialen Katheterbiopsie für die Diagnostik und die Beurteilung der Prognose der kongestiven Kardiomyopathie. Dtsch. Med. Wschr. *100*, 717 (1975)
7. Maron, B.J., Ferrans, V.J., Roberts, W.C.: Ultrastructural features of degenerated cardiac muscle cells in patients with cardiac hypertrophy. Amer. J. Path. *79*, 387 (1975)
8. Meerson, F.Z.: The myocardium in hyperfunction, hypertrophy and heart failure. Circulat. Res. *25*, Suppl. 2 (1969)
9. Oakley, C.M.: Clinical definitions and classification of cardiomyopathies. Postgrad. med. J. *48*, 703 (1972)
10. Oakley, C.M.: The relation between function and causation in cardiomyopathy. Postgrad. med. J. *51*, 271 (1975)
11. Olsen, E.G.J.: Cardiomyopathies in "Clinical-Pathologic Correlations 1". Cardiovascular Clinics. Edwards, J.E. (ed.). Philadelphia: F.A. Davis Company, 1972a, p. 239
12. Olsen, E.G.J.: Pathology of primary cardiomyopathies. Postgrad. med. J. *48*, 1972b, 732
13. Olsen, E.G.J.: The Pathology of the Heart. New York: Intercontinental Medical Book Corporation, 1973, Chap. 2, p. 26
14. Olsen, E.G.J.: Diagnostic value of the endomyocardial bioptome. Lancet *1974/I*, 658
15. Olsen, E.G.J.: Pathological recognition of cardiomyopathy. Postgrad. med. J. *51*, 277 (1975)
16. Olsen, E.G.J.: Pathologie der „primären" Kardiomyopathien. Münch. Med. Wschr. *118*, 735 (1976a)
17. Olsen, E.G.J.: Diagnostic value of the endomyocardial bioptome. (Annotation). Amer. Heart J. *91*, 398 (1976b)
18. Olsen, E.G.J.: Myocardial biopsies. Recent Advances in Cardiology, Chap. 13, p. 349. Churchill Livingstone 1977a

19. Olsen, E.G.J.: Endomyocardial biopsies. Is pathological examination of use? (Abstract). Presented at the Autumn meeting of the British Cardiac Society, 1976. Brit. Heart J. *39*, 349 (1977b)
20. Richardson, P.J.: King's endomyocardial bioptome. Lancet *1974/I*, 660
21. Richardson, P.J., Livesley, B., Oram, S., Olsen, E.G.J., Armstrong, P.: Angina pectoris with normal coronary arteries. Transvenous myocardial biopsy in diagnosis. Lancet *1974/II*, 677
22. Sakakibara, S., Konno, S.: Endomyocardial biopsy. Jap. Heart J. *3*, 537 (1962)
23. Sekiguchi, M., Konno, S.: Diagnosis and classification of primary myocardial disease with the aid of endomyocardial biopsy. Jap. Circulat. J. *35*, 737 (1971)

7. Light-Microscopic Evaluation of Myocardial Biopsies

B. KUNKEL, H. LAPP, G. KOBER, and M. KALTENBACH

Right and left ventricular biopsies were performed during diagnostic heart catheterizations in patients with COCM. In each patient two biopsy samples were taken, one for electron microscopy and a second for light microscopy. Tissue preparation for electron microscopy is time consuming. Histologic sections, however, are available within a short time, and much data which give important information on the patient's myocardium can be thus obtained. Presence and degree of myocardial hypertrophy as well as the amount of interstitial fibrosis can be calculated easily by histologic examination.

Material and Methods

Patients studied were divided into two groups (Table 1). Group I consisted of 32 patients with early COCM. These patients had no clinical signs of cardiac failure at rest. Cardiac volume was slightly to moderately above normal. ECG showed abnormal tracings in all cases, such as left ventricular hypertrophy, arrhythmias, or conduction disturbances. The left ventricular ejection fractions were slightly decreased or normal in a few cases. Left ventricular enddiastolic volumes were mildly or moderately increased.

Group II included 34 patients with advanced COCM. In this group clinical examination revealed signs of cardiac failure. Cardiac volume was markedly

Table 1. Data of patients with early and with advanced COCM.

I. Early COCM	
Congestive heart failure	Absent at rest
Roentgenologic heart volume	Increased (> 800 ml/173 m²)
ECG	Evidence of cardiac hypertrophy, arrhythmia or conduction disturbances
Ejection fraction	Slightly decreased (> 50%), sometimes normal
Enddiastolic volume	Slightly increased, sometimes normal
II. Advanced COCM	
Congestive heart failure	Present
Roentgenologic heart volume	Markedly increased (> 1000 ml/173 m²)
ECG	Predominant path. changes
Ejection fraction	Markedly reduced (< 50%)
Enddiastolic volume	Markedly increased

increased, and the ECG was abnormal in most cases. The enddiastolic volume was markedly increased, and the ejection fraction was substantially reduced.

Tissue samples for light microscopy were fixed with formalin. The sections were cut at 8 μ and stained by the following methods:

1. Hematoxylin-Eosin, for general morphology
2. Goldner for connective tissue
3. PAS for carbohydrates
4. Hart for elastic tissue
5. Congo-red for amyloid.

To quantify the degree of cardiac hypertrophy, cell diameters of 50–80 cross-sectioned cardiac muscle cells were measured in each sample.

The amount of interstitial fibrosis was determined morphometrically: In each of four different sections of one biopsy specimen, 10 randomly sampled areas were studied by using a square counting grid consisting of 25 points which was put into the eye piece. By these means 1000 points were counted in each biopsy sample. The connective tissue content was calculated with the formula

$$V_v = P_p$$

The volume fraction of connective tissue contained in the unit volume of myocardium equals the number of points falling on profiles of connective tissue divided by the total number of test points [2].

Results

Microscopic evaluations of the biopsies revealed alterations of the endocardium and the interstitium, as well as of the cardiac muscle cells. The results obtained in both groups are listed in Table 2. Common findings were hypertrophy of cardiac muscle cells, interstitial fibrosis, interstitial lipomatosis, and areas with active fibrous tissue cells. Although all findings were present in both groups, they varied significantly in severity and quantity, as shown in Table 1.

Focal or diffuse endocardial fibrosis was found in 11.7% of the cases with early COCM (group I) and in 46% of the cases with advanced COCM (Fig. 1). In one patient maximal endocardial thickness reached 150 μ. Both collagen and elastic fiber contents were increased.

Proliferation of smooth muscle cells was present in 8.7% of early CMs and in 12.4% of advanced forms of the disease. Occasionally thick layers of smooth muscle cells ran in different directions (Fig. 2). Fibrocytes and fibroblasts as well as histiocytes and in a few patients single lymphocytes were present in the thickened endocardium.

The interstitium of normal myocardium is narrow and contains capillaries and a few interstitial cells. In our patients with early and advanced CM, however, the subendocardial myocardium showed focal or diffuse interstitial fibrosis of varying severity (Fig. 3). As described above, the collagenous fiber content was quantified morphometrically by a point-counting system. Less than 5% of

Table 2. Microscopic findings in early and advanced COCM.

	Early forms (I) n[a]	Early forms (I) %	Advanced forms (II) n[b]	Advanced forms (II) %
Myocardial hypertrophy Mean muscle cell diameter				
Slight (16–20 μ)	18	52.2	10	31
Moderate (21–25 μ)	4	11.6	14	43.4
Severe (> 26 μ)	1	2.9	7	21.7
Interstitial fibrosis Fibrous tissue content				
Slight (6–10%)	6	17.4	1	3.1
Moderate (11–19%)	6	17.4	8	24.8
Severe (> 20%)	2	5.8	13	40.3
Endocardial fibrosis	4	11.6	15	46.5
Interstitial lipomatosis	3	8.7	1	3.1
Inflammatory infiltrations	2	5.8	2	6.2
Increase in fibrocytes, fibroblasts and histiocytes	3	8.7	9	27.9
Smooth muscle cells	3	8.7	4	12.4
Normal myocardium	4	11.6	–	–

[a] Total n = 34 [b] Total n = 32

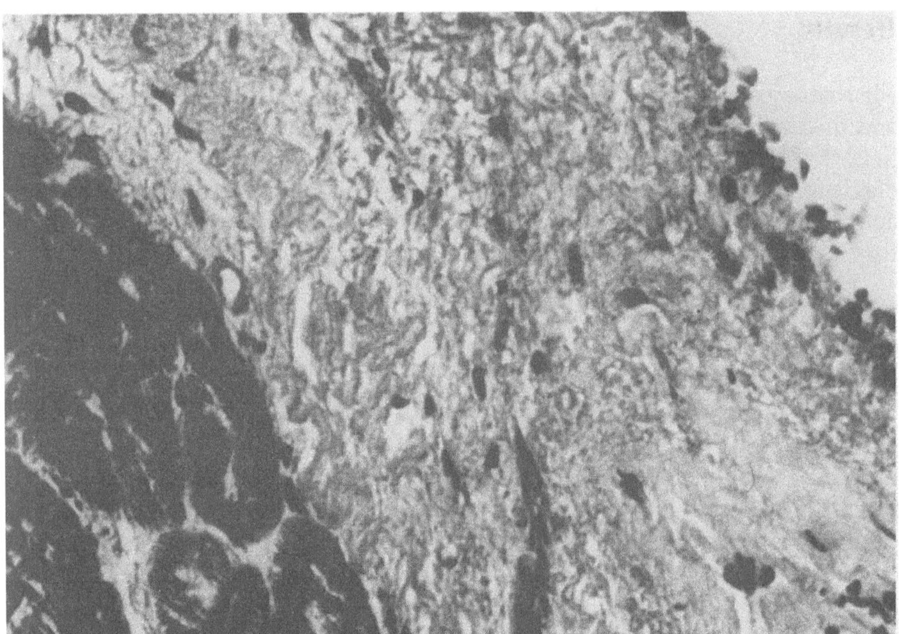

Fig. 1. Marked endocardial fibrosis. Endocardial thickness, 85 μm. Goldner. × 500

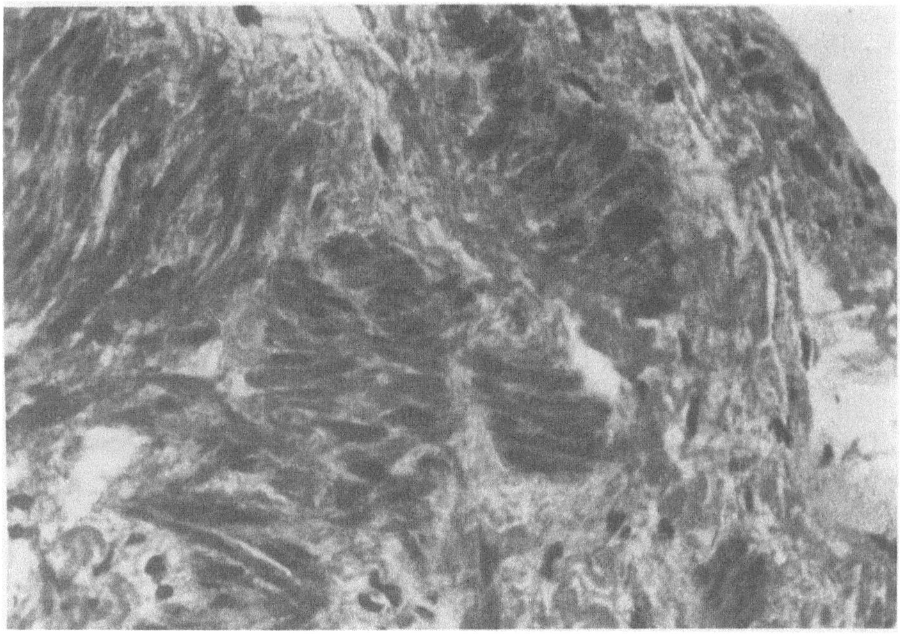

Fig. 2. Endocardial fibrosis. Within the thickened endocardium layers of smooth muscle cells with different orientations. Goldner. × 500

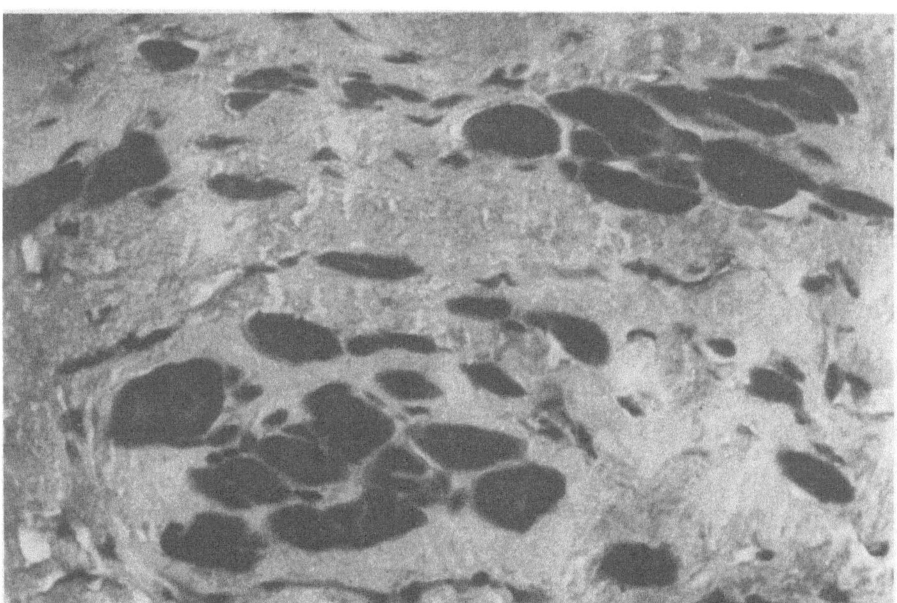

Fig. 3. Severe interstitial fibrosis. Islets of cardiac muscle cells are surrounded by hyalinized collagen tissue. Goldner. × 500

collagenous tissue was considered normal: 6–10% was defined as light fibrosis, 11–19% as moderate, and more than 20% as severe interstitial fibrosis.

Of group I 42.6% showed an increase in connective tissue which was considered mild in 17.4%, moderate in 17.4%, and severe in 5.8%. The latter two cases showed small subendocardial scarring which extended over more than 20% of the biopsy sample. This scar formation however was not believed to be representative for the total myocardium, but it was indicative of an existing myocardial disease (Table 3).

Table 3. Connective tissue content in patients with early and advanced COCM.

Connective tissue content	Early forms n[a]	%	Advanced forms n[b]	%
< 5%	20	58.0	10	31.0
6–10%	6	17.4	1	3.1
11–19%	6	17.4	8	24.8
> 20%	2	5.8	13	40.3

[a] Total n = 34 [b] Total n = 32

Of advanced COCM, 31.2% had a normal amount of collagenous tissue in the biopsy material. An increase in collagenous fiber content was found in 68% of the same patient group (Table 3). Of the latter cases, 3.1% exhibited a mild, diffuse, or focal collagen fiber increase; 24.9% had a moderate and 40.6% a severe interstitial fibrosis. In patients with severe fibrosis small islets of cardiac muscle cells were found in the partially hyalinized collagenous tissue (Fig. 3). Diffuse or focal interstitial fibrosis was a common finding in our patients, whereas subendocardial scars replacing degenerated cardiac muscle were found only in a few cases.

In most biopsies the interstitial fibrous tissue contained only a few fibrocytes. In 8.8% of early CMs and in 28.1% of the cases with advanced forms of the disease, a focal increase in fibrocytes, fibroplastic cells, and histiocytes was observed (Fig. 4).

In both patient groups, cardiac muscle cells showed signs of hypertrophy of varying degree with enlargement of the nucleus and cell diameter (Figs. 5 and 6). The mean cell diameters are listed in Table 4. Five patients with HOCM and one patient with aortic valve stenosis are included for comparison.

Table 4. Mean muscle cell diameter in early and advanced COCM.

Mean cell diameter	Early forms n[a]	%	Advanced forms n[b]	%	HOCM/AS[c] n
< 15	11	31.9	1	3.1	
16–20	18	52.2	10	31.0	4 (HOCM)
21–25	4	11.6	14	43.4	
26–30	1	2.9	6	18.6	1 (AS)
> 30	–	–	1	3.1	

[a] Total n = 34 [b] Total n = 32
[c] HOCM, hypertrophic obstructive cardiomyopathy. AS, aortic valve stenosis

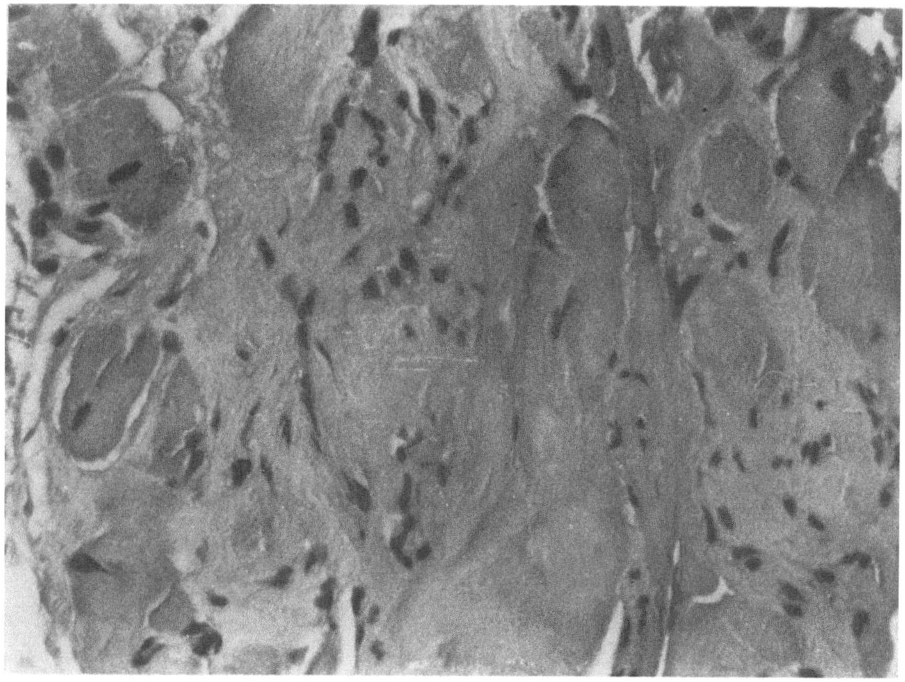

Fig. 4. Interstitial fibrosis. Increase in interstitial connective tissue cells. H & E. ×500

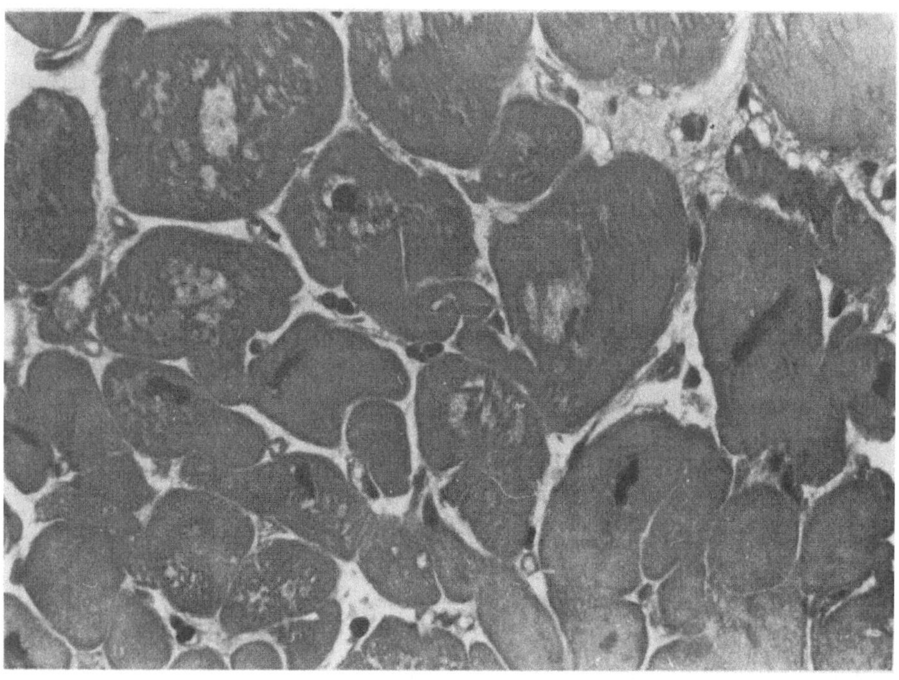

Fig. 5. Severe hypertrophy of cardiac muscle cells. H & E. ×500

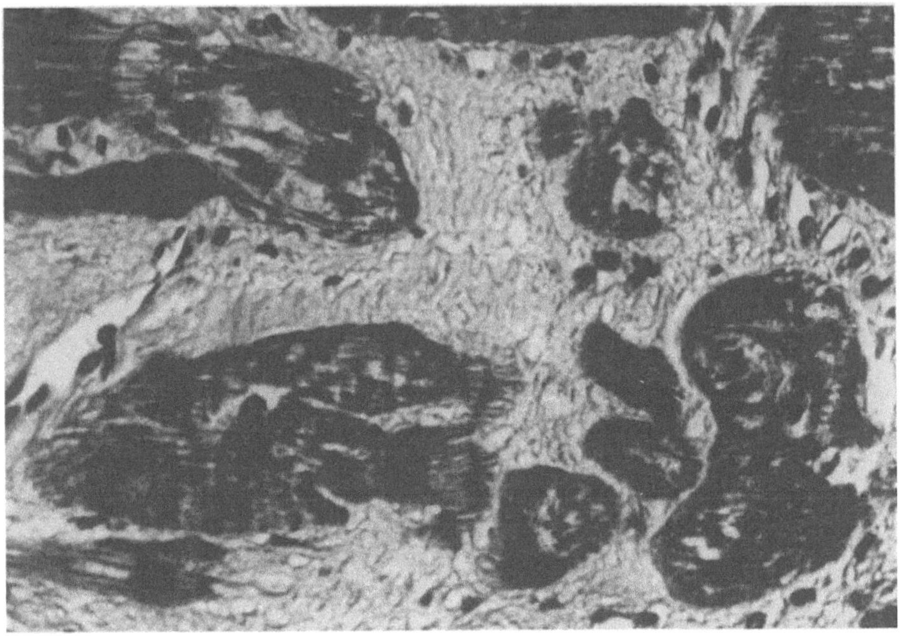

Fig. 6. Severe hypertrophy of cardiac muscle cells and interstitial fibrosis. Cardiac muscle cells exhibit loss of myofibrils. Goldner. × 500

In 31.9% of early CMs normal diameters of cardiac muscle cells were found, whereas 53% of these cases had already a mild and 11.7% a moderate myocardial hypertrophy. Severe hypertrophy of cardiac muscle cells was found in one patient of this group. Normal mean cardiac muscle cell diameters were found in one patient with advanced COCM, and 31% showed a mild enlargement of the mean fiber diameter. Hypertrophy was moderate in 43.7% and severe in 21.8%.

Nuclear changes due to hypertrophy were always present, and in isolated cases were the only indication of cardiac hypertrophy. Such nuclei were enlarged and polymorph in shape with multiple indentations and flattening of the nuclear poles. Some cardiac muscle cells were polynuclear. In many cases degenerative changes such as karyopyknosis and severe loss of myofibrils occurred.

In four patients focal or diffuse, massive interstitial infiltrations with mononuclear inflammatory cells were found (Fig. 7). These cases were defined as chronic myocarditis. Two of these patients had been suffering from severe cardiac failure for several years, whereas only mild cardiac symptoms such as arrhythmias were found in the other two.

Discussion

The diagnosis of COCM is based on clinical and hemodynamic data. Etiology and pathogenesis of the disease seem to be heterogeneous. Some of the cases described were identified as chronic myocarditis by histologic examination of biopsy ma-

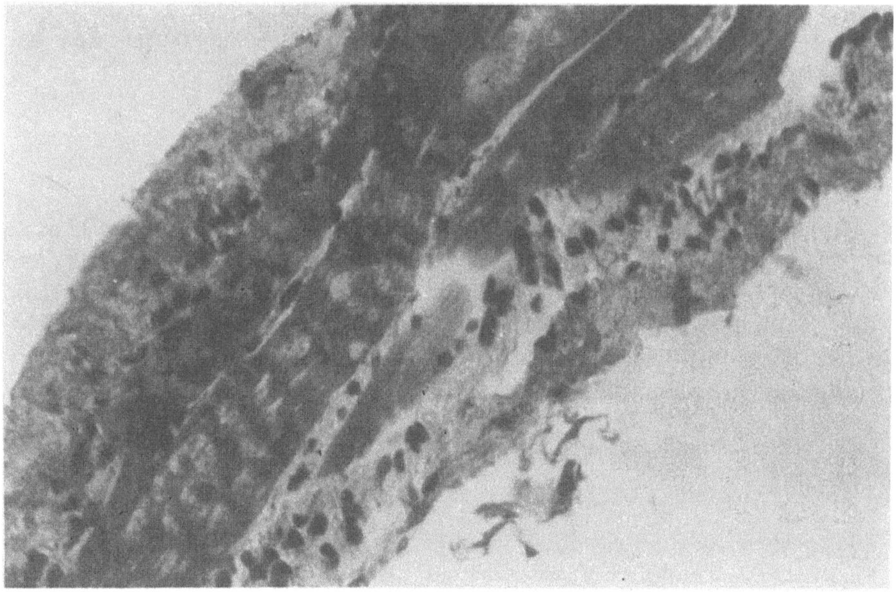

Fig. 7. Chronic myocarditis with diffuse infiltration of lymphocytes. Muscle cells show contraction bands. Goldner. × 500

terial. This examination, however, did not clarify whether the inflammation was caused and maintained by a nonidentified agent, or whether, for example, immunologic factors were the precipitating cause. As known from autopsies, myocarditis is focal in most cases; myocardial biopsy therefore appears not to be an appropriate diagnostic method for establishing the diagnosis.

Myocardial hypertrophy and interstitial fibrosis are characteristic, though nonspecific histologic findings in the remaining patients with early or advanced COCMs [3–7]. In advanced stages of the illness the histologic alterations are much more pronounced; the severe increase of myocardial fibrous tissue in these cases is partially responsible for impairment of ventricular function [1]. On the other hand 32% of these patients with advanced CMs do not exhibit severe myocardial fibrosis [4]. Cardiac failure in these cases is less clear. It may be traced to late stages of hypertrophy which can be diagnosed by electron microscopy or to biochemical impairment of cellular functions.

Patients with early COCMs presented with myocardial hypertrophy and increase in myocardial fibrous tissue less severe than in patients with advanced stages of the disease. These changes indicate an underlying myocardial disease before impairment of ventricular function occurs.

The diagnosis of COCM cannot be made by microscopic examination of biopsy material [7]. Similar changes can be found in many other cardiac diseases [1, 3]. Quantified histologic changes, however, correspond well with the severity of the disease.

The cause of cardiac hypertrophy – the predominant histologic finding in COCM – is still unknown. It remains to be clarified whether an initial degenerative process leads to cardiac damage which in turn is compensated by hypertrophy or whether the hypertrophy is primary and in its late stages causes cardiac failure.

Summary

A qualitative and quantitative histologic study in 34 cases with early and 32 cases with advanced COCM was carried out. In both groups cardiac hypertrophy and interstitial fibrosis of varying degree were the predominant though nonspecific histologic findings. Quantitative analysis showed good correlation with the severity and of the histologic changes the stage of the disease. A few cases could be identified as chronic myocarditis.

References

1. Büchner, F., Weyland, R.: Die Insuffizienz des hypertrophierten Herzmuskels im Lichte seiner Narbenbilder. Munich: Urban & Schwarzenberg 197
2. Elias, H., Hennig, A., Schwarz, D.E.: Stereology: Applications to biomedical research. Physiol. Rev. *51*, 158 (1971)
3. Mc Kinney, B.: Endomyocardial fibrosis and cardiomegaly of unknown origin: A comparative histologic study. In: Cardiomyopathies. Bajusz, E., Rona, G. (eds.). Munich: Urban & Schwarzenberg, 1974
4. Okada, R.: A morphological classification of the idiopathic cardiomyopathy and allied cardiac disease. Jap. Circulat. J. *35*, 755 (1971)
5. Olsen, E.G.J.: Pathology of primary cardiomyopathies. Postgrad. med. J. *48*, 732 (1972)
6. Olsen, E.G.J.: Pathologie der primären Kardiomyopathien Münch. med. Wschr. *118*, 735 (1976)
7. Roberts, W.C., Ferrans, V.J.: Pathologic anatomy of the cardiomyopathies. Hum. Path. *6*, 287 (1975)

8. Electron-Microscopic Findings in Congestive Cardiomyopathy

H.-J. Knieriem

In Chapters 6 and 7 various macroscopic, histologic, histochemical and some ultrastructural findings in cases of COCM have been discussed. This chapter primarily concerns the electron-microscopic findings. There is now substantial evidence that electron-microscopic studies of myocardial biopsy specimen can increase understanding of the disease and the course of COCM, especially if the ultrastructural findings are correlated with clinical data.

In collaboration with the First Medical Clinic B (Department of Cardiology) of the University of Düsseldorf we have studied biopsy specimen of 182 patients, 48 cases of which were COCM (for clinical data see Ch. 11). The biopsy specimens were obtained by transvenous and/or transarterial catheter biopsy using the Konno and the Kings College bioptome (Olympus). The myocardial tissues were fixed in buffered 4% glutaraldehyde solution, postfixed in osmium and embedded in araldite. Ultrathin sections were studied under a Siemens electron microscope 101.

The biopsy specimens were usually large enough that many myocardial fibers and their relation to each other could be studied without too many contraction bands, which sometimes occur during biopsy.

By light microscopy of semithin sections, stained with toluidine blue, we could determine the size and shape of the myocardial cells, the degree of hypertrophy and the extent of interstitial and endocardial fibrosis. We also could evaluate the endothelium of the capillaries, the wall thickness of small arteries and arterioles, as well as the occurance of interstitial cellular inflammatory infiltrations. As pointed out in Chapter 9, semithin sections may be used to measure the thickness of myocardial cells for grading the stage of hypertrophy and the degree of interstitial fibrosis in relation to the myocardial cells. The changes of the nucleus depend on the stage of hypertrophy. If severe hypertrophy is present enlargement of the nuclei corresponding to increased amounts of DNA (Pfitzer 1971, 1972) are found. The chromatin substance is often irregularly distributed along the nuclear membrane; sometimes two or even three nucleoli can be observed. Various deep indentations of the membranes and inclusions of sarcoplasmic components (Figs. 1 and 2) were observed on the enlarged nuclei.

The behavior of the myocardial fibers can be evaluated by light microscopy as well as by electron microscopy. In cases of COCM we find in most biopsy specimens an abnormal branching. However, in contrast to HOCM, the hypertrophic myocardial cells are not in bizarre and whorl-like disarray, but rather are usually longer – not as plump, short and extremely enlarged as in HOCM [6, 19, 22, 21].

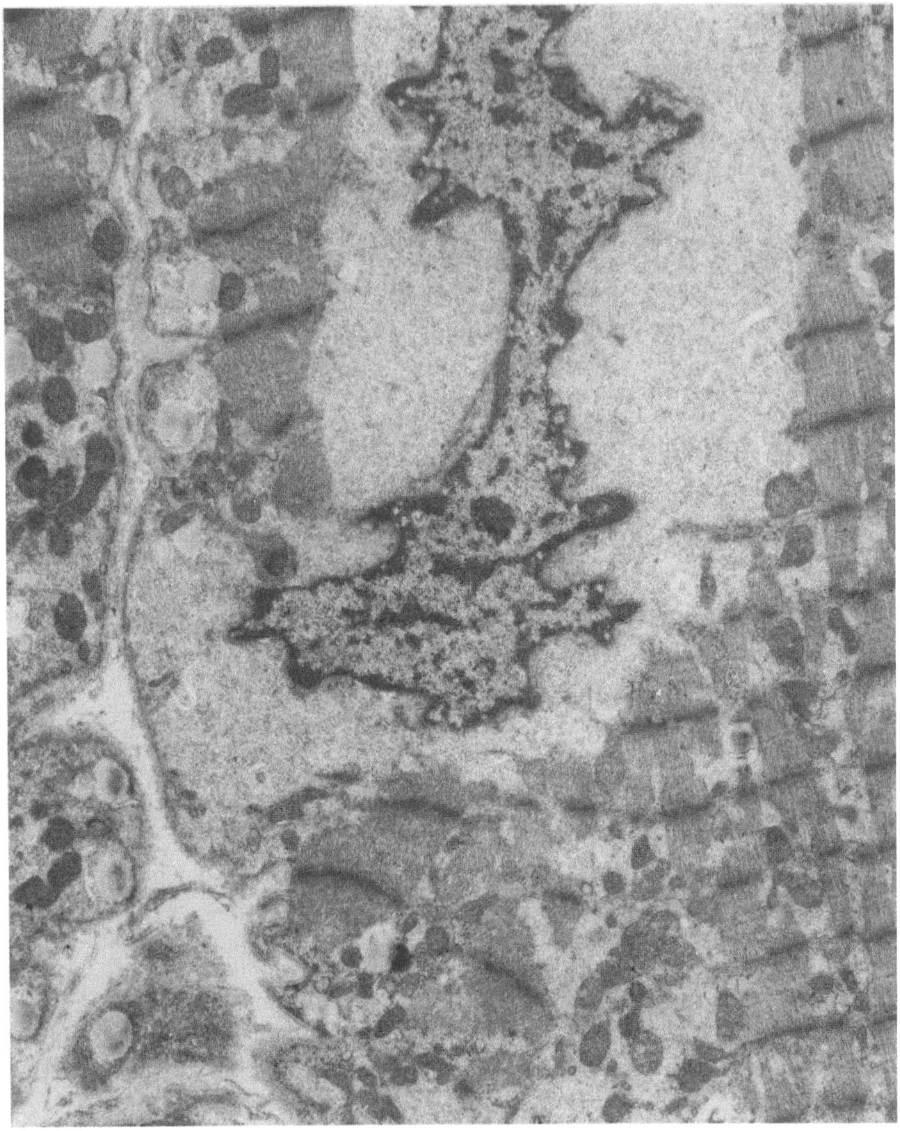

Fig. 1. Enlarged wing-like nucleus with irregular distribution of chromatin substance. Within the sarcoplasm of the myocardial cell several lipid droplets. ×7200

Electron microscope studies show COCMs to exhibit the disarrangement and abnormal branching of the moderately hypertrophied muscle cells and of their myofibrils within the single cells (Fig. 3). The myofibrils show at times a three-dimensional structure, the nucleus surrounded by myofibrils, contracting against each other as in cases of HOCM [5, 7, 9]. Furthermore, the disarray of myofibrils can be found near the growth zone of the intercalated discs (Fig. 4). Finally the

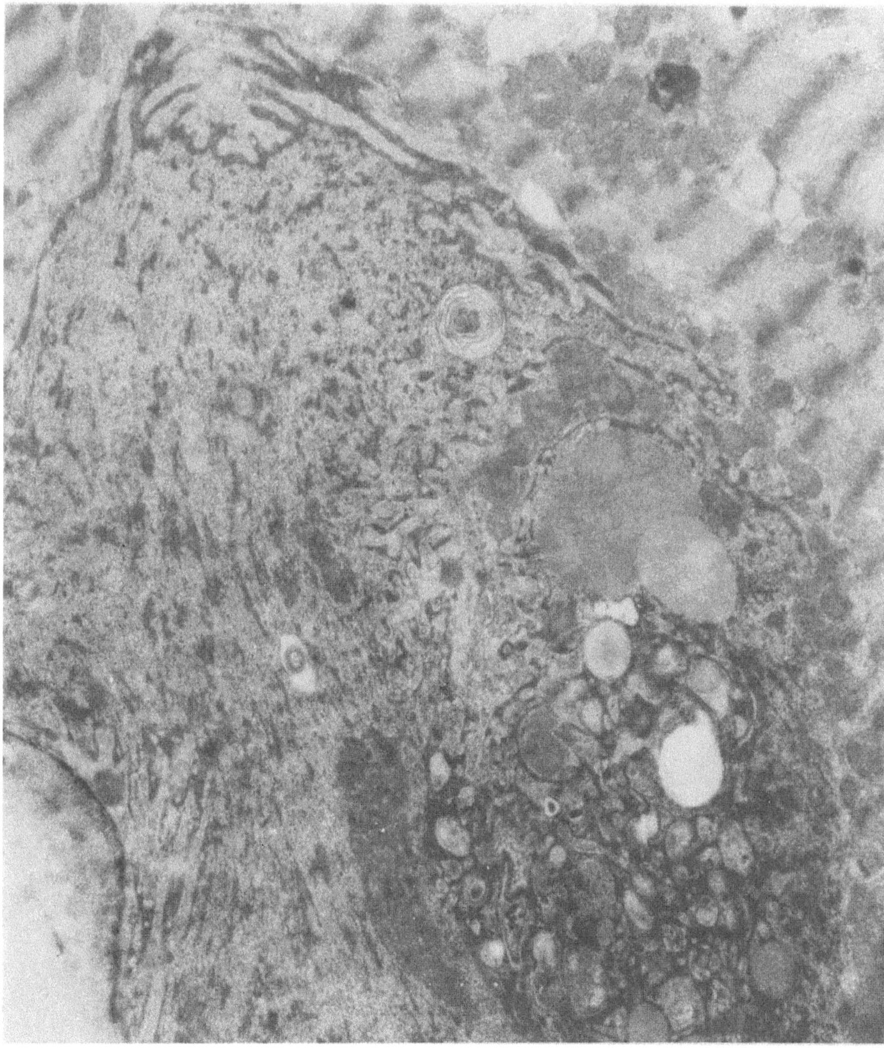

Fig. 2. Part of enlarged nucleus with multiple indentations of the nuclear membrane and inclusions of lipid vacuoles and myelin figures. × 7200

subunits of the myofibrils, the myofilaments, may exhibit brush-like derangements and disarray within the cytoplasm of the myocardial cells (Fig. 5). Sometimes the disarray is combined with newly formed myofilaments without organizations of the Z bands and regular sarcomeres. Additional abnormalities of the Z band material can be observed in a few cases of COCMs (Fig. 6). Band- and string-like formation of Z-band material can even imitate myofilaments structures of smooth muscle cells (Fig. 7), but it should be stated that such abnormalities are rare findings in COCM.

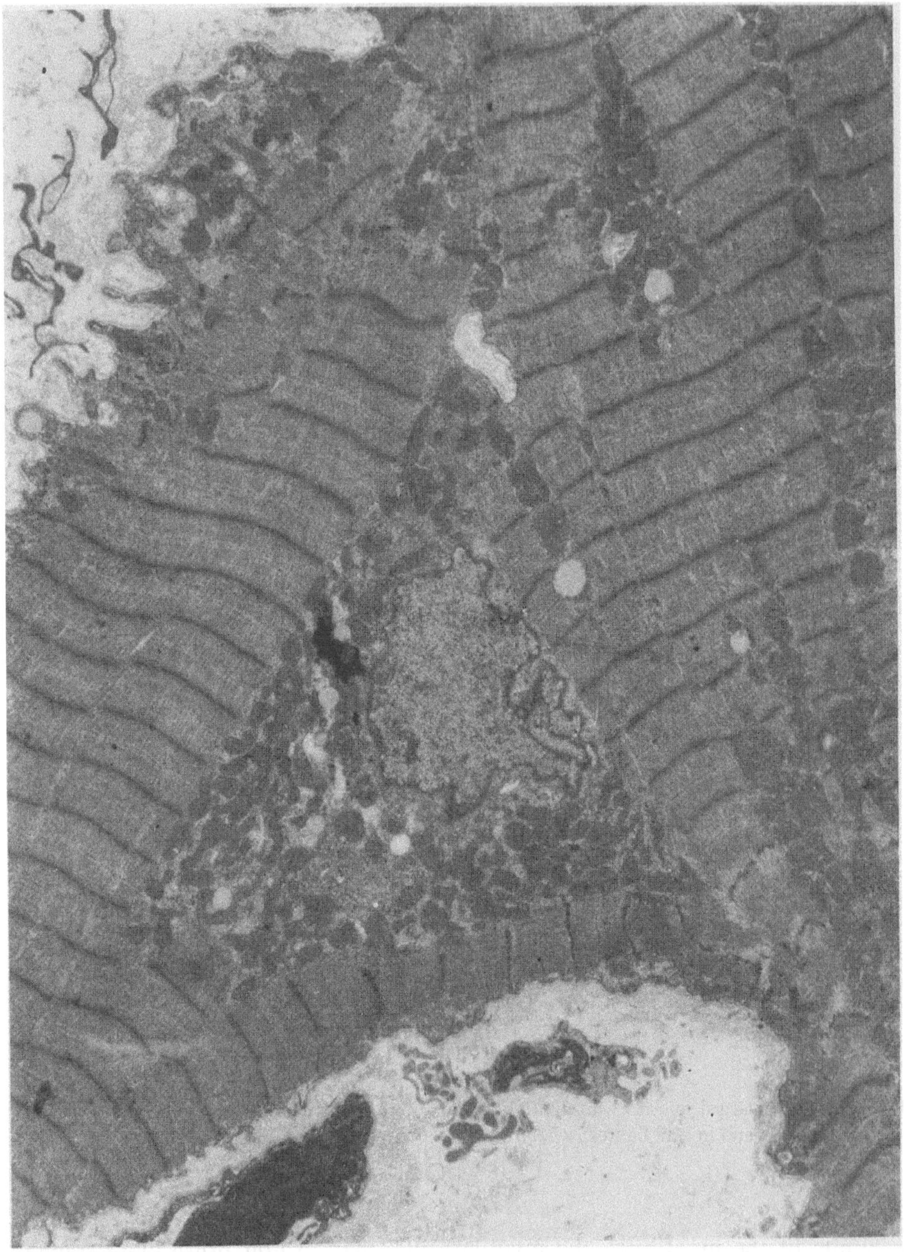

Fig. 3. Three-dimensional branching of the myofibrils within myocardial cell surrounding the nucleus and perinuclear mitochondria. Moderate interstitial fibrosis. × 5760

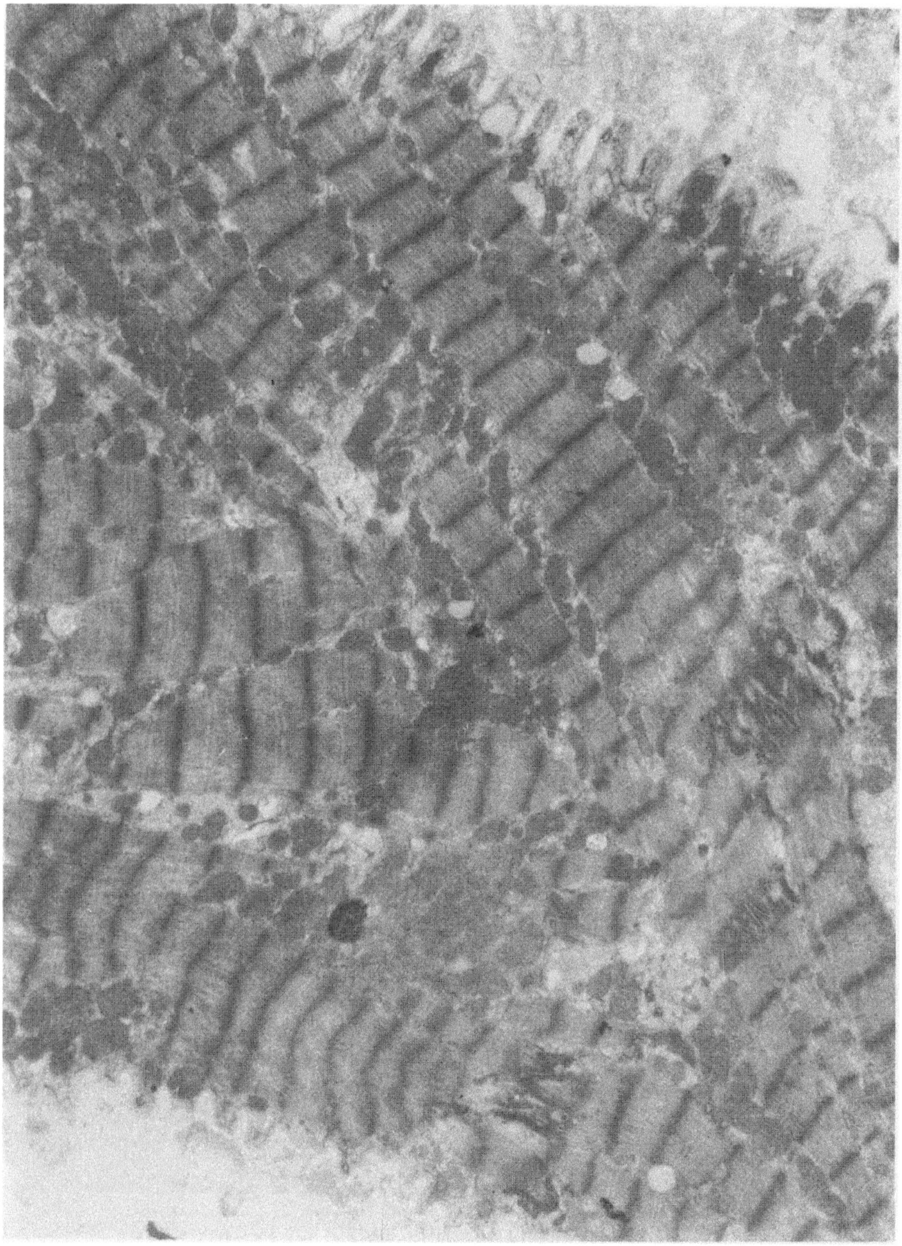

Fig. 4. Disarray of myofibrils within myocardial cell in the immediate vicinity of the growth zone of the intercalated disc. ×4000

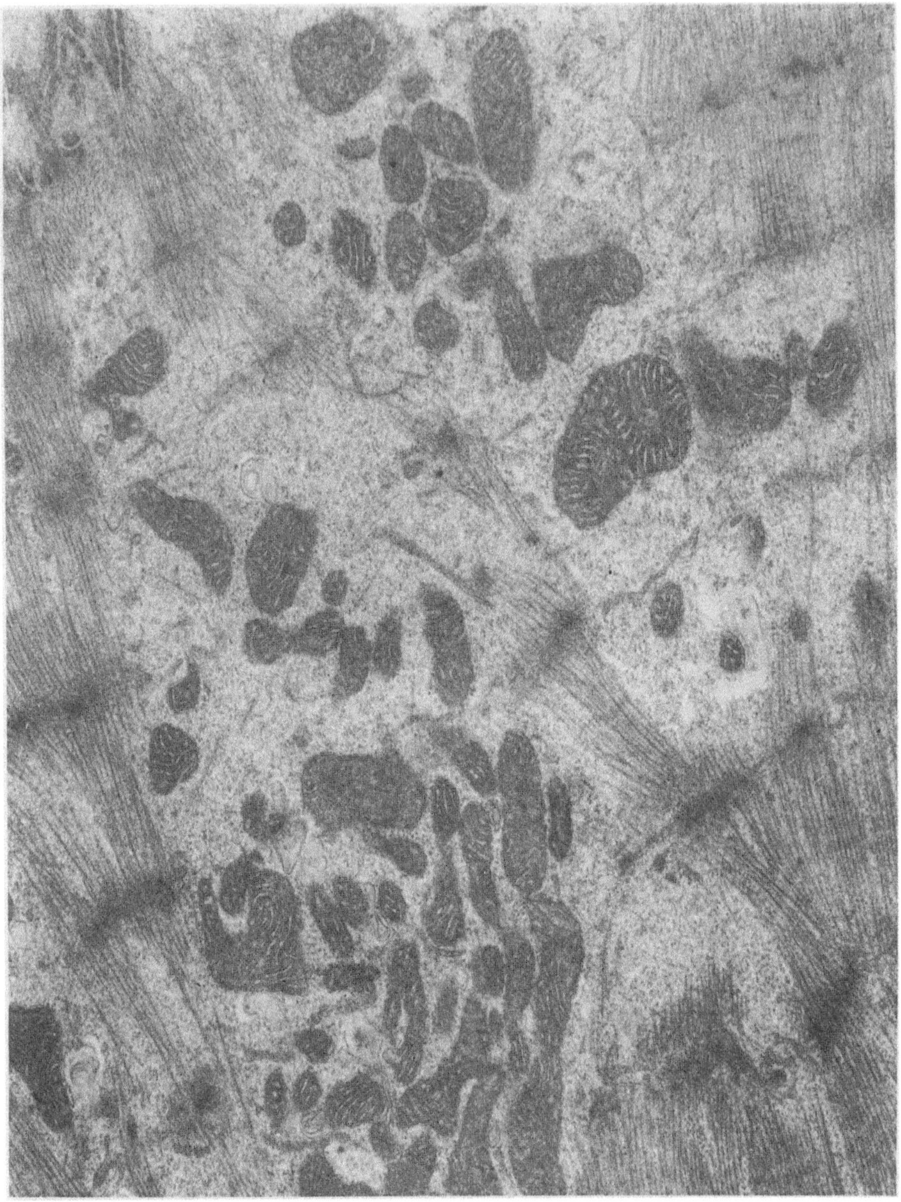

Fig. 5. Disarray and brush-like formation of myofilaments combined with loss of Z-band material and loosening of sarcomere structures. Within the myocardial sarcoplasm are small degenerated mitochondria. × 18 700

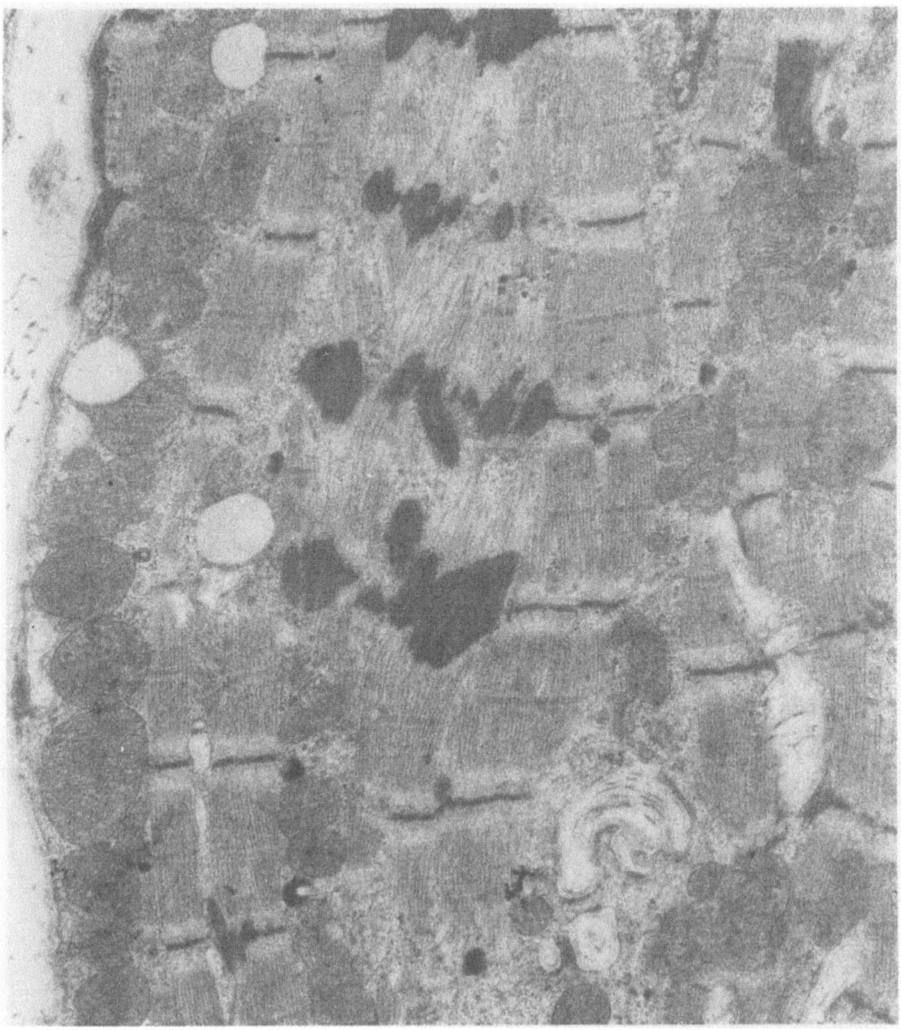

Fig. 6. Abnormal formation of electron-dense Z-band material within myocardial cells combined with disarrangement of the original sarcomere texture. Between the mitochondria a few lipid droplets are present. ×10800

Different experimental models of pressure and volume load hypertrophy [17, 1] have shown that changes of the mitochondria depend on the stage and severity of the hypertrophy. In the early stages, an augmentation of usually large but otherwise intact mitochondria are found, often referred to as "mitochondriosis" [4]. Such an increase in mitochondria number can be interpreted as an adapted or still compensated stage of hypertrophy. In cases of COCM, mostly in late stages of the disease, small and degenerated mitochondria (Fig. 8) are found. The ratio of mitochondria to myofibrils is decreased, shifting unfavorably toward a decrease

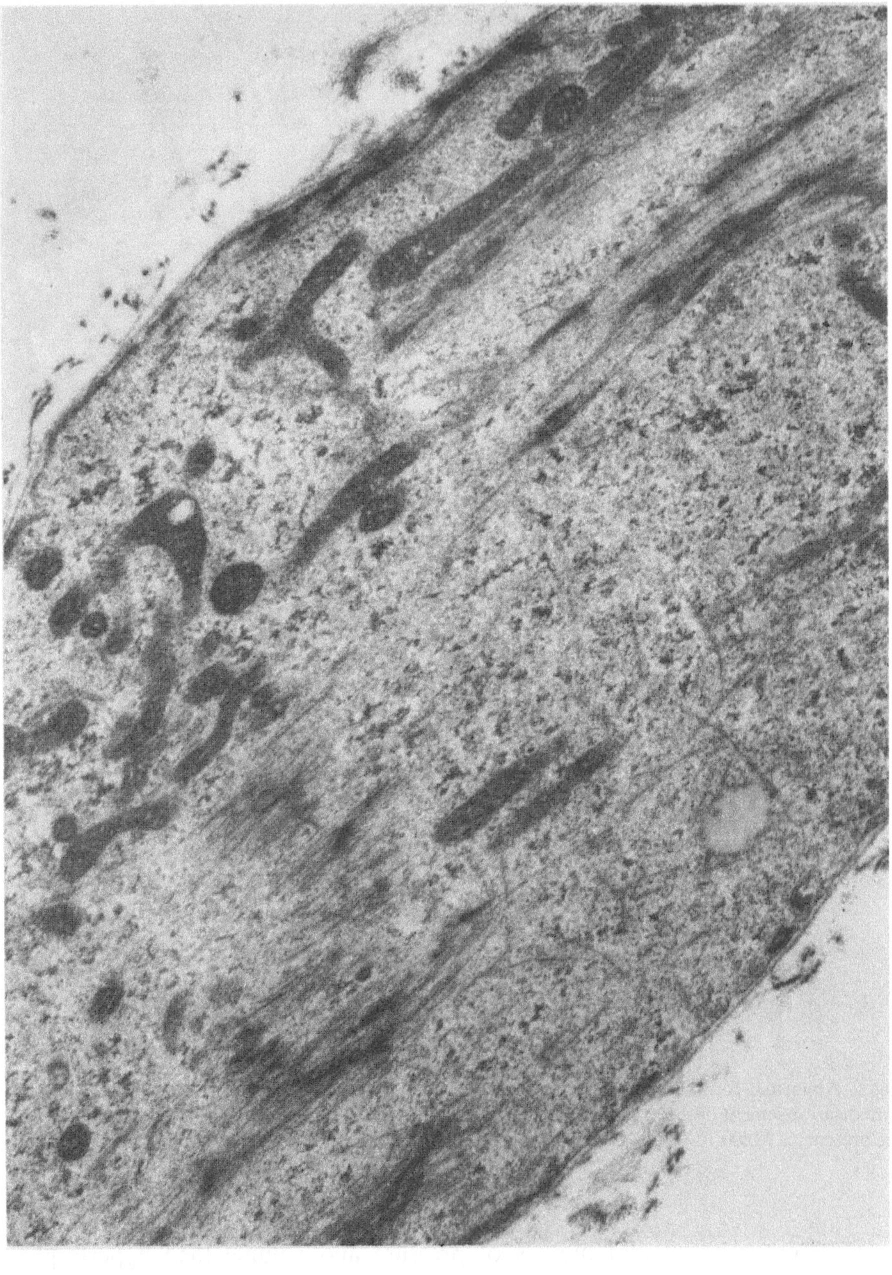

Fig. 7. Extreme loss of myofilaments and ordinary sarcomere structures with smooth muscle-like transformation of a myocardial cell. × 14400

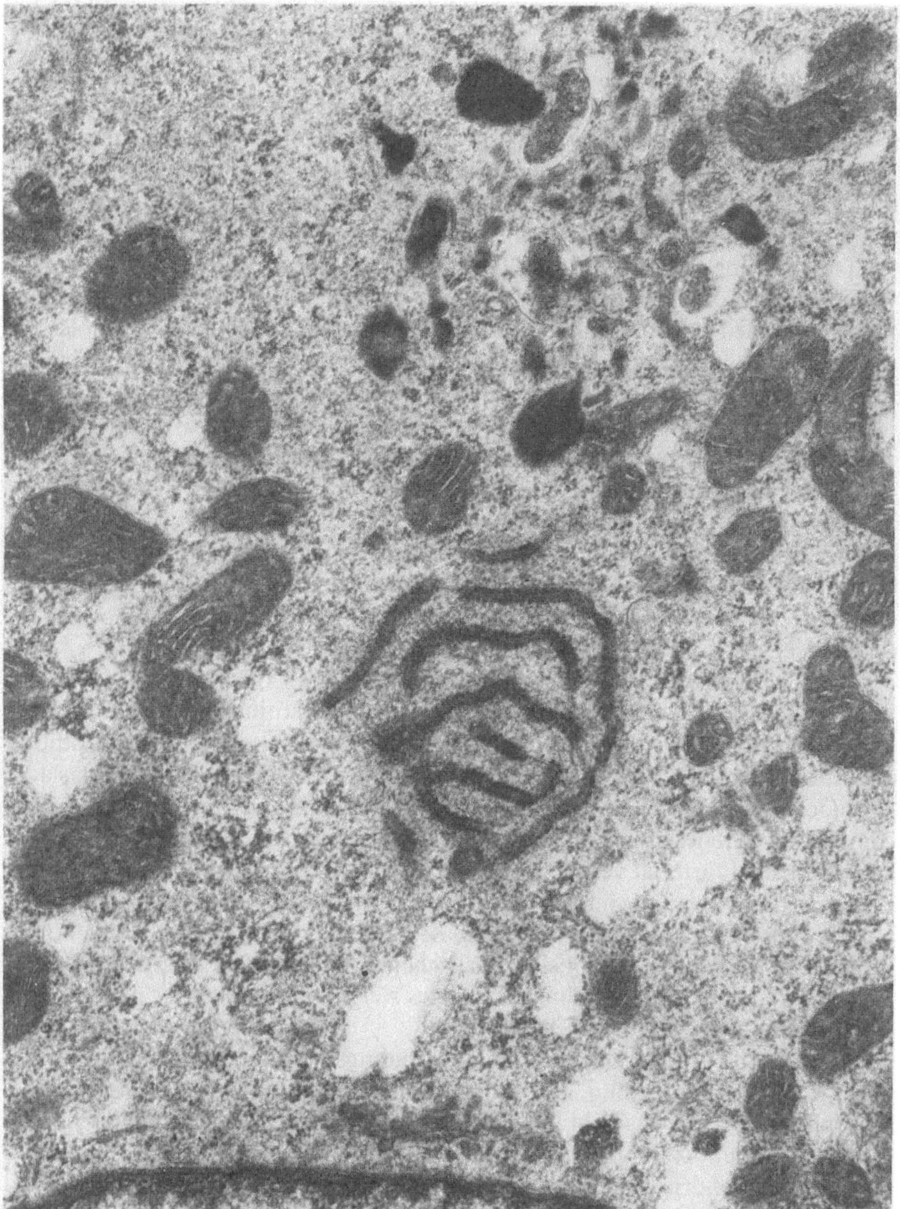

Fig. 8. Occurrance of rough endoplasmic reticulum within the perinuclear sarcoplasm. Numerous small degenerated mitochondria, foci of lysosomal granules and augmentation of free ribosomes. ×21 600

of mitochondria. The mitochondrial matrix shows increased density with fusion of the mitochondrial cristae.

Changes in other organelles include the content of free ribosomes, the occurance of ergastoplasmic lamellae, or rough endoplasmic reticulum which is usually not present in normal myocardium (Fig. 8). Furthermore, enlargement of the Golgi apparatus and moderate dilatation of the sarcoplasmic reticulum are found. The amount of glycogen is usually decreased in cases of COCMs, in contrast to hypertrophic CMs [6, 19].

The most important finding in COCM is the occurance of degenerative changes within the myocardial cell. Different forms of lysosomes, myelin-figures sometimes combined with degenerated mitochondria and cytoplasmic vacuoles are observed (Fig. 9). In some cases sequestration of necrotic material from the myocardial cells could be demonstrated (Fig. 10).

Hypoxic changes of mitochondria are not seen in all of our myocardial biopsy specimens but they occur quite often in surgically resected material, particularly from open heart surgery and coronary perfusion procedures (see Ch. 13).

In evaluating the prognosis of cases with COCM, degenerative cell changes have been of special significance [2, 13]. Degenerative changes can also be seen in the late stages of hypertrophic CM or ischemic lesions, but they occur at an early stage in COCM. They are a serious indication for the poor prognosis of the disease (see also Ch. 22).

Interstitial fibrosis is another characteristic sign of COCM which has already been stressed in Chapters 6 and 9. Within the interstitium increased amounts of collagen fibers surround myocardial cells and capillaries (Fig. 10). In addition endocardial fibrosis can be present, sometimes combined with hyperplasia of subendocardial smooth muscle cells (Fig. 11). Within the fibrotic areas, small compressed adrenergic nerve fibers can be observed. The endothelium of capillaries and small arterial vessels are usually unchanged. No thrombi were found. In a few cases with severe interstitial fibrosis, thickening of the basement membrane was present (Fig. 12). However, the degree of vascular changes was not so severe that it could be responsible for ischemic lesions of myocardial cells. Inflammatory mononuclear cellular infiltrates were seen in only four patients, and are therefore not included in this group.

In order to correlate our morphologic findings with the clinical data in cases of COCMs, the following morphologic changes have been selected for the "morphologic score" used in Chapter 22: degenerative changes (e.g. lysosomes, increased amounts of lipofuscin granules, myelin figures, lipid droplets), changes of the mitochondria, myofibrillar changes with disorientation and abnormal branching, interstitial fibrosis, and the different degrees of hypertrophy.

The morphologic findings alone are certainly nonspecific, but in combination with clinical data they have proved to be of great value (see Ch. 22). In addition the number and size of mitochondria and the thickness of myofibrils, as well as measurements of the endoplasmic reticulum in 20 biopsy specimen, did not reveal further significant changes. It should be emphasized that the observation of severe "qualitative" cell changes in one specimen proved to be of more significance than the occurance of only a few small or slight changes in the overall evaluation of multiple specimens.

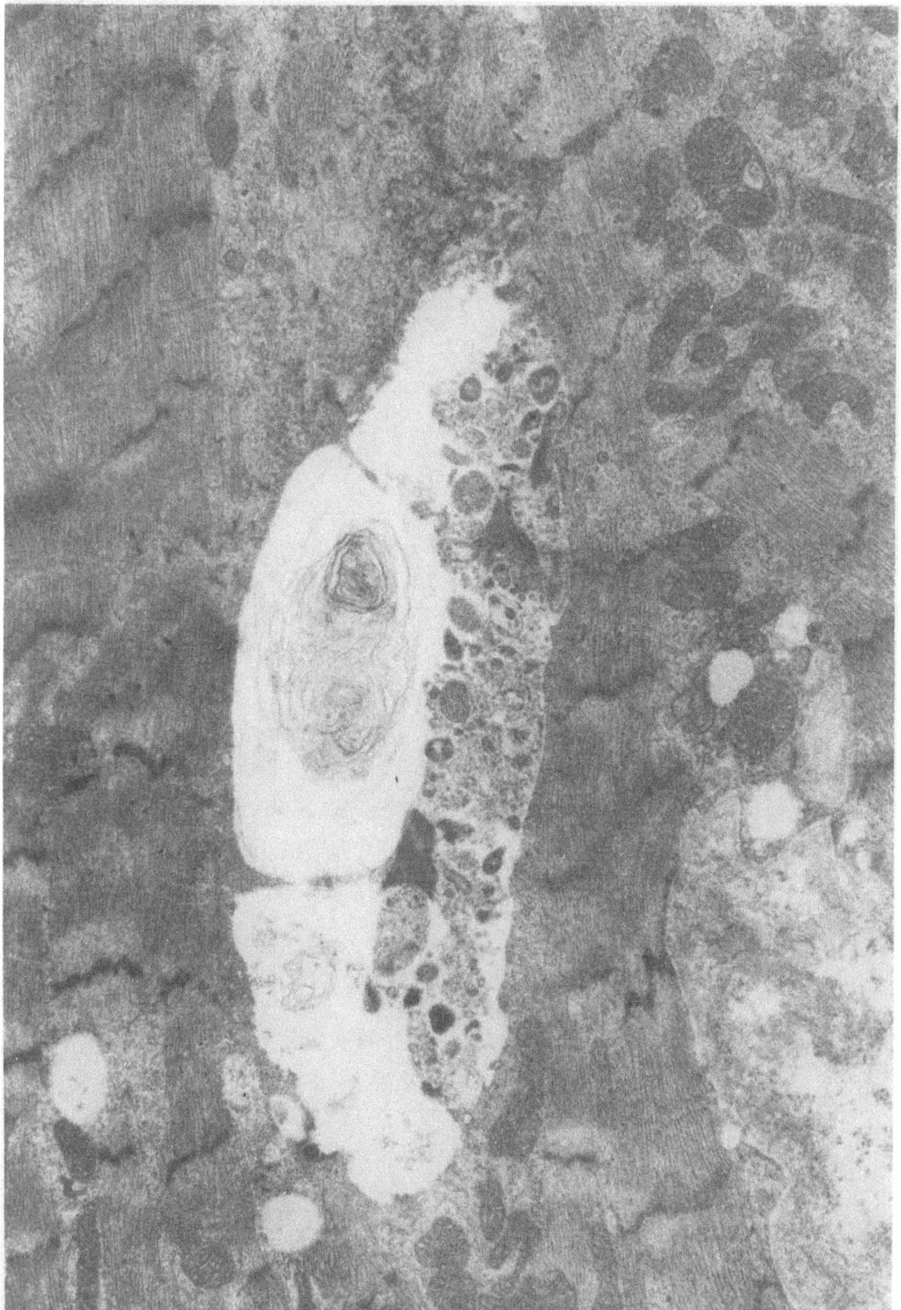

Fig. 9. Focus of degenerated cell changes within a myocardial cell with myelin figures and multiple lysosomal granules and vacuoles. In addition intracellular lipid depositions are present between mitochondria and myofibrils. × 8400

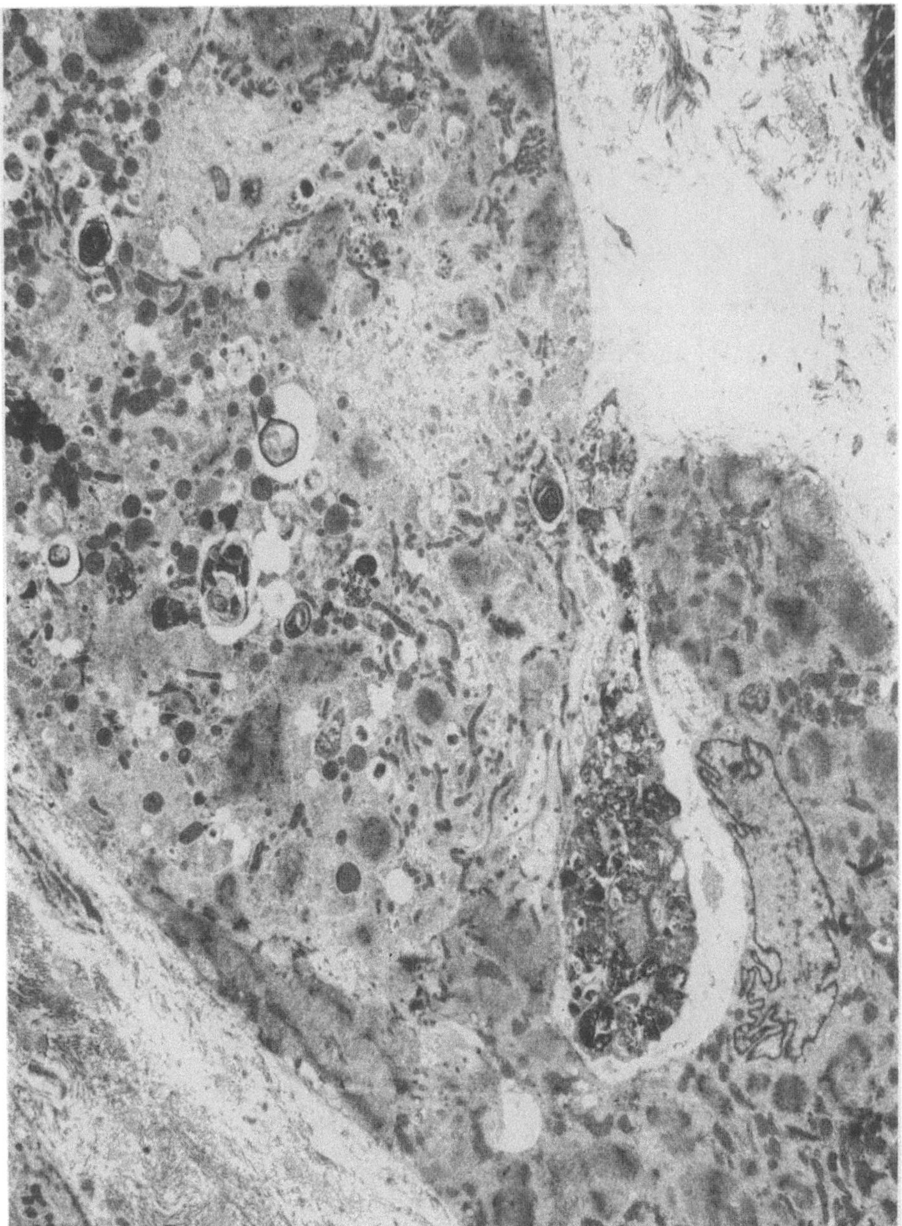

Fig. 10. Severe necrobiotic cell changes with numerous myelin figures, lysosomal granules and sequestration of cell debris. Marked interstitial fibrosis surrounding the myocardial cell. ×4400

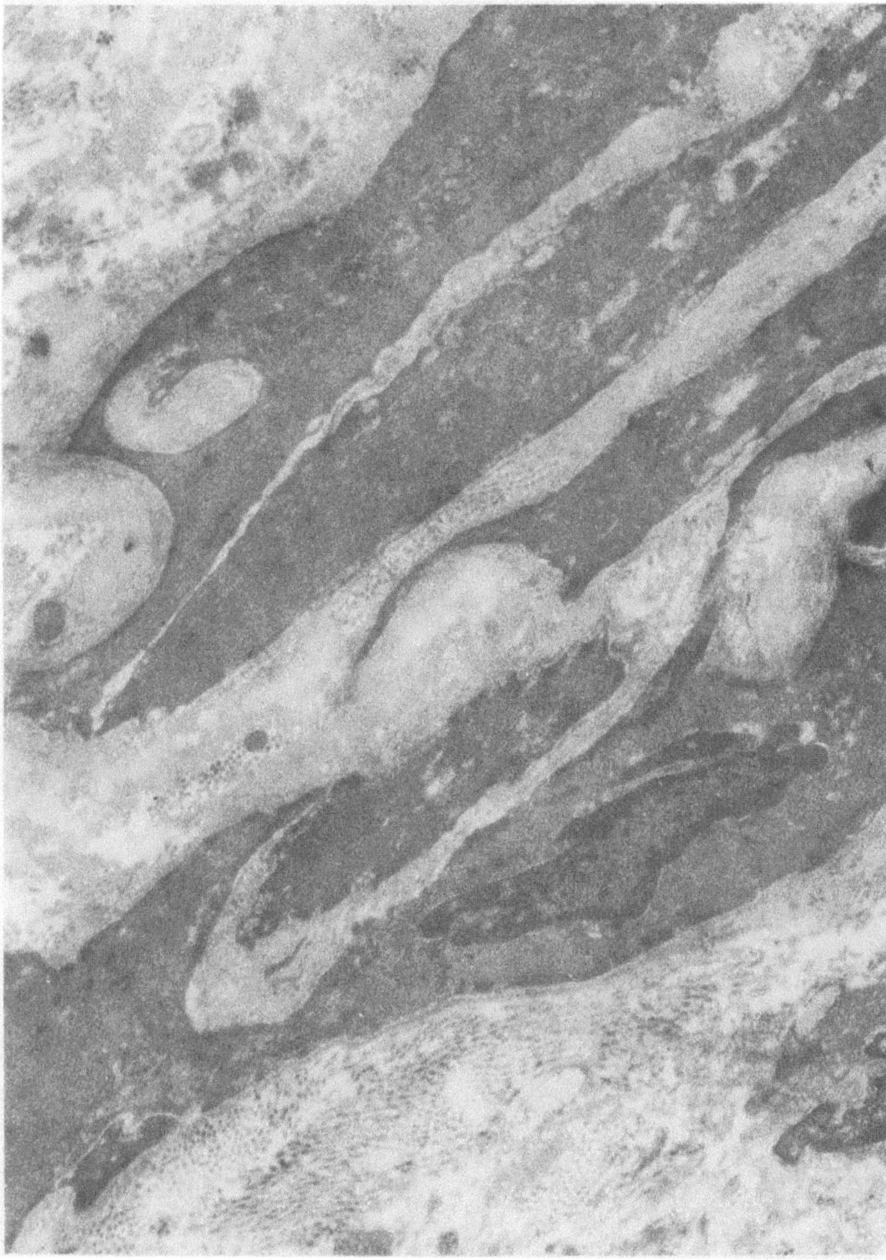

Fig. 11. Endocardial fibrosis with hyperplasia of smooth muscle cells. Between the smooth muscle cells increased collagen fibers and immature elastic matrix is present. ×12000

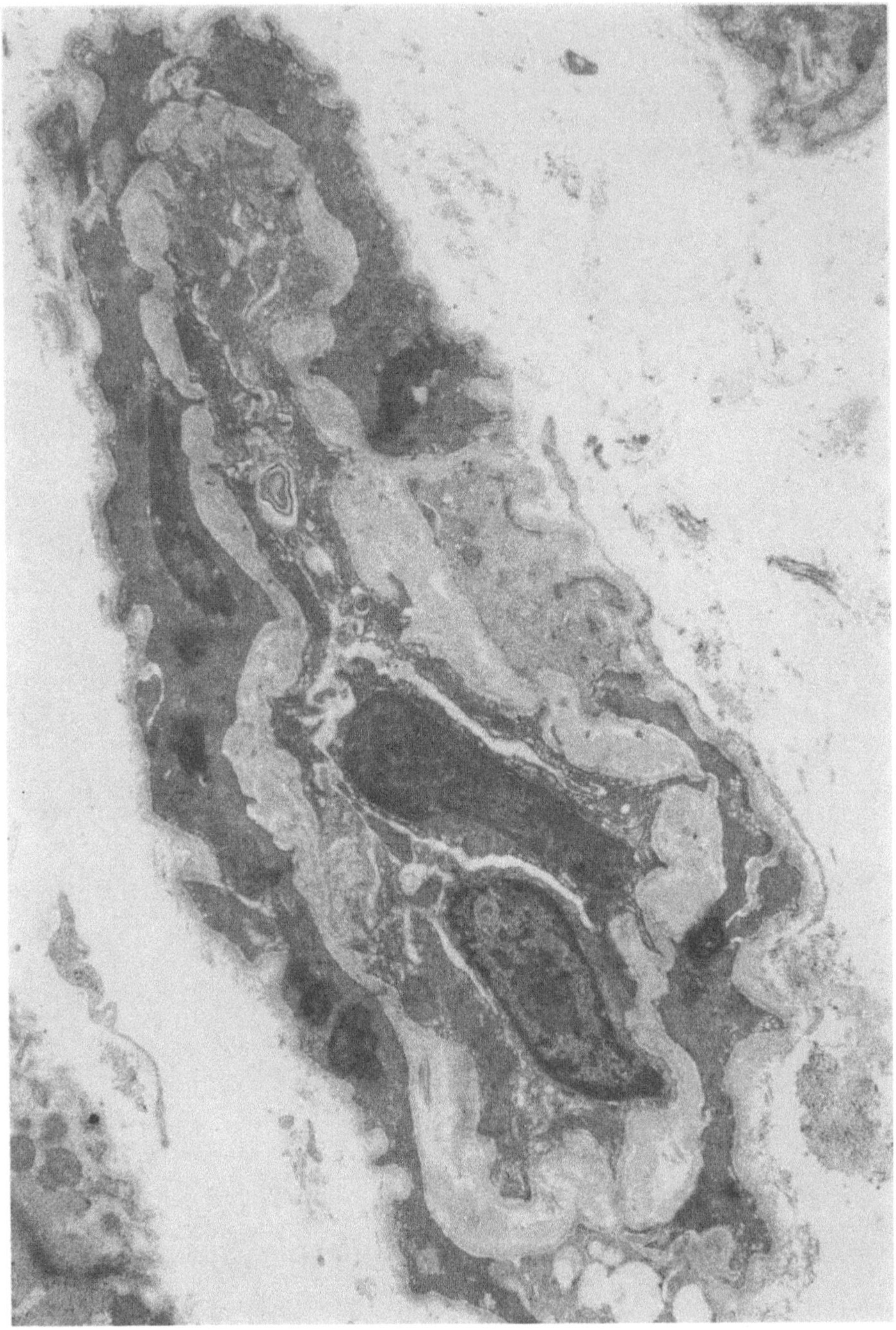

Fig. 12. Arteriole within fibrosed interstitium with proliferated endothelial cells and thickening of the basement membrane. Slight vacuolization of surrounding smooth muscle cells. ×7200

Conclusions

1. The combination of hypertrophy and interstitial fibrosis and degenerative changes of the myocardial cells correspond with the poor prognosis of cases with COCM. Light microscopic examination alone is not sufficient for the evaluation of the disease.
2. Although the morphologic findings alone are unspecific, they can be of significant diagnostic and prognostic value after correlation with clinical data.
3. Therefore, the morphologic findings, especially the ultractructural findings in myocardial biopsy specimen, can support the clinical diagnosis of COCM.
4. The close correlation of ultrastructural findings of myocardial biopsy specimens with clinical data may lead to a better understanding of the disease and the course of the still idiopathic COCMs. The different data should also be correlated with postmortem findings of previously biopsied patients.

References

1. Bozner, A., Meessen, H.: Die Feinstruktur des Herzmuskels der Ratte nach einmaligem und wiederholtem Schwimmtraining. Virchows Arch. Abt. B Zellpath. *3*, 248 (1969)
2. Breithardt, G., Knieriem, H.-J., Kuhn, H., Loogen, F., Gleichmann, U.: Comparison of clinical data and ultrastructural findings in myocardial biopsies of patients with congestive cardiomyopathies. Int. Study Group for Res. Cardiac Structure and Metabolism, Prag 1974. Munich-Berlin-Vienna: Urban u. Schwarzenberg 1977
3. Büchner, F., Onishi, S.: Herzhypertrophie und Herzinsuffizienz in der Sicht der Elektronenmikroskopie. Munich-Berlin-Vienna: Urban u. Schwarzenberg 1970
4. Doerr, W., Roßner, J.A., Dittgen, R., Rieger, P., Derks, H., Berg, G.: Cardiomyopathie. Berlin-Heidelberg-New York: Springer Verlag 1977
5. Ferrans, V.J., Massumi, R.A., Shugoll, G.I., Ali, N., Roberts, W.C.: Ultrastructural studies of myocardial biopsies in 45 patients with obstructive or congestive cardiomyopathy. In: Cardiomyopathies. Bajuz, E., Rona, G. (eds.). Munich-Berlin-Vienna: Urban u. Schwarzenberg 1974
6. Ferrans, V.J., Morrow, A.G., Roberts, W.C.: Myocardial ultrastructure in idiopathic hypertrophic subaortic stenosis. A study of operatively excised outflow tract muscle in 14 patients. Circulation *45*, 769 (1972)
7. Knieriem, H.-J.: Morphologische Grundlagen der Herzhypertrophie. Verh. dtsch. Ges. Kreisl.-Forsch. *38*, 1 (1972)
8. Knieriem, H.-J.: Zur Differentialdiagnose zwischen Myokarditis und idiopathischer Kardiomyopathie aus pathologisch-anatomischer Sicht. Therapiewoche *24*, 1054 (1974)
9. Knieriem, H.-J., Kuhn, H., Breithardt, G.: Morphologische Befunde bei Myokardbiopsien. Verh. dtsch. Ges. Path. *59*, 570 (1975)
10. Knieriem, H.-J., Kuhn, H., Breithardt, G.: Zur Diagnostik der primären Kardiomyopathien mit Hilfe der Myokardbiopsie. Z. Kardiol., Suppl. *2*, 26 (1975)
11. Knieriem, H.-J., Kuhn, H., Breithardt, G.: Correlation of clinical data and electron-microscopic findings of myocardial biopsies in congestive and hypertrophic cardiomyopathies. 7th Europ. Congr. Cardiol., Amsterdam (1976)
12. Knieriem, H.-J., Stroobandt, R., Meyer, H., Bourgeois, M.: Hypertrophic nonobstructive cardiomyopathy caused by disorder of the myofiber texture. Virchows Arch. Abt. A path. Anat. u. Hist. *367*, 209 (1975)
13. Kuhn, H., Breithardt, G., Knieriem, H.-J., Loogen, F., Both, A., Schmidt, W.A., Stroobandt, R., Gleichmann, U.: Die Bedeutung der endomyokardialen Katheterbiopsie für die Diagnostik und Beurteilung der Prognose bei congestiver Cardiomyopathie. Dtsch. med. Wschr. *100*, 717 (1975)
14. Meessen, H.: Structural bases of myocardial hypertrophy. Brit. Heart J., Suppl. *33*, 94 (1971)
15. Meessen, H.: Morphologie der Myokardhypertrophie. Verh. dtsch. Ges. inn. Med. *77*, 43 (1971)

16. Meessen, H., Poche, R.: Beiträge zur pathologischen Anatomie der Fallotschen Fehler und zur idiopathischen Herzhypertrophie. Anglo-German med. Rev. *4*, 73 (1967)
17. Novi, A.M.: Beitrag zur Feinstruktur des Herzmuskels bei experimenteller Herzhypertrophie. Beitr. path. Anat. *137*, 19 (1968)
18. Olsen, E.G.J.: Morbid anatomy and histology in hypertrophic obstructive cardiomyopathy. In: Ciba Foundation Symposium, London, 1971
19. Olsen, E.G.J.: Pathology of hypertrophic obstructive cardiomyopathy. In: Cardiomyopathies. Bajusz, E., Rona, G. (eds.). Munich-Berlin-Vienna: Urban u. Schwarzenberg 1974
20. Olsen, E.G.J.: Die Pathologie der primären Kardiomyopathien. Z. Kardiol. Suppl. *2*, 1 (1975)
21. Pearse, A.E.G.: The histochemistry and electron microscopy of obstructive cardiomyopathy. In: Cardiomyopathies. Ciba Foundation Symposium. Wolstenholme, G.E.W., O'Connor, M. (eds.). Boston: Little Brown u. Co. 1964
22. Van Noorden, S., Olsen, E.G.J., Pearse, A.E.G.: Hypertrophic obstructive cardiomyopathy. A histological, histochemical and ultrastructural study of biopsy material. Cardiovasc. Res. *5*, 118 (1971)

9. Ultrastructural Evaluations in Early and Advanced Congestive Cardiomyopathies

B. Kunkel, H. Lapp, G. Kober, and M. Kaltenbach

The results of light-microscopic evaluations were reported in Chapter 7. This chapter presents the electron-microscopic findings of the biopsy material.

Material and Methods

Endomyocardial biopsies from 75 patients were studied. The patients were divided into two groups: Group I included 33 patients with early congestive CM. In these patients, heart volumes were slightly or moderately increased, they showed marked ECG changes, enddiastolic volumes were slightly to moderately increased, and ejection fractions slightly reduced.

Group II included 42 patients with typical advanced congestive CM. In these patients, enddiastolic left ventricular volumes were markedly increased, ejection fractions were reduced more than 50%, and left ventricular enddiastolic pressures at rest were usually elevated.

The biopsy specimens were fixed with cold 2.5% glutaraldehyde in 0.1 *M*. phosphate buffer, postfixed with sucrose, and embedded in Vestopal. The ultrathin sections were stained with lead citrate and uranylacetate.

Results

The incidence of electron-microscopic changes is listed in Table 1. Both groups showed similar ultrastructural alterations which, however, are more frequent and more pronounced in patients with advanced congestive CM. These changes are related to hypertrophy, to degeneration of cardiac muscle cells, or to interstitial fibrosis of the myocardium. Most common are alterations of the nuclei, followed by changes of mitochondria, myofibrils, Golgi's apparatus, T-system, and the sarcoplasmic reticulum, as well as of other cell structures.

Nuclear changes of cardiac muscle cells were observed in 39% of group I and in all patients of group II (Figs. 1 and 2). The nuclei were enlarged, lobulated or crenalated, and polymorphic in shape. Nuclear membranes were deeply invaginated and sometimes formed pseudoinclusions. Prominent nucleoli were often found. Frequently binucleated cardiac muscle cells were seen in cases with severe hypertrophy. In some cases with pronounced cardiac hypertrophy, irregular arrangement of nuclear chromatin was observed.

Myofibrils were more numerous in hypertrophic cardiac muscle cells. In 29% of the patients in group I and in 71% of those in group II varying degrees of

Table 1. Electron-microscopic findings in patients with early (n = 33) and advanced (n = 42) congestive cardiomyopathy.

	Early forms		Advanced forms	
	n	%	n	%
Nuclear changes	13	39.3	42	100
Myofibrillolysis / loss of myofibrils	9	27.2	30	71
Z-band abnormalities	9	27.2	19	45.2
Myofibrillar disarray	12	36.3	24	57.1
Mitochondriosis	36	78.7	42	100
Loss of mitochondria	4	12.4	16	38
Abnormal variability in mitochondrial size	11	33,3	35	83
Mitochondrial degeneration	13	39.3	28	66.6
Myelin figures	11	33.3	23	54.7
Dilatation of T-tubules	13	39.3	24	57.1
Hypertrophy of sarcoplasmatic reticulum	4	12.1	14	33.3
Dilatation of sarcoplasmatic reticulum	14	42.6	19	25.2
Hypertrophy of the Golgi apparatus	19	57.5	25	59.5
Rough endoplasmatic reticulum	11	33.3	16	38.0
Increase in glycogen content	10	30.3	20	47.6
Increase in lipid droplets	10	30.3	21	49.9
Increase in lipofuscin granules	13	39.3	25	59.9
Increase in lysosomes	4	12.1	17	40.4
Interstitial fibrosis	8	24.2	26	61.9
Increase in interstitial cells	2	9.0	23	54.7

destruction of actin and myosin filaments were found. Some cells exhibited a significant loss of myofibrils (Fig. 3). In these "clarified" muscle cells, myofibrils may be replaced by proliferated sarcoplasmic reticulum or mitochondria, or glycogen granules (Fig. 11).

Myofibrilar disarray was originally thought to be characteristic of HOCM. Its occurrence in congestive CM was described minimal. In the present study it was found that myofibrillar disarray occurs in 36% of early congestive CM and in 57% of advanced cases (Fig. 4). In contrast to the findings in HOCM, myofibrillar abnormalities in both groups were focal and only found in a few cardiac muscle cells. Changes were predominantly localized near the intercellular junctions, which were often merkedly twisted.

Alterations of Z-band material were observed in 27% of patients in group I and in 45% of the group II patients (Figs. 4 and 5). These alterations consisted of widening, clumping, and splitting. Z-band abnormalities were often found in areas of myofibrillar disarray, in combination with myofibrilysis.

Mitochondrial accumulation was found not only in all cases of advanced congestive CM, but also in 78% of patients with early forms of disease. With increasing severity of cardiac hypertrophy some cardiac muscle cells exhibited

Fig. 1. Nucleus of a hypertrophied cardiac muscle cell showing invaginations of the nuclear membrane. (×4000) ▷

Fig. 2. Part of a binucleated cardiac muscle cell. (×3000)

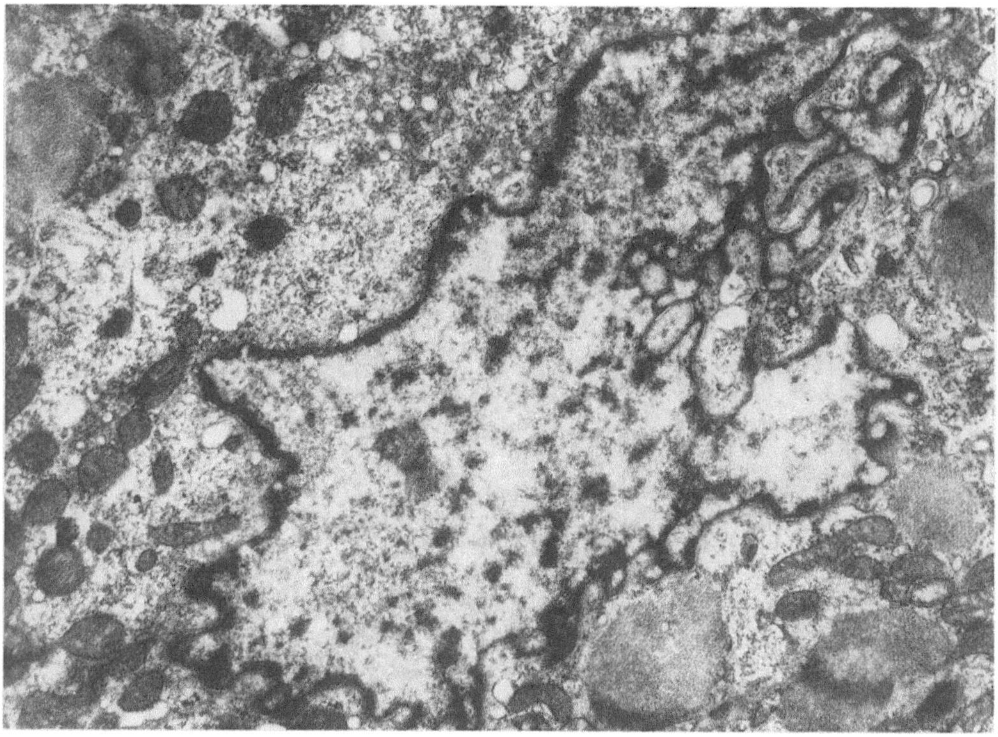

1

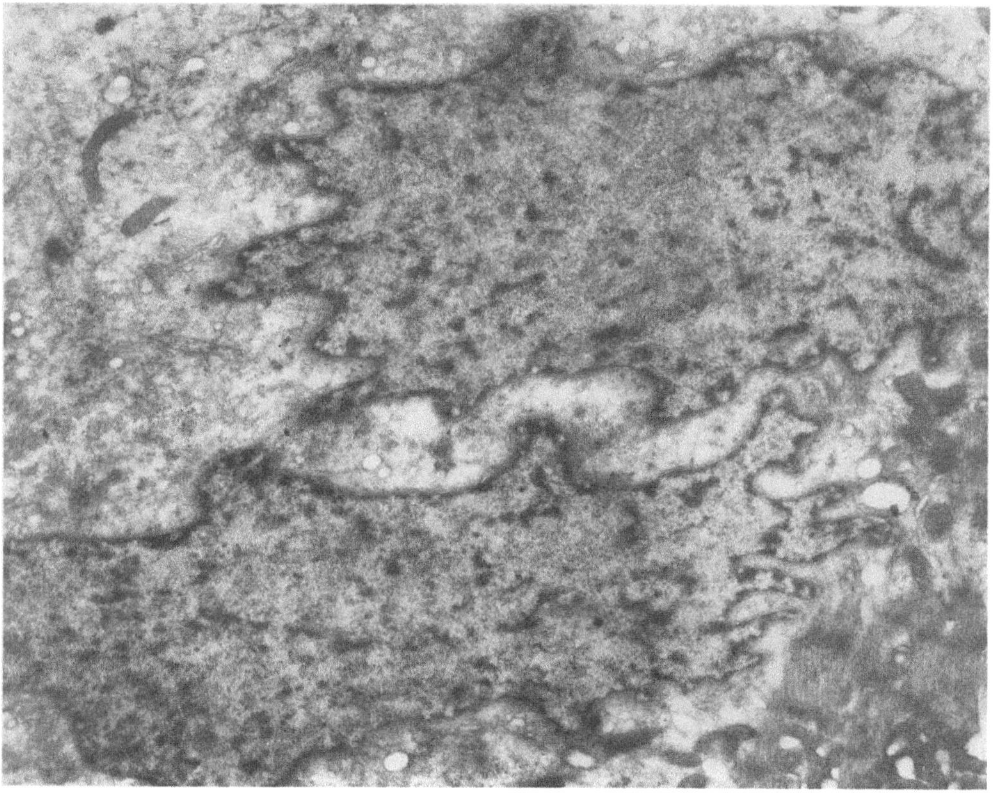

2

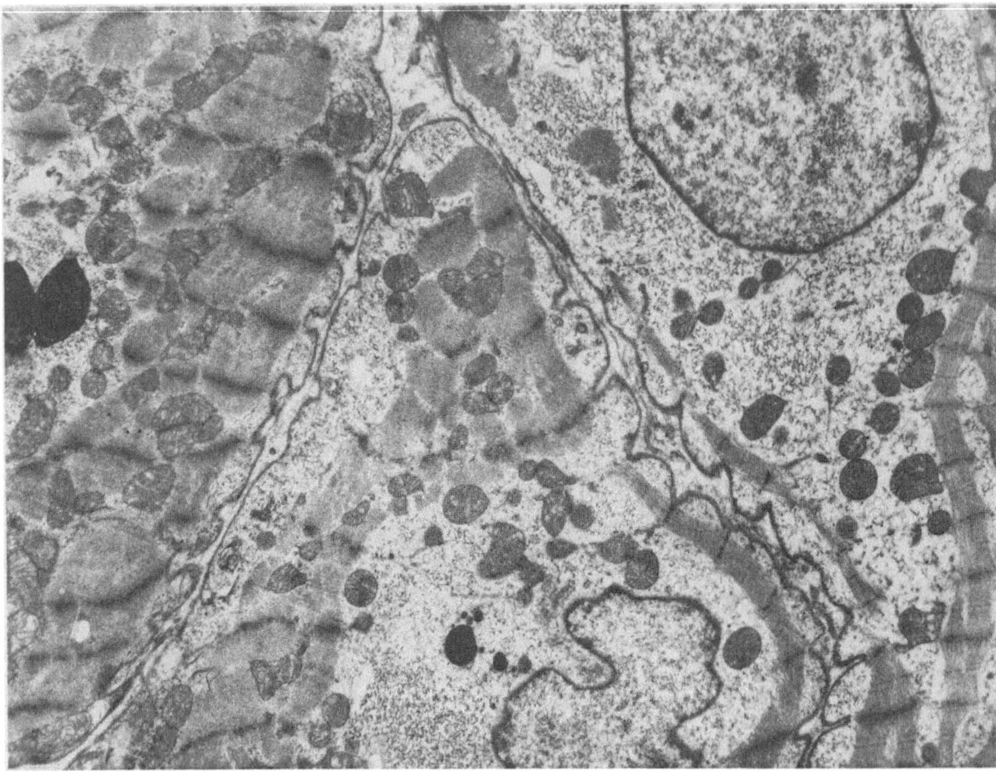

3

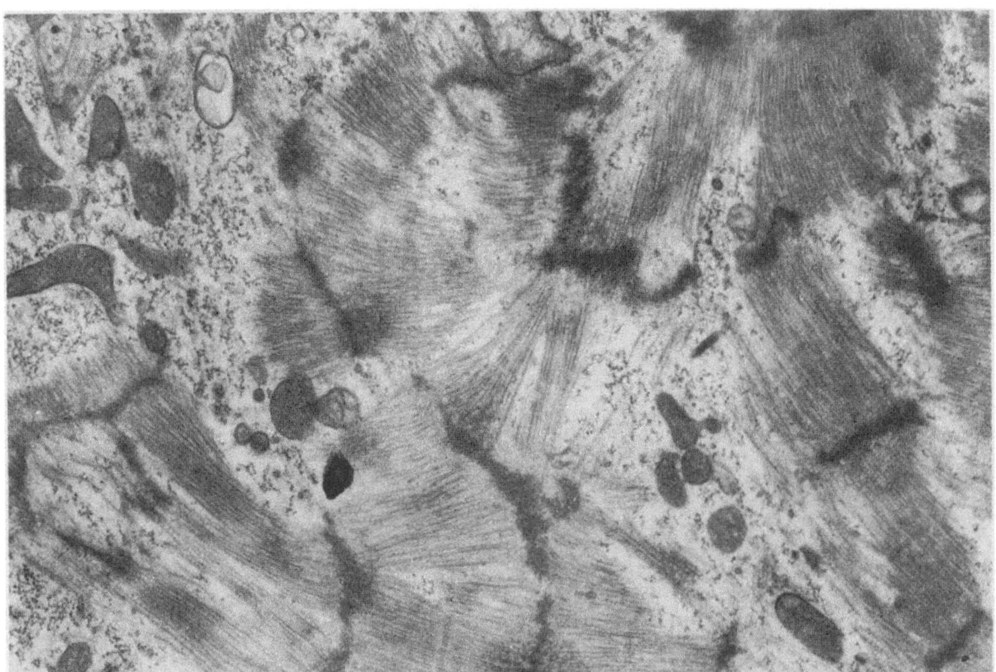

4

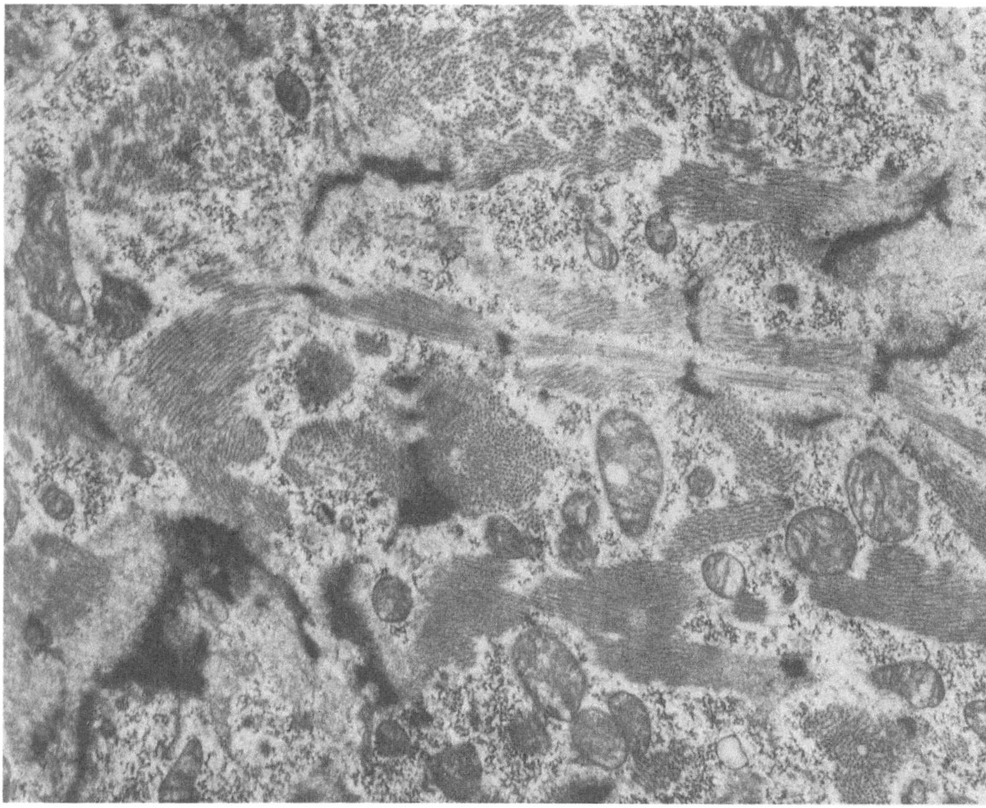

Fig. 5. Accumulation and irregular arrangement of Z-band material. Myofibrillolysis and abnormal orientation of myofibrils. (×9000)

loss of mitochondria. This was found in 12% of group I patients and in 38% of group II patients (Fig. 6).

In addition to the increase in number, pronounced variations in mitochondrial size were also observed (Fig. 7). Abnormally small mitochondria were predominant in some cardiac muscle cells and were found in 33% of the patients with early congestive CM and in 83% of those with advanced diseases. Such small mitochondria may have a normal structure, but often the number of cristae was reduced or the cristae were arranged in concentric lamellae. Other degenerative mitochondrial changes were seen, predominantly in group II: electron-dense inclusions, formation of myelin figures from mitochondria, and cristolysis and clarification of the matrix (Figs. 6 and 8). Myelin figures were increased in 33%

◁ Fig. 3. Severe loss of myofibrils. The cardiac muscle cell on the left side shows normal content of myofibrils. (×3500)

Fig. 4. Marked myofibrillar disarray combined with myofibrillolysis and Z-band abnormalities. (×12000)

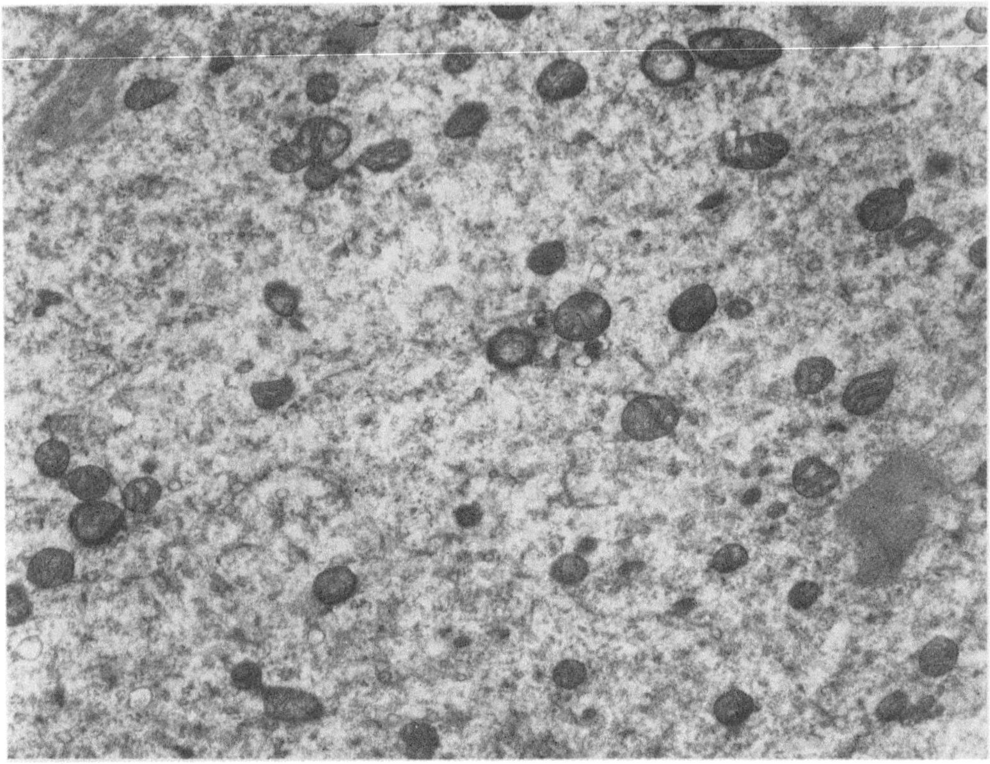

6

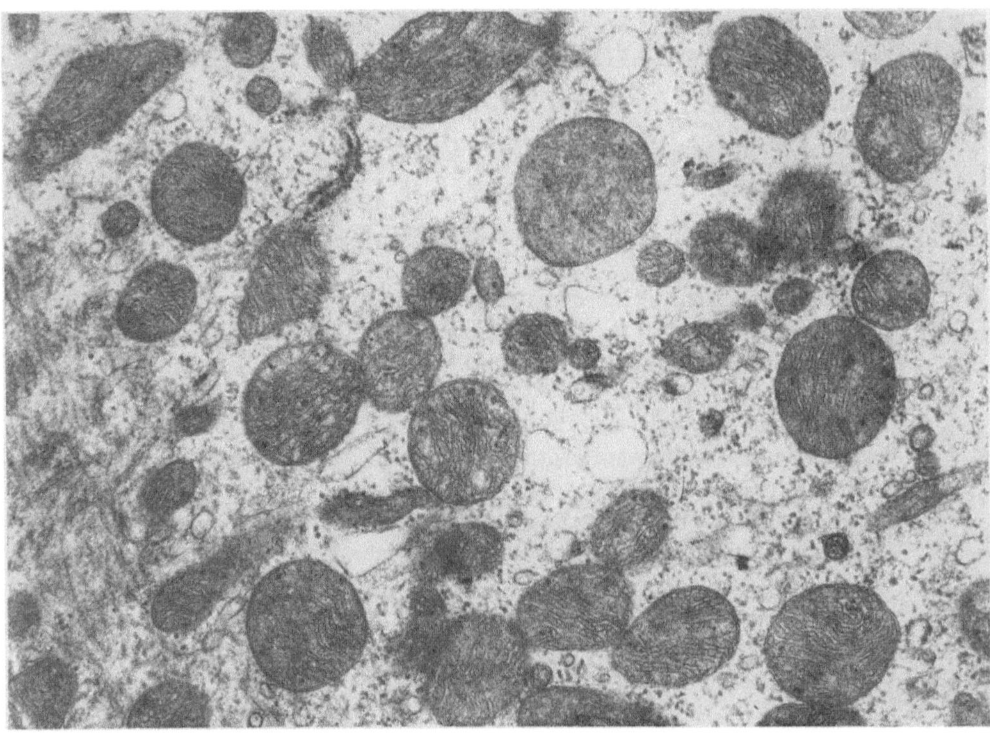

7

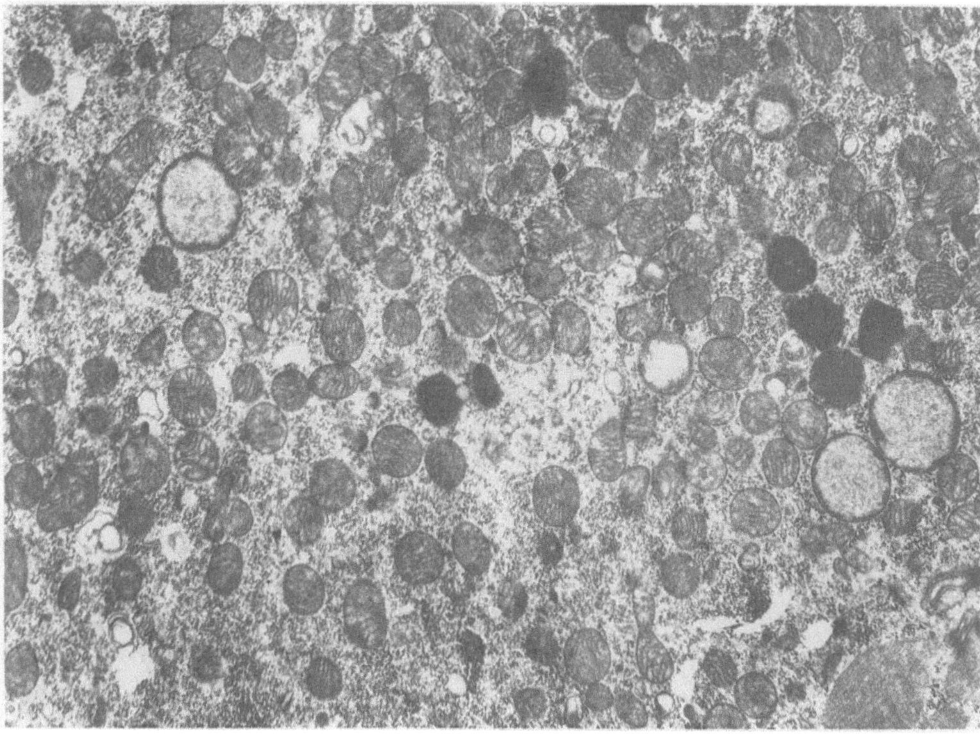

Fig. 8. "Mitochondriosis". Single mitochondria exhibit complete loss of cristae. (×6000)

of patients with early forms of the disease and in 54% of patients with advanced congestive CM (Fig. 9).

In both groups Golgi structures were increased in size and in number, and spiral lamellae of rough sarcoplasmic reticulum were localized near the nuclear poles in about 50% of the cases in both groups (Figs. 10 and 13).

The glycogen content of cardiac muscle cells showed wide variations. However, there was no clear correlation between the severity of hypertrophy and the cellular glycogen content.

In individual cardiac muscle cells a large number of lipid droplets was observed in 30% of the cases with mild clinical symptoms and in 49% of the severe cases.

The sarcoplasmic reticulum was dilated in 42% of early congestive CM and in 25% of the advanced forms. Sometimes the sarcoplasmic reticulum proliferated markedly in degenerated cardiac muscle cells with loss of myofibrils and mitochondria (Fig. 11). A proliferation or dilation of T-tubules was found in 34% of the patients in group I and in 52% of the cases of the second group.

◁ Fig. 6. Loss of myofibrils and mitochondria. Remaining mitochondria are small and the number of cristae is reduced. (×4000)

Fig. 7. Marked variations in mitochondrial size. (×14000)

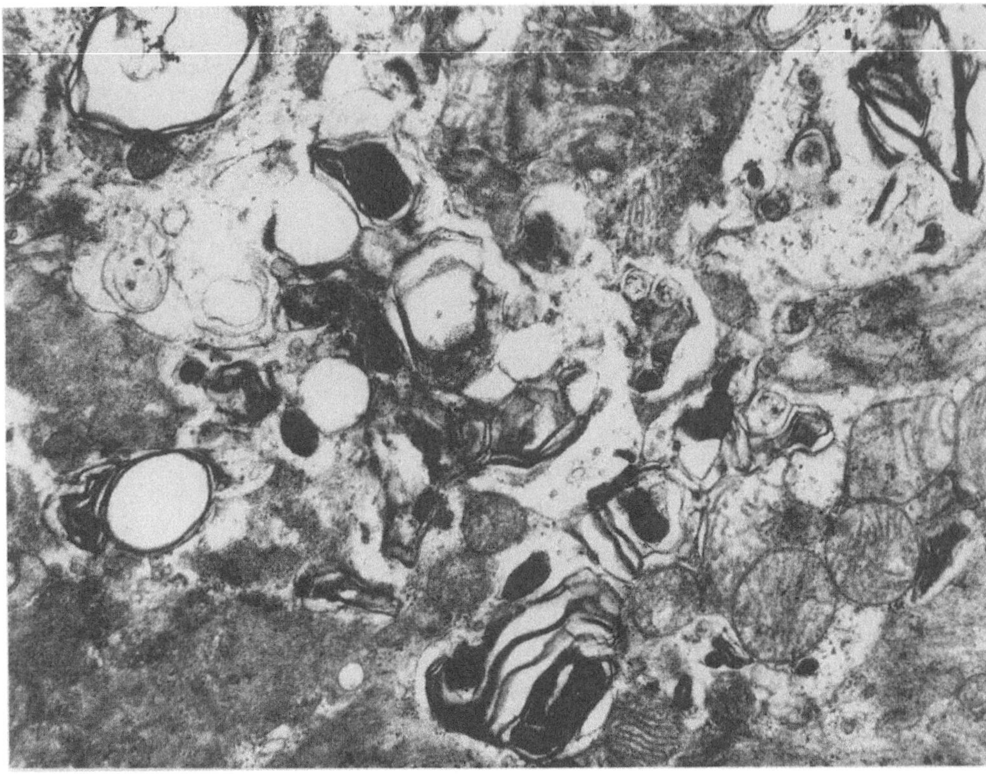

9

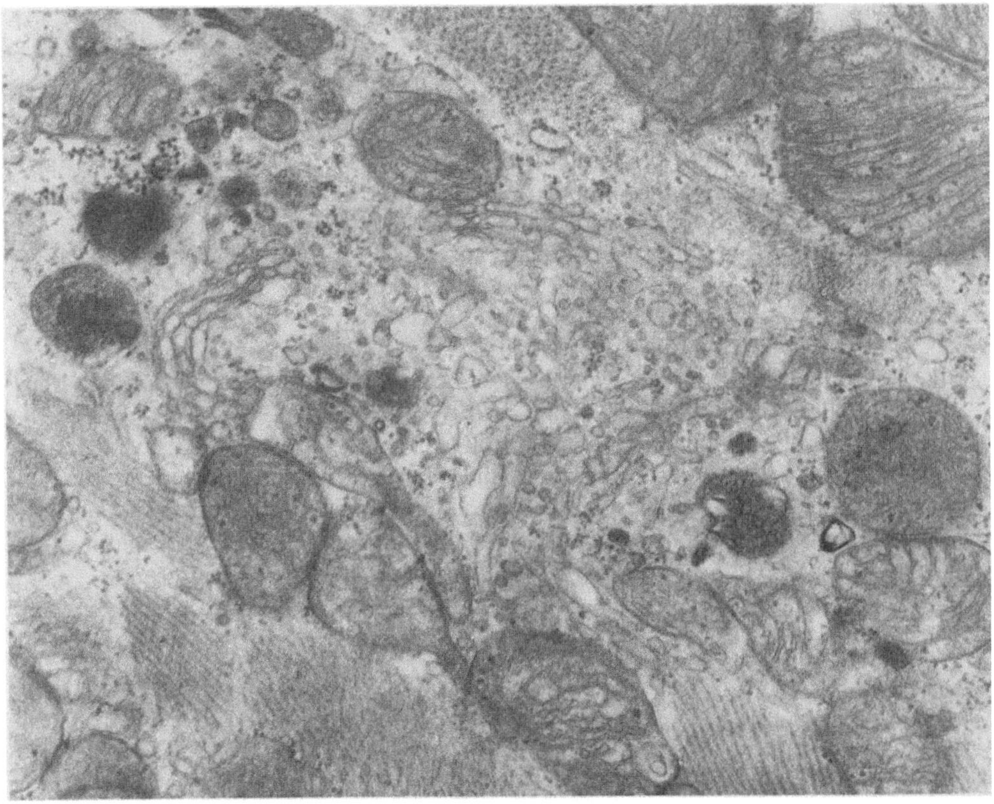

10

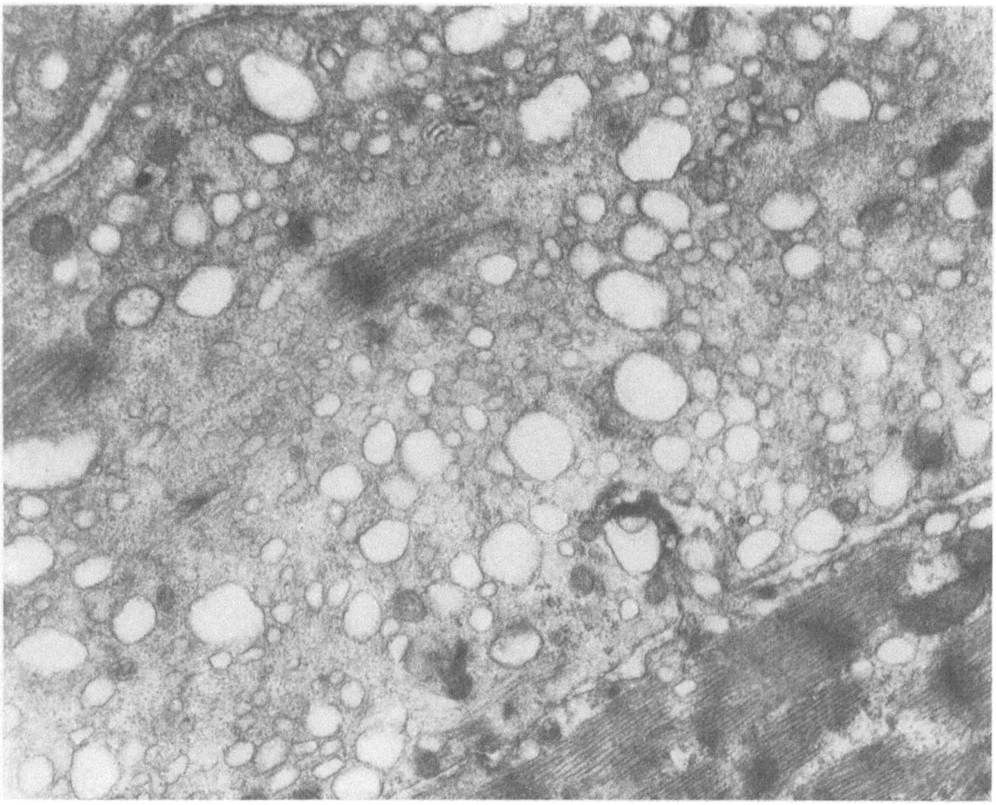

Fig. 11. Marked proliferation and dilation of the sarcoplasmatic reticulum in a cardiac muscle cell which shows nearly complete loss of myofibrils and mitochondria. (× 1000)

Numerous lipofuscin granules were localized near the nuclear poles of cardiac muscle cells in both groups (Fig. 12). Lysosomes were found close to Golgi structures and to lipofuscin granules in 12.5% of group I and in 40% of the patients of group II (Fig. 13).

The subendocardial layers of myocardium which are excised during biopsy showed an interstitial fibrosis in 24% of the early and in 61% of the advanced forms of congestive CM. In 9.1% of the cases with mild disease and in 54% of advanced CM, increases in fibrocytes and fibroplastic cells as well as in singular macrophages and lymphocytes were present (Fig. 14).

◁ Fig. 9. Myelin figures in a markedly degenerated cardiac muscle cell. (× 11000)

Fig. 10. Hypertrophied Golgi structure in a hypertrophied cardiae muscle cell. (× 13000)

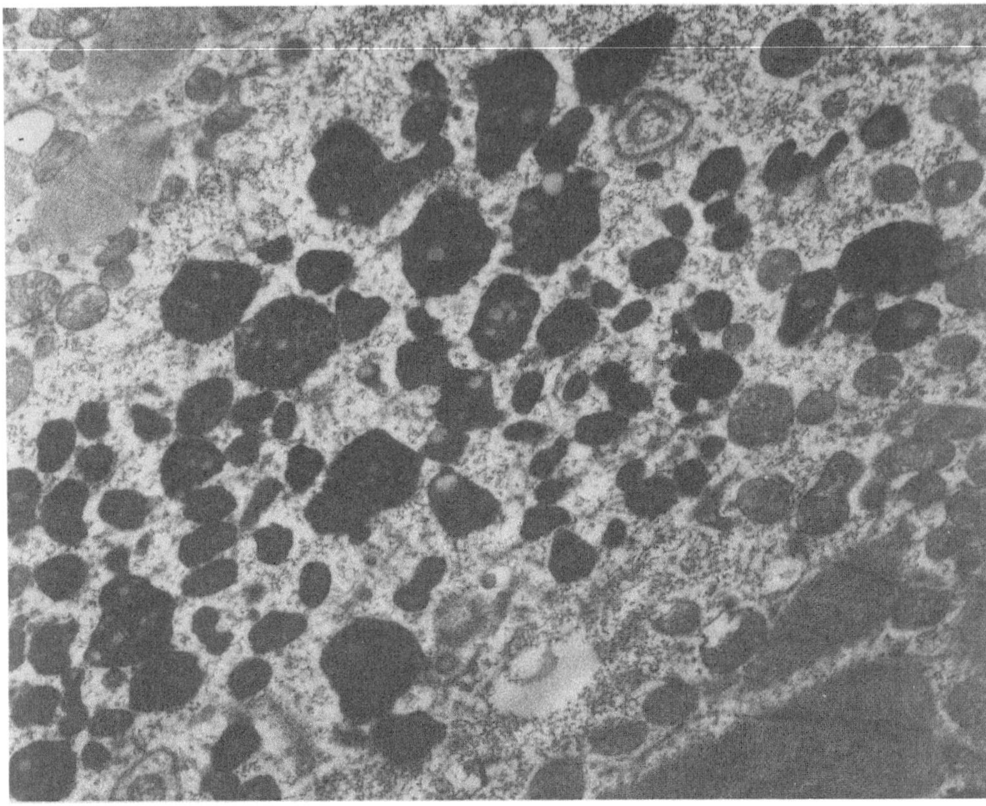
12

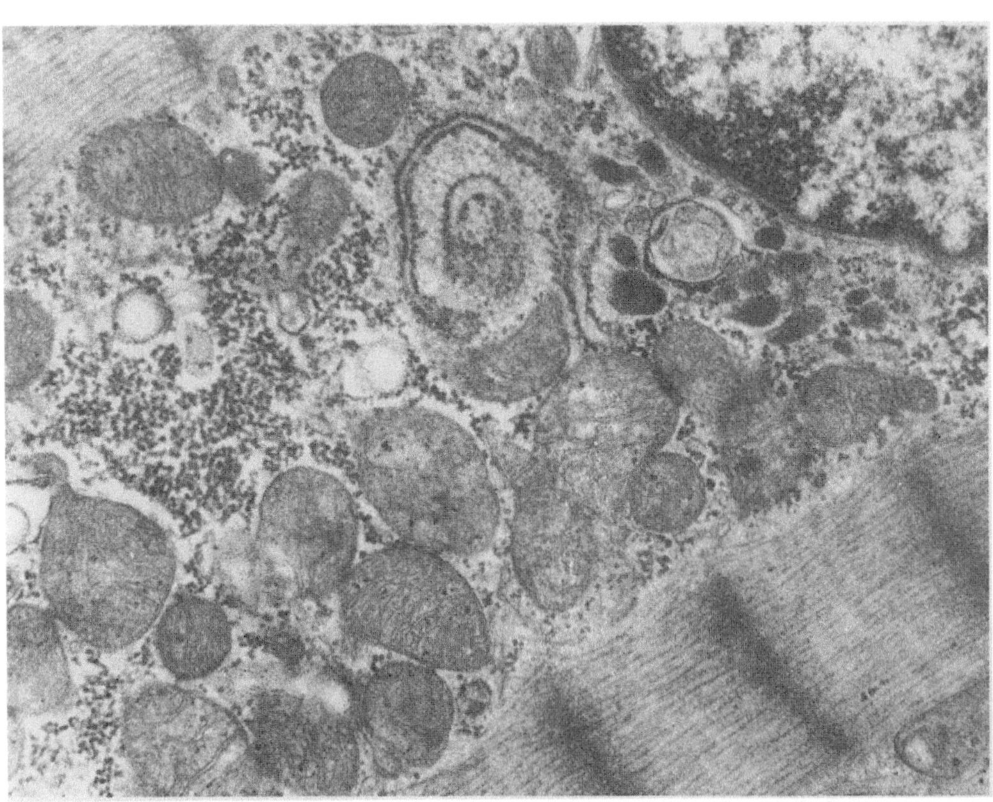
13

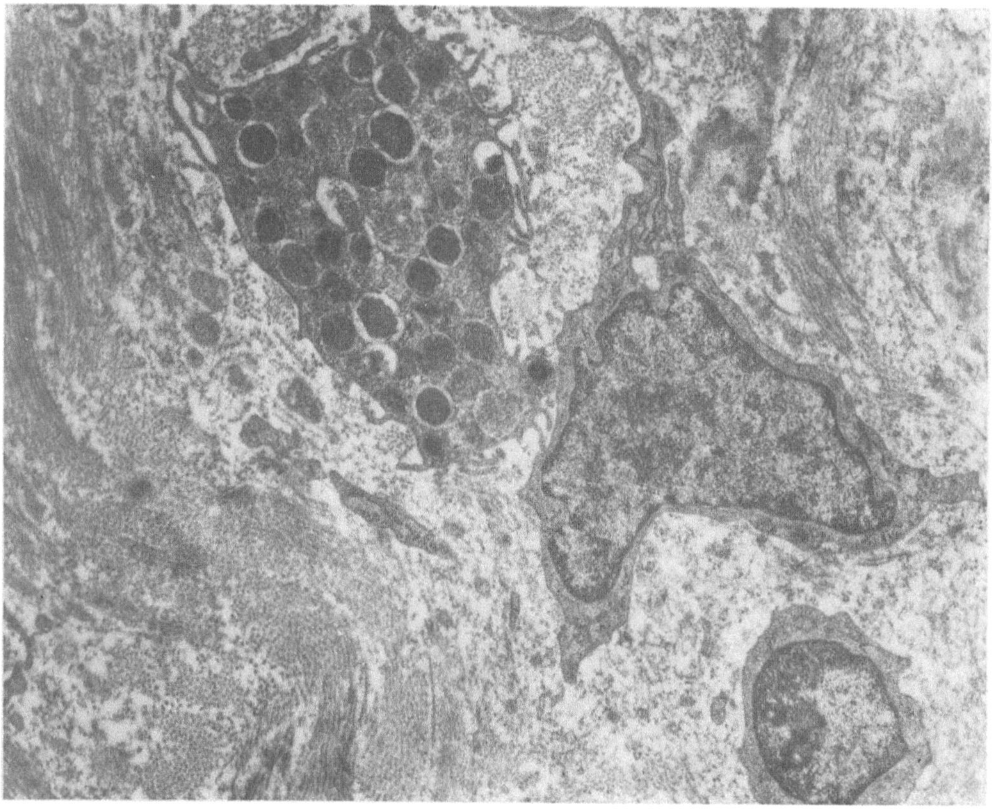

Fig. 14. Area of interstitial fibrosis containing a Mast cell, a fibrocyte and a lymphocyte. (× 6000)

Discussion

Identical ultrastructural changes of cardiac muscle cells were observed in early and advanced congestive cardiomyopathy, occurring more frequently and more severely in the latter. It is of considerable interest that these ultrastructural changes in COCM develop even before the onset of clinical cardiac failure.

Many of those changes are caused by myocardial hypertrophy which in various degrees is already present in most patients with early COCM.

Severe cellular damage such as that in COCM has also been seen in various other forms of heart disease associated with advanced hypertrophy [3, 6]. Cardiac hypertrophy thus appears to be responsible for a great number of degenerative ultrastructural changes.

◁ Fig. 12. Accumulation of lipofuscin granules. (× 6000)

Fig. 13. Rough surfaced endoplasmatic reticulum. Small lysosomes surrounding a myelin figure. (× 17000)

In contrast, in several cases of early COCM, cellular damage was much more pronounced than would have been anticipated from the degree of cardiac hypertrophy. Hence, myocardial damage in COCM seems to be the result both of cardiac hypertrophy and primary cell degeneration.

Myofibrillar disarray is a typical finding in hypertrophic CM [1,5,7,8]. Ferrans reported this phenomenon in congenital heart disease with outflow tract obstruction [3]. We observed myofibrillar irregularities in a patient with combined aortic valve disease. In patients with congestive CM, myofibrillar disarray was thought to occur only very rarely. Ferrans observed abnormalities of myofibrillar orientation in 3 of 31 patients with congestive CM [1]. Kuhn *et al.* described myofibrillar disarray in 12 of 19 patients with congestive CM [4]. In our biopsy material myofibrillar disarray was found in 57% of the cases with advanced and in 36% of the patients with early congestive CM.

In contrast to cases with HOCM, myofibrillar disarray in congestive CM affects only a few cells. The origin of this phenomenon is still unknown. In most cases severe hypertrophy is present. Therefore, myofibrilar disarray might be a sequence of hypertrophy. In some early forms, however, myofibrilar disarray is present without remarkable hypertrophy of cardiac muscle cells. Hence, a primary cellular disorder is a possible explanation.

The amount of connective tissue present in most cases of early and advanced congestive CM can be quantitated more reliably by light than by electron microscopy. Normal myocardial interstitium only contained a few fibrocytes, while in many cases with congestive CM a substantial increase in fibrocytes, fibroblasts, and macrophages was noted – at times accompanied by single lymphocytes. This increase in interstitial cells was considered indicative of progressive interstitial fibrosis.

Since identical ultrastructural changes were found in various other forms of heart disease, such as aortic valve disease, none of the alterations in heart muscle cells were specific.

The cause of cardiac hypertrophy as the predominent finding still remains unknown. As opposed to cardiac valve disease or arterial hypertension, it cannot be interpreted as a consequence of hemodynamic overload. A possible stimulus for development of cardiac hypertrophy, however, may be some functional deficiency within the contractile system of the heart muscle cell.

Summary

Ultrastructural changes of early and advanced congestive CM were studied in 75 patients. The changes of cells were unspecific. They can be related to the amount of hypertrophy and cellular degeneration. In both patient groups identical ultrastructural alterations occurred. They were, however, more frequent and more pronounced in patients with advanced forms of the disease.

References

1. Ferrans, V.J., Massumi, R.A., Shugoll, A.N., Roberts, W.C.: Ultrastructural studies of myocardial biopsies in 45 patients with obstructive or congestive cardiomyopathy. In: Cardiomyopathies. Bajusz, E., Rona, G. (eds.). Munich: Urban und Schwarzenberg 1974
2. Hatt, P.Y., Berjal, G., Moravec, J., Swynghedauw, B.: Heart failure: An electron microscopic study of the left ventricular papillary muscle in aortic insufficiency in the rabbit. J. mol. cell. Biol. *1*, 235 (1970)
3. Jones, M., Ferrans, V.J., Morrow, A.G., Roberts, W.: Ultrastructure of crista supraventricularis muscle in patients with congenital heart diseases associated with right ventricular outflow tract obstruction. Circulation *51*, 39 (1975)
4. Kuhn, H., Breithardt, G., Knieriem, H.-J., Loogen, F., Both, A., Schmidt, W.-A.K., Strobandt, R., Gleichmann, U.: Die Bedeutung der endomyokardialen Katheterbiopsie für die Diagnostik und Beurteilung der Prognose der kongestiven Kardiomyopathie. Dtsch. med. Wschr. *100*, 717 (1975)
5. Maron, B., Ferrans, V.J., Henry, W., Clark, C.E., Redwood, D., Roberts, W.C., Morrow, A.G., Epstein, S.: Differences in distribution of myocardial abnormalities in patients with obstructive and nonobstructive asymmetrical septum hypertrophy. Circulation *50*, 436 (1974)
6. Maron, B.J., Ferrans, V.J., Roberts, W.C.: Myocardial ultrastructure in patients with chronic aortic valve disease. Amer. J. Card. *35*, 725 (1975)
7. Olsen, E.G.J.: Pathology of hypertrophic obstructive cardiomyopathy. In: Cardiomyopathies. Bajusz, E., Rona, G. (eds.). Munich: Urban und Schwarzenberg 1974
8. Van Noorden, S., Olsen, E.G.J., Pearce, G.E.: Hypertrophic obstructive cardiomyopathy, a histological, histochemical and ultrastructural study of biopsy material. Cardivasc. Res. *5*, 118 (1971)

10. Myocardial Ultrastructure in Human Cardiac Hypertrophy

V. J. Ferrans

Summary

Degenerative changes observed in biopsies of ventricular myocardium from 111 patients with heart disease of various types are described. Criteria are given for the classification of degenerative changes as mild, moderate, and severe, and the significance of these changes is discussed.

Meerson and co-workers have developed the concept that cardiac muscle evolves through three different functional stages during the time course of hypertrophy [1]. Hypertrophy begins to develop during the first stage, in which there is an increase in energy production and protein synthesis. A stable state of cardiac hyperfunction exists during the second stage. The third stage is characterized by gradual exhaustion of the ability of the heart to synthesize proteins, by failure to renew myofibrils and mitochondria, and by myofibrillar damage and cellular atrophy. While it has long been known that irreversible myocardial failure eventually develops in many humans and experimental animals with cardiac hypertrophy of long standing, in the last few years electron-microscopic observations have elucidated the sequence of complex morphologic changes that occur in human cardiac hypertrophy of various causes. A summary of these observations is presented in this communication, which is based on electron-microscopic studies of a large number of myocardial biopsies from patients with various types of heart disease.

Materials and Methods

The ultrastructural studies that are described in this communication were made of right or left ventricular myocardium from 111 patients. These patients were classified according to the nature of their lesions into the following four groups: a) 75 patients with congenital heart diseases characterized by right ventricular hypertrophy and by obstruction to right ventricular outflow (with or without intracardiac shunts) in whom crista supraventricularis muscle was obtained at open heart operation; b) 16 patients with hypertrophic CM (asymmetric septal hypertrophy, ASH) in whom ventricular septal muscle was resected at the time of left ventricular myotomy–myectomy; c) 16 patients with aortic valvular disease (6 with predominant aortic stenosis, 5 with pure aortic regurgitation, and 5 with combined aortic stenosis and regurgitation) in whom biopsies of the left ventricular free wall were obtained at the time of aortic valvular replacement (14 patients) or aortic commissurotomy (2 patients); and d) 4 patients with combined mitral and aortic valvular disease in whom biopsies of the left ventricular free wall were obtained at the time of double valve replacement.

All tissues were fixed with cold 3% glutaraldehyde in 0.1 *M* phosphate buffer, pH 7.2, washed with several changes of cold 5% sucrose in 0.1 *M* phosphate buffer, pH 7.2, dehydrated with ethanol and propylene oxide, and embedded in Maraglas [2]. Semithin sections were stained with alkaline toluidine blue and examined with a light microscope to select areas for ultrathin sectioning. Ultrathin sections were stained with uranyl acetate and lead citrate.

Results

Hypertrophied, Nondegenerated Cardiac Muscle Cells

The majority of cardiac muscle cells in the tissues of all patients were hypertrophied, with transverse diameters ranging from 15–70 μ (normal, 10–15 μ). As described below, clearly atrophic cells (< 10 μ in diameter in adult hearts) were seen only in patients with long-standing hypertrophy and with evidence of myocardial degeneration. In ventricular myocardium of all patients with aortic or mitral valvular disease, the muscle cells were parallel and joined by end-to-end intercellular junctions (intercalated discs). Intercellular junctions joining the sides of adjacent cells also were common, frequently demarcating lateral projections of cytoplasm that projected from the side of one cell into that of the adjacent cell (Fig. 1). The junctions in these lateral projections have been named multiple intercalated discs [3–5] because they frequently involve two or more sides of the lateral projections. It has been postulated [5] that these cytoplasmic processes form as a result of mechanical forces exerted on normally occurring lateral junctions and that such processes have an interlocking effect between adjacent cells that tends to prevent the slippage of adjacent layers of ventricular muscle cells.

In the ventricular septum of all patients with hypertrophic CM, many hypertrophied muscle cells had bizarre shapes and exhibited a disorganized arrangement, often forming whorls. The contractile elements of such cells also were disorganized, with myofibrils coursing in different directions within a given cell and often radiating from Z bands in a diverging manner (Fig. 2). In patients with HOCM, these changes were much more prevalent in the ventricular septum than elsewhere, whereas in patients with nonobstructive hypertrophic CM, they were much more widespread, with foci of disarray of cells located throughout the free walls of both ventricles [6]. Cells with the features just described were present in rare, minute foci in crista supraventricularis muscle from 14 (18%) of the 75 patients with congenital heart diseases associated with obstruction to right ventricular outflow. The incidence of these changes in these patients according to age was as follows: 1 (3%) of 36 patients aged 10 months–10 years; 6 (27%) of 22 patients aged 11–20 years; 4 (10%) of 10 patients aged 21–29 years, and 3 (38%) of 8 patients aged 30–53 years.

In all patients with cardiac hypertrophy, enlarged, nondegenerated muscle cells contained numerous compact myofibrils that were separated by mitochondria

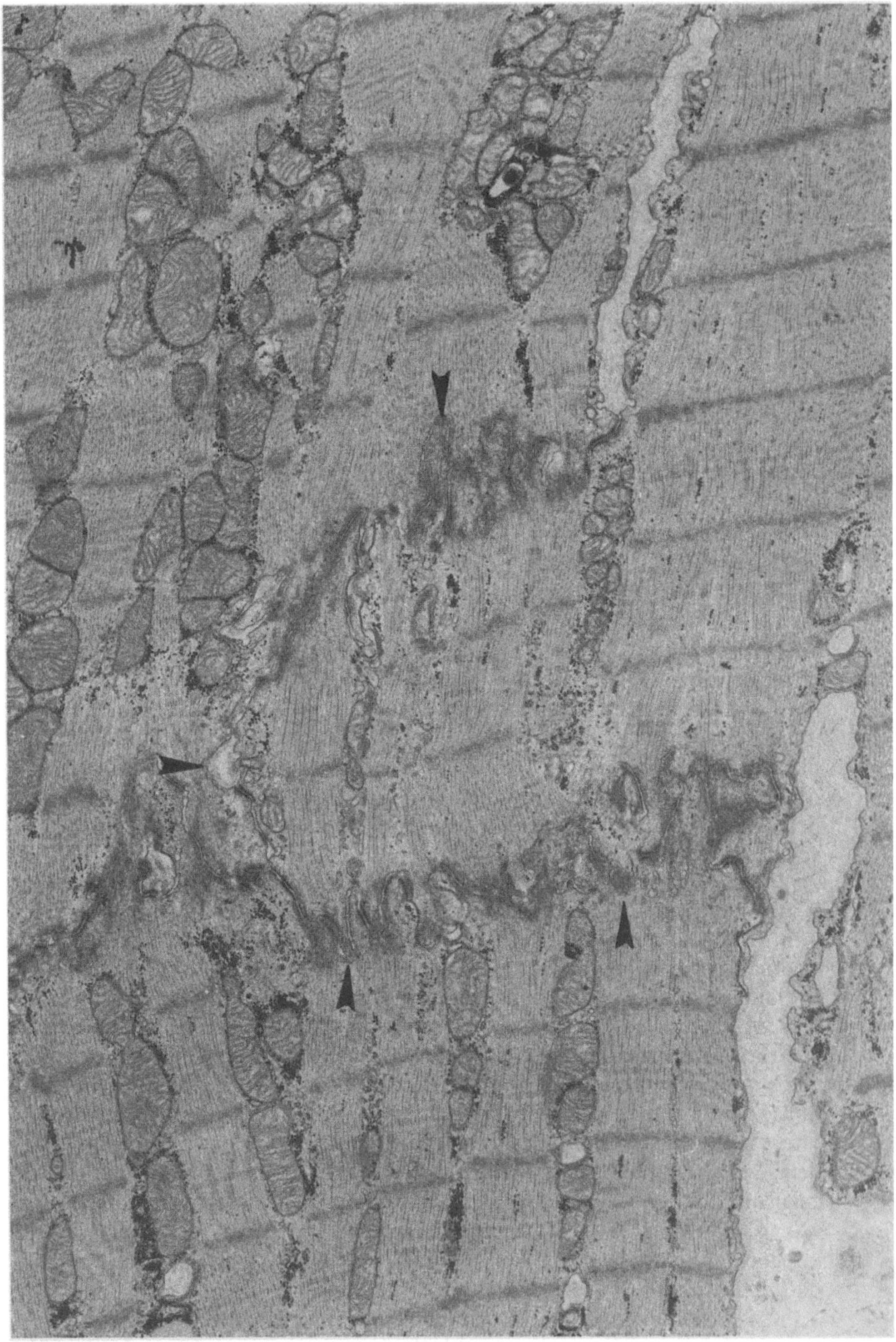

and glycogen particles. Adjacent to the nuclei were conical-shaped myofibril-free areas that contained enlarged Golgi complexes and numerous glycogen particles and lipofuscin granules. The size of these perinuclear areas usually was proportional to that of the nuclei. Perinuclear areas of the type just described were most prominent in cells that had large nuclei with blunt or square tips. The mitochondria showed marked variations in size, some much smaller (1500 Å in diameter) than normal (Fig. 3A). Mitochondria occasionally contained inclusions of glycogen (Fig. 3B), either in the α or β form, located in the outer mitochondrial compartment [7]. More rarely, spherical inclusions of material resembling lipid were present in the inner (matrix) mitochondrial compartment (Fig. 3C). Some of the lipid-like inclusions had stippled, electron-dense areas of unknown composition.

Mild, focal thickening of Z bands was common in hypertrophied, non-degenerated cells. Small accumulations of Z band material, often continuous with actual Z bands, often were adjacent to the sarcolemma. Increased numbers of ribosomes were found in hypertrophied cells, either free in the cytoplasm or attached to the membranes of endoplasmic reticulum. Nuclei usually were enlarged and showed marked irregularities of membrane contours. Some T tubules were dilated. These morphologic features of hypertrophy without degeneration are summarized in Table 1.

Degenerated Cardiac Muscle Cells

During the course of the studies summarized herein, it became evident that a certain population of cardiac muscle cells in some of our patients showed changes that could not be considered to be simple manifestations of the hypertrophy process. The features of such changes and their similarity to changes occurring in experimental animals under controlled conditions (see [8] for review) suggested that these alterations are degenerative in nature; this conclusion was supported by analysis of the clinical setting in which these changes were found. Using the occurrence of myofibrillar lysis as the ultimate criterion for the recognition of myocardial cellular degeneration, we found degenerated cardiac muscle cells in left ventricular myocardium in 2 of the 5 patients with pure aortic regurgitation and 4 of the 5 patients with combined aortic stenosis and regurgitation, but in none of the 6 patients with predominant aortic stenosis [9]; in ventricular myocardium of 6 of the 16 patients with hypertrophic CM [8] and in crista supraventricularis muscle of 11 of the 75 patients with congenital heart diseases associated with obstruction to right ventricular outflow. All the latter 11 patients were over age 10 (1 of 22 patients aged 11–20 years; 2 of 10 patients aged 21–29 years, and each of the 8 patients aged 30–53 years). None of the 36 patients with congenital heart disease who were less than 10 years of age showed myofibrillar lysis. The degenerative changes in the various groups of patients were qualitatively similar [8–11]. We classified degenerative changes according to their severity as mild,

◁ Fig. 1. Crista supraventricularis muscle from 30-year-old patient with tetralogy of Fallot, showing multiple intercalated disc (*arrowheads*) limiting cytoplasmic process that extends from the cell on right towards the center. × 17 500

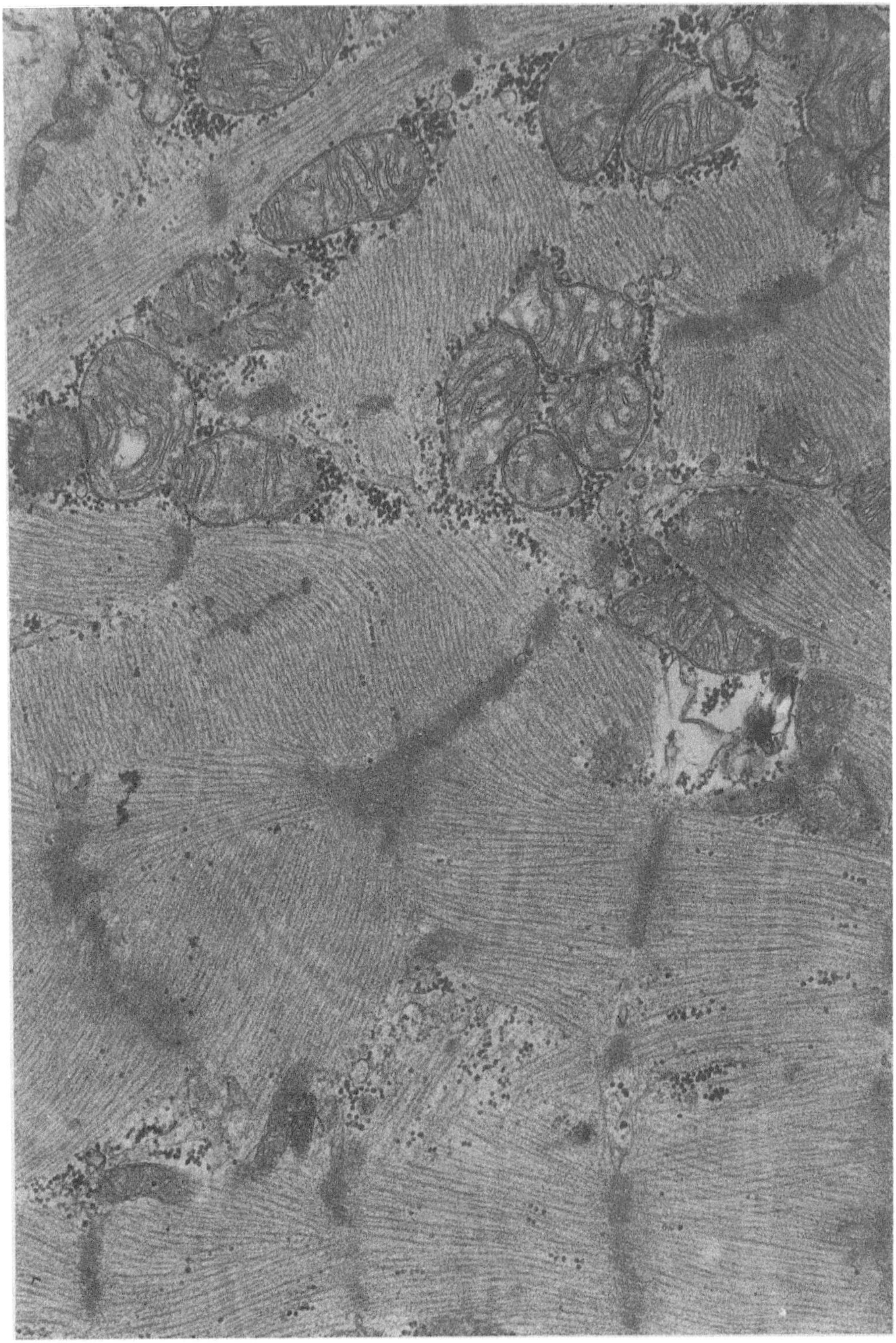

Table 1. Ultrastructural features of hypertrophied or degenerated cardiac muscle cells[a].

Morphologic feature	Hypertrophy without degeneration	Mild degeneration	Moderate degeneration	Severe degeneration
Cell size	↑	N or ↑	N or mildly ↑	↓
No. of myofibrils/cell	↑	N or ↑	↓	↓↓
Changes in myofilaments	0	Focal ↓ affecting thick > thin filaments	↓↓ Affecting thick > thin filaments	↓↓ Affecting thick > thin filaments
No. of cytoskeletal (100 Å) filaments	↑ (Focal)	↑ (Focal)	↑ (Disorganized)	↑ (Disorganized)
Changes in Z-band material: Focal thickening; marked proliferation; subsarcolemmal accumulations	+	+	Rare	0
Elongated masses in center of cell; streaming, clumping, fragmentation	0	+	+	+
Foci of proliferation of SR	0	Sparse	Extensive	Extensive
No. of T tubules	N	N	Variable	↓ or absent
Changes in intercellular junctions	Marked convolutions	Marked convolutions	Partial dissociation	Extensive dissociation
Presence of intracytoplasmic junctions	Very rare	Rare	+	+
Changes in glycogen:				
No. of β particles	↑	↑	Variable	Variable
Presence of α particles	+ (focal)	+ (focal)	+ (focal)	+ (focal)
Presence of glycogen-like basophilic degeneration material	0	0	+ (focal)	+ (focal)
Size of Golgi complexes	↑	↑	↓	0
No. of ribosomes (free or membrane-bound)	↑	↑	↓	↓
Changes in mitochondria:				
Number	↑	↑	Variable	Variable
Size	Variable	Variable	Variable	Variable
Presence of myelin figures	0	0	+	+
Nuclear size	↑	↑	↑	↑
No. of lipofuscin granules	↑	↑	Variable	Variable
Spherical microparticles	Very rare	Rare	Common	Common
Thickness of basement membranes	N	N or ↑	↑↑	↑↑
Amount of interstitial fibrous tissue	N	↑	↑↑	↑↑
Dissociation of cells	0	0	+	+

[a] +, present; 0, absent; ↑, increased; ↑↑, markedly increased; ↓, decreased; ↓↓, markedly decreased; N, normal; SR, sarcoplasmic reticulum

◁ Fig. 2. Ventricular septal muscle from patient with HOCM. The myofibrils show severe disarray, and myofilaments radiate in all directions from widened Z band at lower center. ×30000

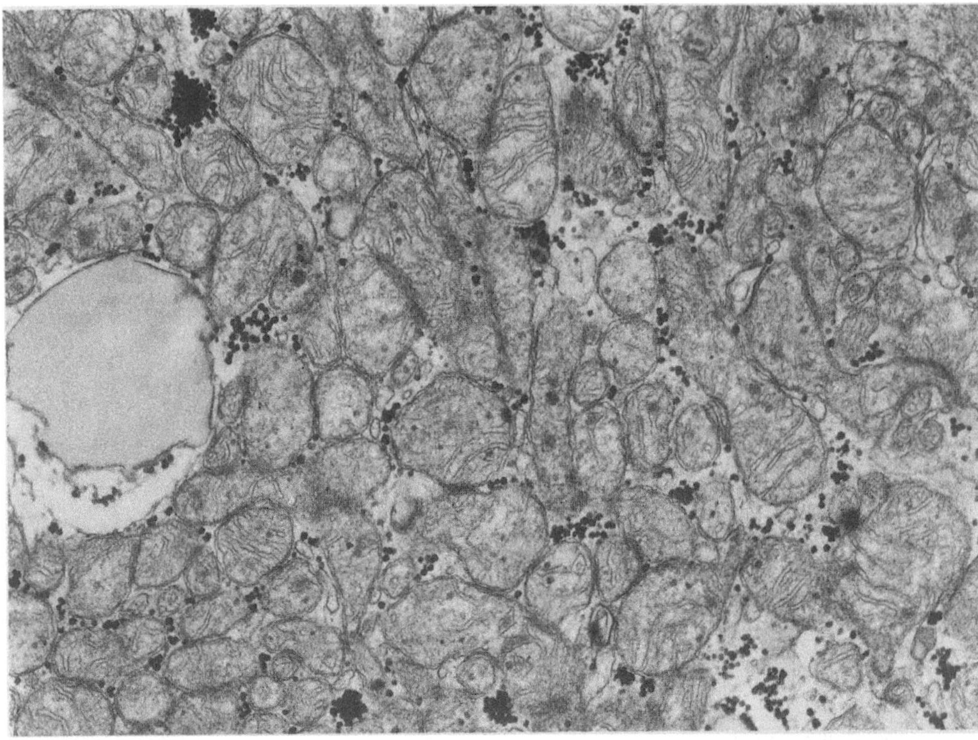

A

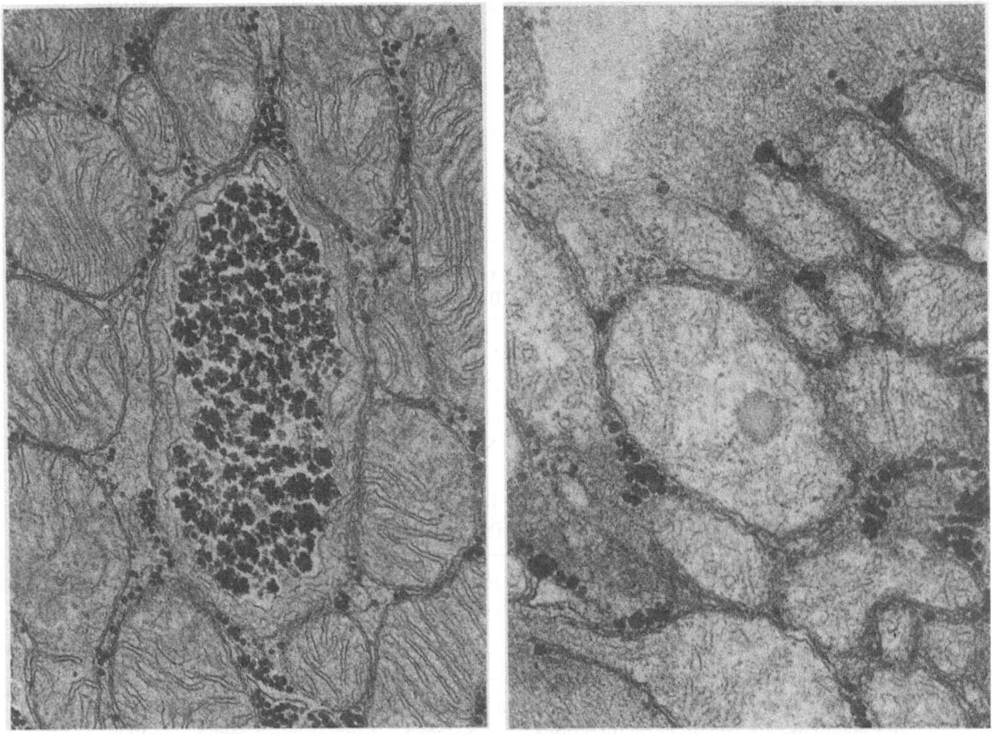

B

moderate or severe. Criteria used for this classification are given below and are summarized in Table 1.

Cardiac muscle cells with *mild degeneration* were either hypertrophied or normal sized, and by light microscopy they were indistinguishable from nondegenerated cells. Cells with mild degeneration exhibited changes in the contractile elements and the sarcoplasmic reticulum. The myofibrils showed streaming and fragmentation of Z bands and spread of Z band material into adjacent areas of the sarcomeres. Elongated, subsarcolemmal accumulations of Z-band material, similar to those in hypertrophied but nondegenerated cells, also were common. Cells with early degeneration also had small focal areas of clumping and streaming of Z bands and lysis of myofilaments. In such areas the loss of thick (myosin) filaments exceeded that of thin (actin) filaments. Because of this, cells showing this change had areas in which the thin filaments were present but unaccompanied by their normal complement of thick filaments. Alterations in the sarcoplasmic reticulum in cells with mild degeneration consisted of dilatation and/or proliferation of tubules of free sarcoplasmic reticulum, which formed small interconnected meshworks in interfibrillary and perinuclear areas.

Cardiac muscle cells with *moderate* or *severe degeneration* (Figs. 4–9) usually were either normal-sized or atrophic (less than 10 μ in diameter). These cells usually were present in areas of fibrosis (Fig. 4), and often had lost most or all of their connections with adjacent cells. They contained decreased numbers of myofibrils, and by light microscopy appeared pale-staining. The surfaces of these

---

◁ Fig. 3. A. Marked variation in mitochondrial size and some very small mitochondria are shown in this review of part of left ventricular muscle cell from a 43-year-old man with aortic stenosis and regurgitation. ×35000. B. Intramitochondrial glycogen deposits (α-rosettes) are present in crista supraventricularis muscle from same patient as in Fig. 1. ×53000. C. Lipid-like intramitochondrial inclusion in left ventricular muscle cell from 46-year-old man with aortic regurgitation. ×60000

Fig. 4. Degenerated cardiac muscle cell in crista supraventricularis of 45-year-old patient with tetralogy of Fallot is surrounded by fibrous tissue and remains connected by an intercellular junction (*lower left*) to a more normal-appearing cell. The degenerated cell has lost virtually all of its contractile elements, of which only a few clumps of electron-dense Z-band material remain in subsarcolemmal locations; the cytoplasm contains a few, small mitochondria and several lipid droplets. ×10800

Fig. 5. View of part of severely degenerated left ventricular muscle cell from same patient as in Figure 3A. Note lipid droplets, numerous tubules of sarcoplasmic reticulum, myelin figures and remnants of myofibrils. ×24000

Fig. 6. Intracytoplasmic junction that resembles a desmosome is present at the surface (*lower left*) of degenerated, atrophic muscle cell in crista supraventricularis of 11-year-old male with double outlet right ventricle and infundibular pulmonic stenosis. Large masses of highly organized Z-band material are associated with thin myofilaments – only a few thick (myosin) filaments (*arrowheads*) remain in this cell. ×54000

Fig. 7. View of dissociating intercellular junction that connects two left ventricular muscle cells (same patient as in Fig. 3C). Note: several clusters of spherical microparticles in area of widening of the space between the apposed plasma membranes; a nexus (*arrowheads*) that still connects two small areas of the surfaces of the cells; a scattering of microfibrils in the widened disc space, and an area of normal apposition of the disc membranes (*lower right*). ×62000. *Inset* shows minute nexus (*arrowheads*) connecting two hemispherical vesicles in another widened disc space. ×60000

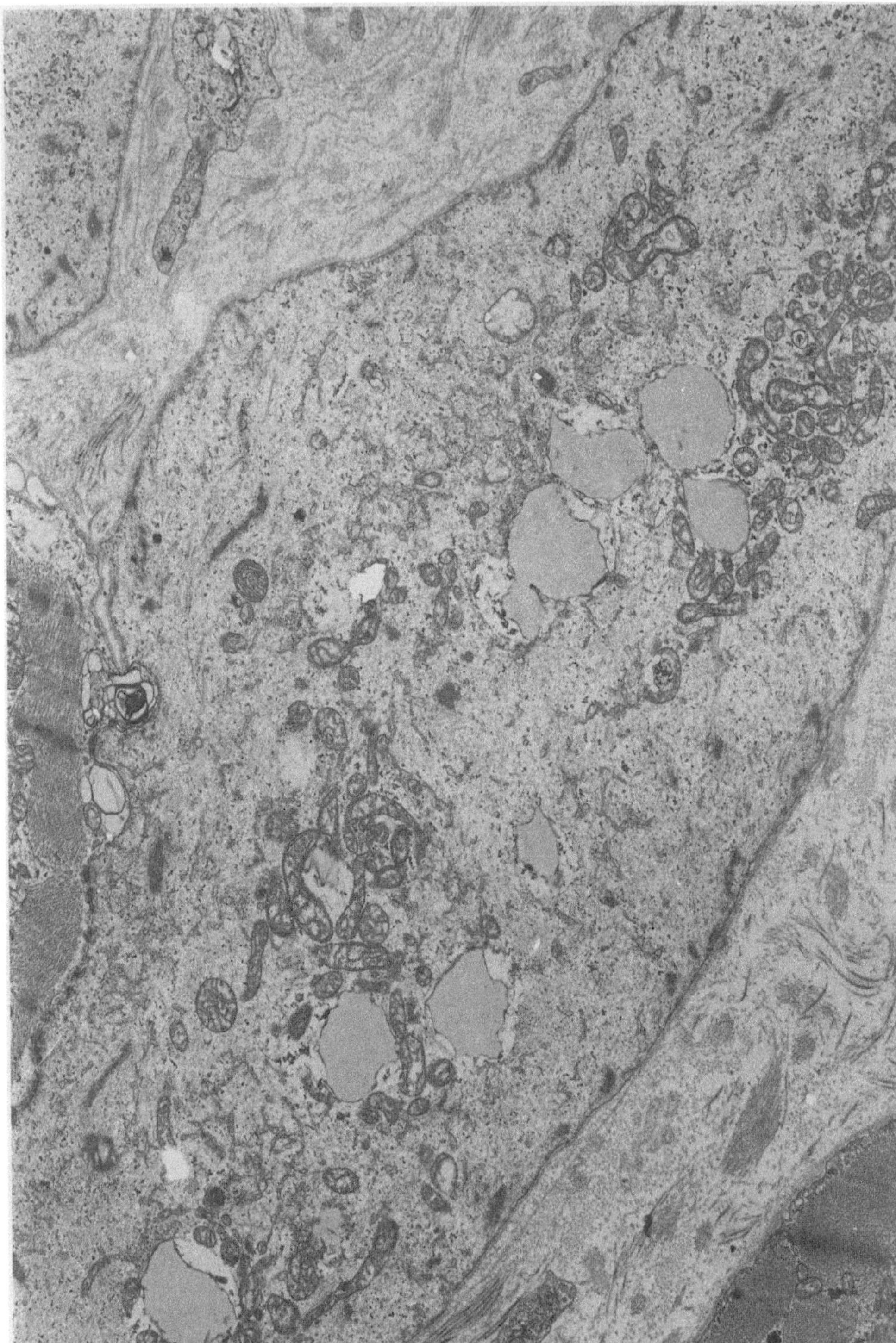

4

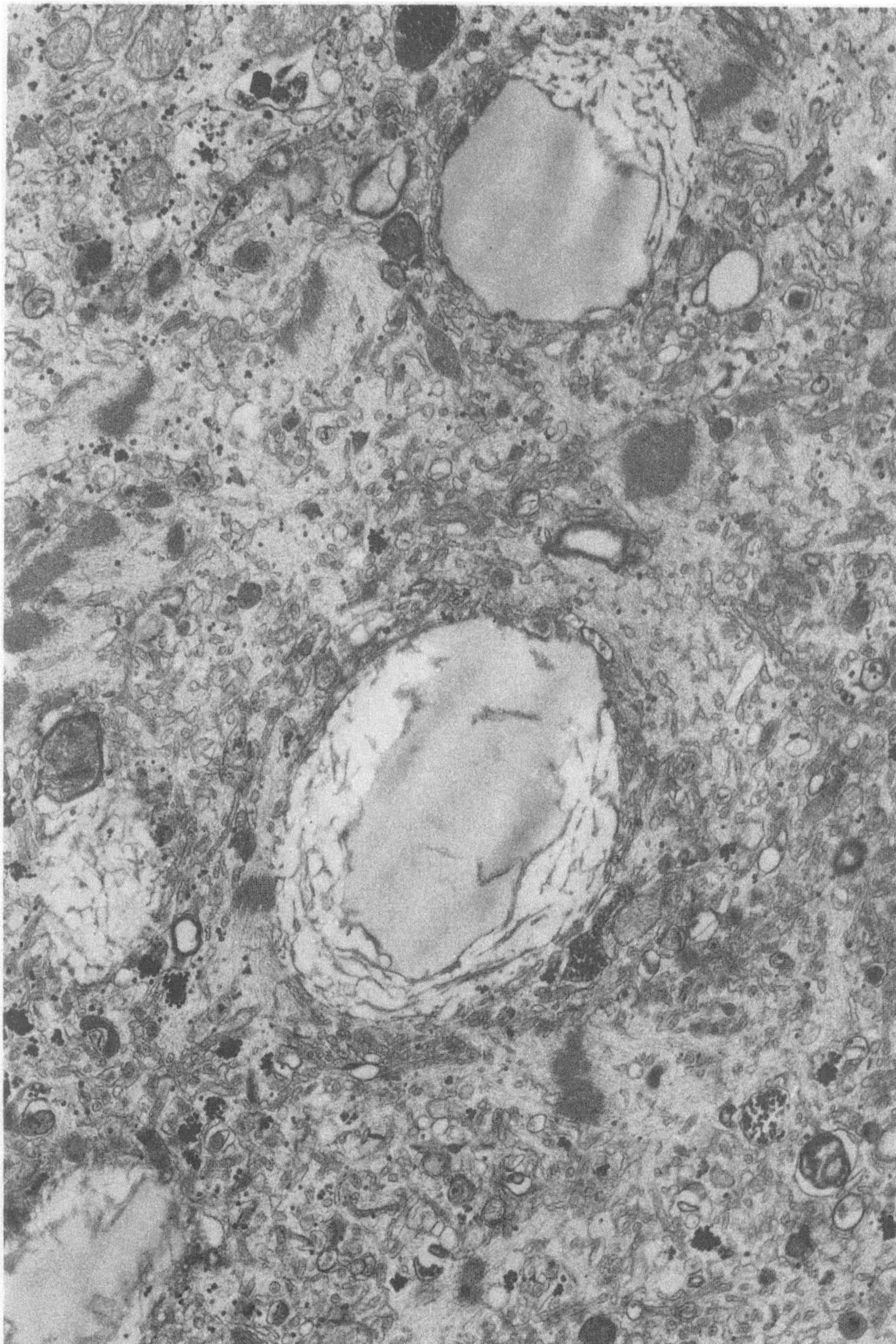

5

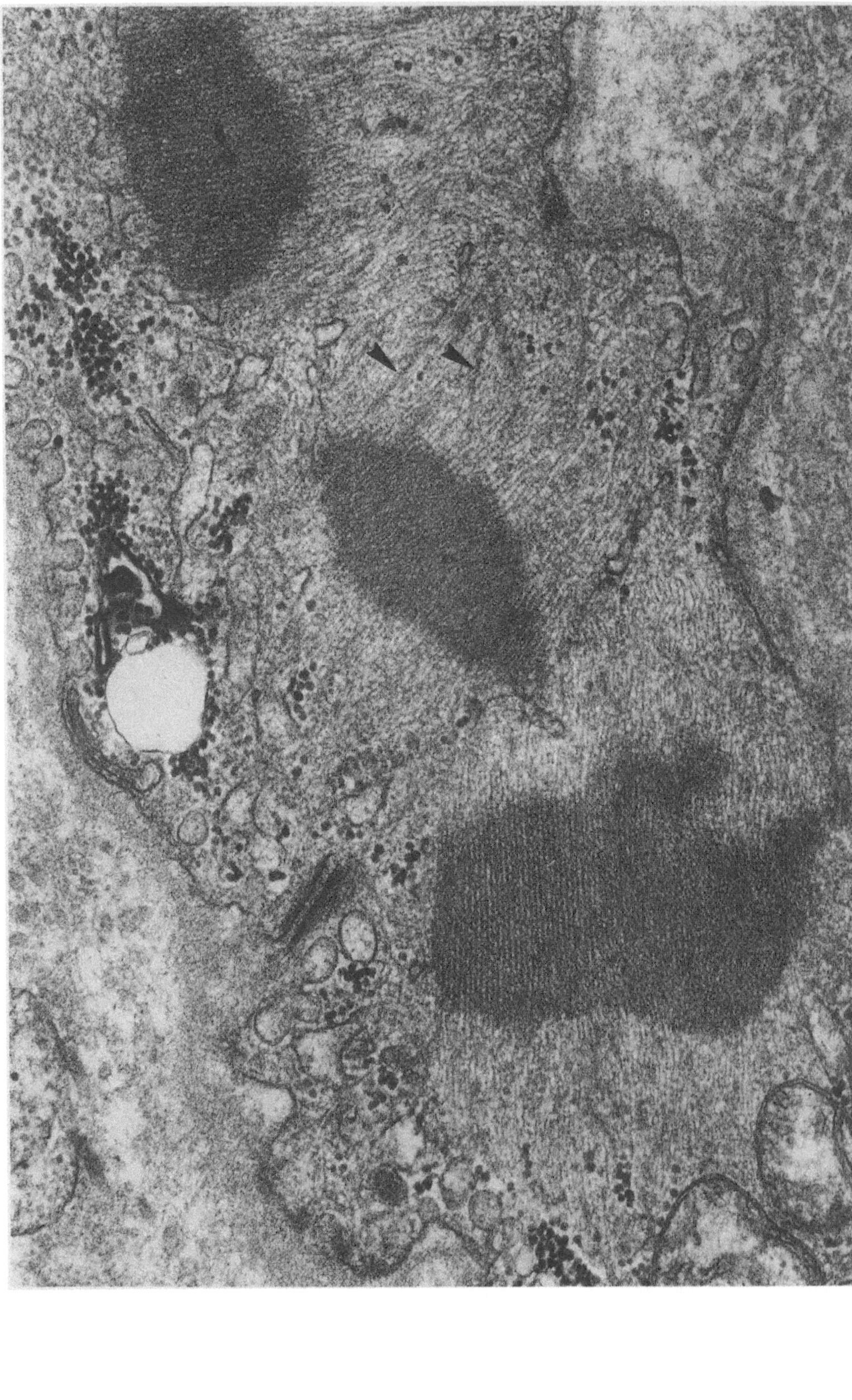

6

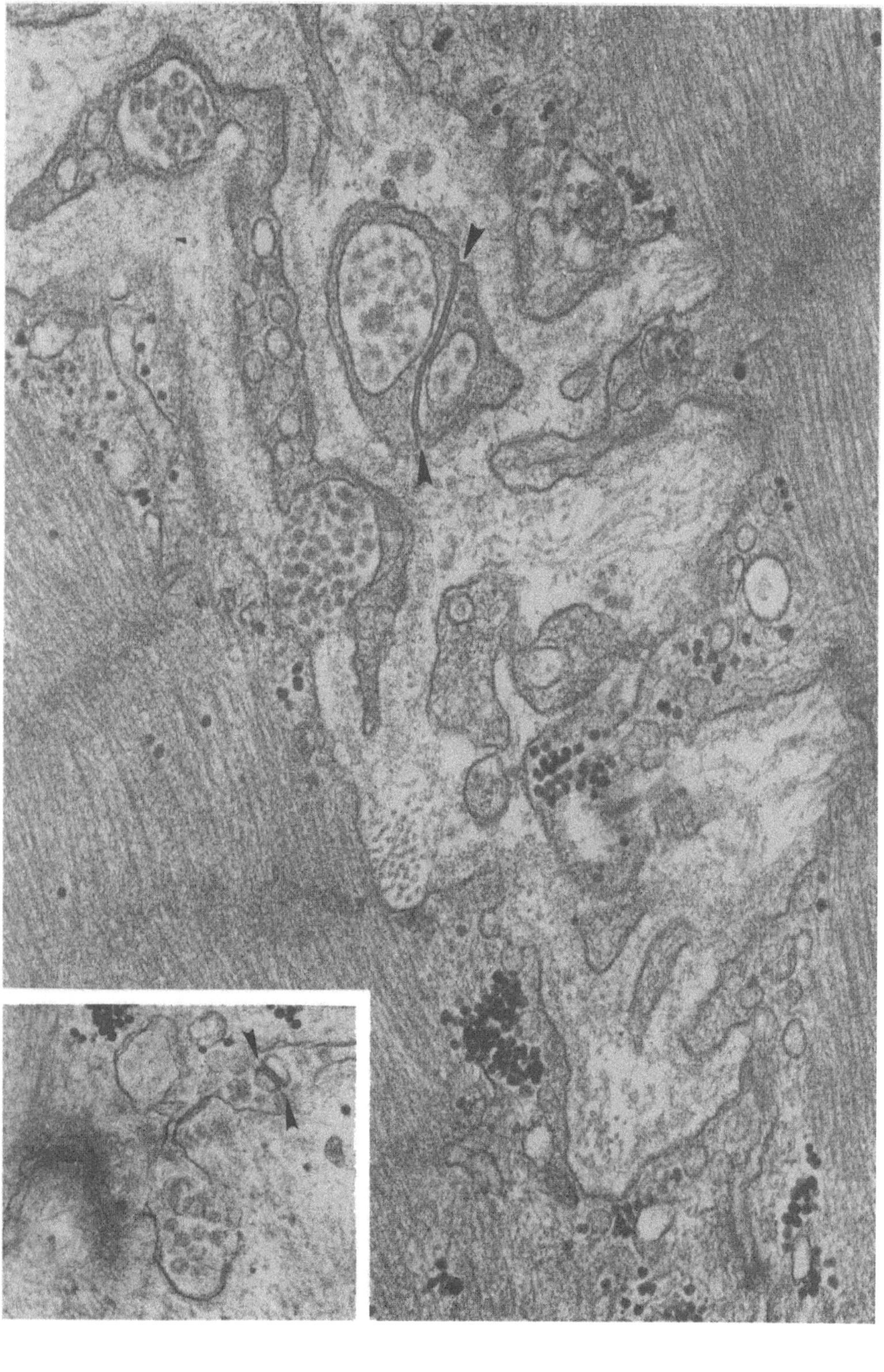

7

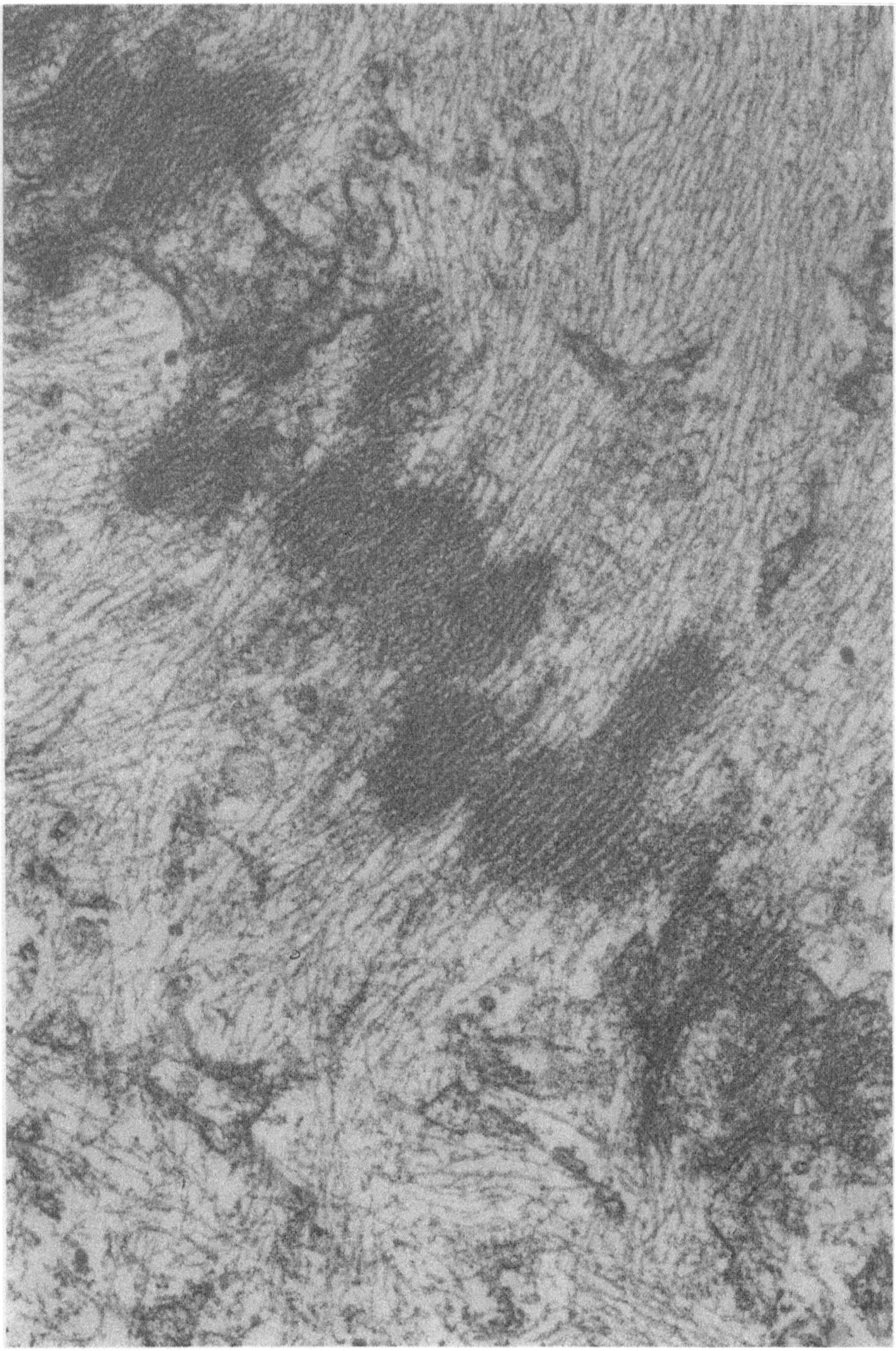

cells often showed marked irregularities in contour (particularly at their free ends) and thickening of their basement membranes. The surfaces of such cells showed two other changes that probably result from the membrane remodeling that occurs when degenerated cells lose their intercellular contacts: the formation of intracytoplasmic junctions (Fig. 6) [12] and of microspherical particles (Fig. 7) [13].

Intracytoplasmic junctions (Fig. 6) are junctional structures formed by the apposition of two areas of the plasma membrane of the same cell. Some of these junctions consisted of desmosome-like structures, whereas others were more complex and resembled parts of intercalated discs. These junctions usually were present in the peripheral areas of cytoplasm at the ends or sides of the cells. Among the 75 patients with congenital heart diseases, intracytoplasmic junctions were found only in 1 of the 67 patients under 29 years of age and in 3 of the 8 patients aged 30–53 years. Possible mechanisms involved in the formation of intracytoplasmic junctions have been discussed in detail by Buja *et al.* (12).

Spherical microparticles (Fig. 7), averaging 500 Å in diameter, were composed of electron-dense cores surrounded by trilaminar membranes, and usually were found in clusters. Spherical microparticles occurred in extracellular locations along the sides and free ends of muscle cells in areas of fibrosis and in the widened spaces between the membranes of partially dissociated intercellular junctions; within muscle cells they were found only within cytoplasmic vesicles of phagocytic origin (Fig. 7). Spherical microparticles frequently were joined together by minute nexuses (Fig. 7) that were structurally similar to those forming parts of intercellular junctions in muscle cells. Among the 75 patients with congenital heart diseases, spherical microparticles were found in 7 of the 8 patients aged 30–53 years and in none of the younger patients. As described elsewhere, spherical microparticles were encountered most frequently in the dilated left atria from patients with mitral valvular disease [13].

Cardiac muscle cells with moderate or severe degeneration showed further progression of the process of myofibrillar loss that began in early degeneration. The four features that characterized these myofibrillar changes were: 1. decreased numbers of myofibrils (Figs. 4 and 5); 2. presence of large numbers of thin myofilaments not associated with thick myofilaments (Figs. 6 and 8); 3. large masses of Z band material scattered throughout the cytoplasm in a disorganized fashion, often with a periodic substructure with a complex lattice, and traversed by thin, parallel filaments (Figs. 6 and 9), and 4. disorganized arrangement of cytoskeletal filaments (100 Å in diameter) which had lost their usual association with Z bands. Myofibrils were virtually absent in the most severely degenerated cells. These cells often assumed characteristic appearances, which depended upon the selective proliferation of certain organelles, such as mitochondria, tubules of sarcoplasmic reticulum, glycogen particles, or large, heterogeneous residual bodies, that filled areas previously occupied by myofibrils. In ventricular muscle, the proliferation of sarcoplasmic reticulum led to the formation of two types of aggregates of

◁ Fig. 8. Longitudinal section showing widened Z band and adjacent thin myofilaments (thick myofilaments are completely absent) in degenerated cardiac muscle cell from crista supraventricularis muscle (same patient as in Fig. 6). ×82500

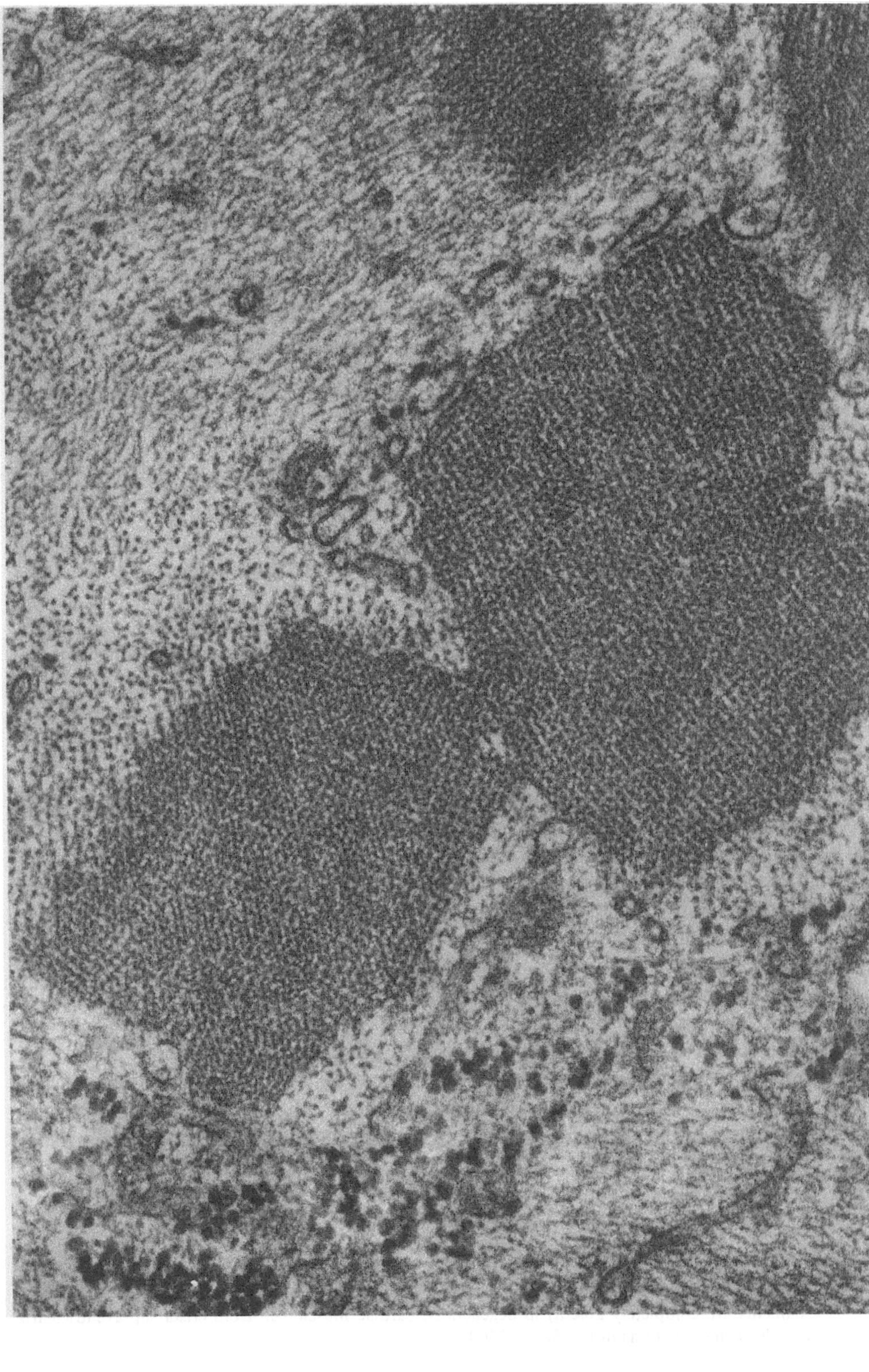

tubules (see [14] for details). The nuclei of degenerated cardiac muscle cells usually showed marked convolutions of their membranes. In some cells, such convolutions were associated with two types of intranuclear tubules (Fig. 10), which we also have described in detail elsewhere [15]. In all patients with myocardial fibrosis, the interstitial spaces contained large numbers of microfibrils (Fig. 11) in addition to collagen fibrils. In some areas, the microfibrils were the predominant element of connective tissue.

Discussion

The observations reviewed herein show that a) degenerated cardiac muscle cells are commonly found in hypertrophied ventricular myocardium from patients with a variety of types of heart diseases; b) in patients with congenital heart diseases associated with right ventricular hypertrophy and obstruction to right ventricular outflow, the incidence of degenerative changes rises markedly with increasing age of the patients; and c) these changes do not differ qualitatively among patients with cardiac hypertrophy of various causes. Although in our limited experience, these changes are more severe in patients with aortic regurgitation than in patients with aortic stenosis [9], the significance of these observations is not clear because these two groups of patients undergo cardiac operations for different medical reasons and at different times in the course of their illnesses.

We believe that the degenerative changes that we observed in association with cardiac hypertrophy represent a final common pathway of cellular damage rather than specific manifestations of any given type of heart disease. This concept is supported by the fact that many of the alterations observed in this study, such as myofibrillar loss, proliferation of sarcoplasmic reticulum, and formation of residual bodies with concentric electron-dense lamellae, also occur in other conditions in humans and in experimental animals (see [8] for review).

The loss of myofibrils that occurs in degenerated cardiac muscle cells is associated with survival of other cellular organelles, including the nuclei and mitochondria. These features distinguish this type of degeneration from cardiac muscle cell necrosis. It is not clear at the present time whether the myofibrillar loss is mediated by an increase in myofibrillar degradation, by a decrease in the synthesis of contractile proteins, by disaggregation of the contractile proteins from a filamentous to a nonfilamentous form, or by a combination of these factors. Nevertheless, it seems reasonable to conclude that the loss of contractile elements from cardiac muscle cells has deleterious effects on cardiac function.

The morphologic changes associated with hypertrophic CM constitute an easily recognizable feature of this disease. However, with respect to these changes, two important points must be remembered: First, the changes are focal, so that they can be missed on examination of only very small pieces of tissue; secondly, they do not provide an absolute "yes" or "no" answer for the

◁ Fig. 9. Cross section through several widened Z bands in same tissue as in Fig. 8. These Z bands show a complex but basically tetragonal lattice. Thick myofilaments are again absent. ×90000

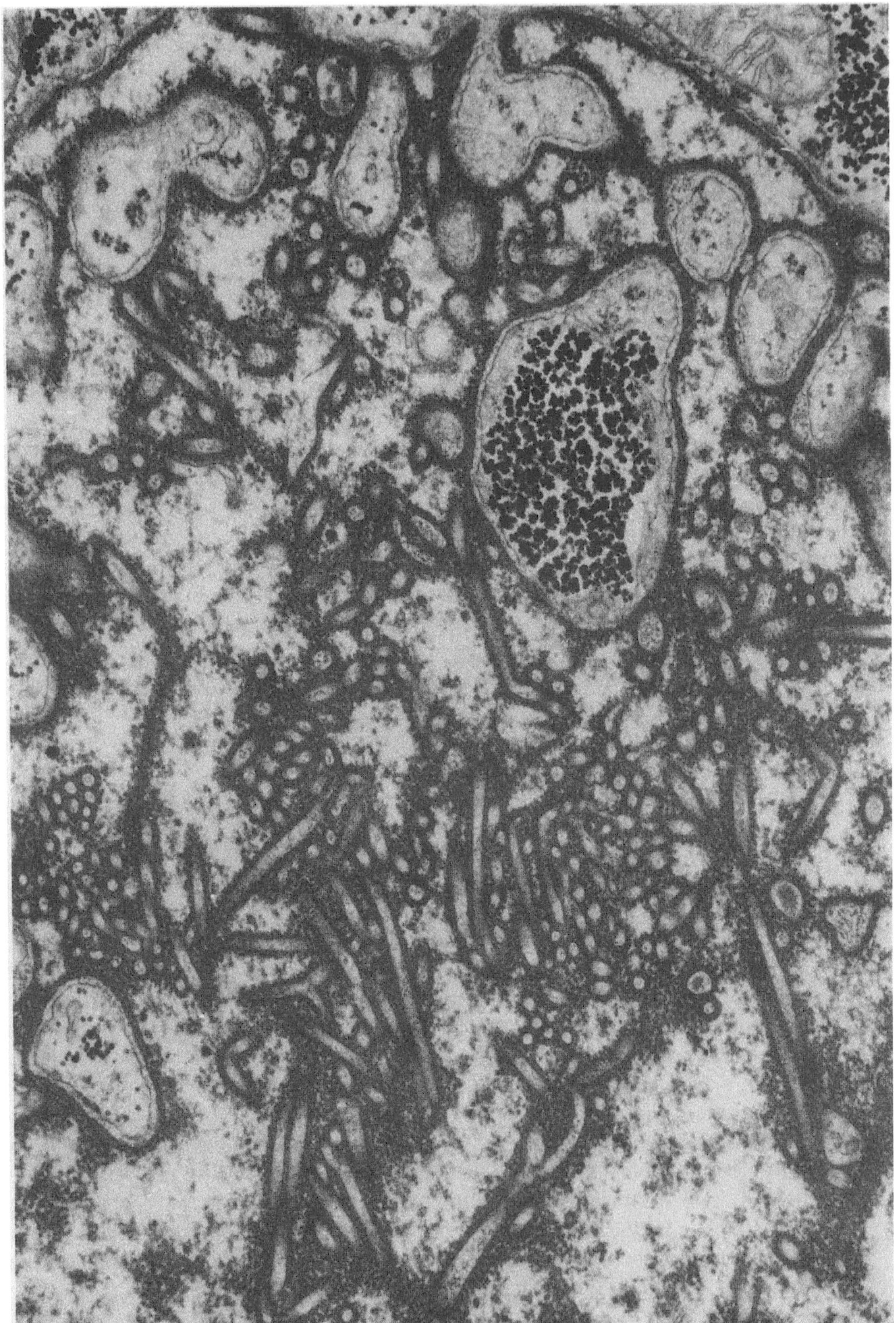

diagnosis of the disease. We have found widespread disarray of cells in patients with hypertrophic CM [16], but we have also found small foci of this type of change in 10% of patients with COCM [17] and in 18% of patients with congenital heart diseases associated with right ventricular hypertrophy and obstruction to right ventricular outflow. Becú *et al.* [18] have found similar features in approximately 50% of patients with isolated pulmonary valvular stenosis (a frequent ocurrence among the latter patients was a dysplastic process that involved vascular connective tissues). Furthermore, disarray of contractile components has been described in cardiac muscle cells under unusual or abnormal conditions, including tissues of normal atrioventricular conducting system, muscle cells at the edges of infarcts, muscle cells of invertebrates, embryonic tissue and in salamander hearts grown in organ culture (see [16, 18, 19] for review). These findings indicate the need for great caution in trying to diagnose hypertrophic CM only on the basis of cardiac biopsy.

Alterations in Z bands and accumulations of Z-band-like material adjacent to the sarcolemma were present in hypertrophied, nondegenerated cells as well as in cells with early degeneration. Streaming or clumping of Z bands appeared to be indicative of early myofibrillar lysis because of the common association of these Z band changes with disruption and loss of myofilaments. Thickening of Z bands, symmetric expansions of Z band material into adjacent regions of the sarcomeres, and subsarcolemmal accumulations of Z band material have been regarded as indicative of the formation of new sarcomeres. However, we have found such changes in degenerated and nondegenerated cells and therefore believe that these alterations are not useful in distinguishing between hypertrophy and degeneration [8]. We regard these alterations as indicative of relative imbalances in the synthesis of different sarcomeric components, so that the synthesis of Z band material is not followed by proper assembly of sarcomeres. Thus, we regard these changes as evidence highly suggestive of arrested or abortive sarcomerogenesis. The formation of intracytoplasmic junctions [12] and of spherical microparticles [13] is related to the cellular surface remodeling that occurs when interstitial fibrosis and cellular dissociation develop. We have presented in detail evidence showing that both of these phenomena also occur in tissues other than myocardium in a variety of conditions [12, 13]. It remains to be determined whether or not the release of intracellular components, in the form of spherical microparticles, into the interstitium can serve as an antigenic stimulus to the development of autoimmune reactions.

Cardiac muscle cells with advanced degeneration appear incapable of normal contractile function. The markedly decreased numbers of myofibrils and the alterations in the sarcoplasmic reticulum and T tubules in these cells probably preclude the generation of normal tensions. Cells with advanced degeneration

---

◁ Fig. 10. Large cluster of nuclear tubules (formed by invaginations of the inner nuclear membranes, so that the lumen of these tubules is continuous with the space between the inner and outer nuclear membranes) and a glycogen-rich nuclear pseudoinclusion (formed by invagination of both inner and outer nuclear membranes and by a corresponding protrusion of a small area of cytoplasm) are seen in left ventricular myocardium of 29-year-old woman with nonobstructive hypertrophic CM. ×33500

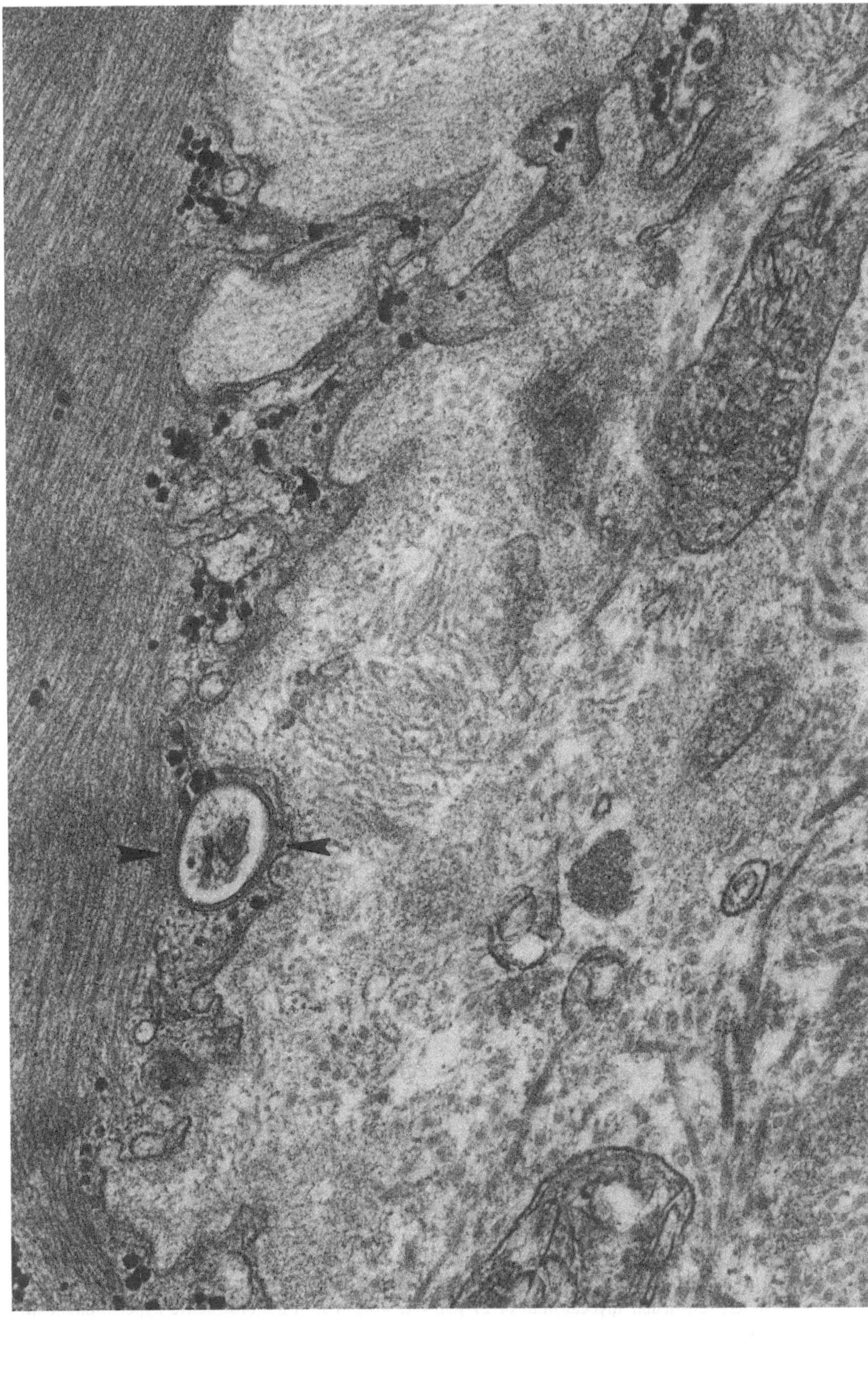

are also surrounded by fibrous tissue, have lost their intercellular connections with adjacent cells, and, therefore, no longer have the capacity to transmit electrical activation to other areas of myocardium. Furthermore, the markedly thickened basement membranes probably also contribute to the isolation of these cells by inhibiting the exchange of nutrients between the intra- and extracellular environments. The process of myocardial fibrosis remains poorly understood, and the reason for extensive participation of microfibrils in this process remains to be elucidated.

Conclusion

It is evident from the observations reviewed here that cardiac muscle cells in the late stages of hypertrophy lose, through mechanisms that remain unclear at present, the control of the synthesis of balanced amounts of different subcellular constituents. It appears likely that the function of nuclear DNA is compromised. Such loss of control of synthetic events can lead to serious disturbances of cellular function. The consequences of this are made particularly severe by the inability of cardiac muscle cells to reproduce themselves. For this reason, it would seem that this damage may be irreversible. Such a damage is clinically evident in patients with long-standing cardiac hypertrophy in whom complete surgical correction of their cardiac lesions does not result in reversal of cardiac dysfunction. Thus, our observations support the viewpoint that patients with surgically correctable heart disease should be operated on before myocardial degeneration develops. Our studies show that myocardial degeneration is not manifested until after 10 years of age in patients with congenital heart diseases characterized by right ventricular hypertrophy and obstruction to right ventricular outflow.

References

1. Meerson, F.Z.: The myocardium in hyperfunction, hypertrophy and heart failure. Circulat. Res. *25*, Suppl. II, 1–163 (1969)
2. Freeman, J., Spurlock, B.O.: A new epoxy embedment for electron microscopy. J. cell. Biol. *13*, 437–443 (1962)
3. Laks, M.M., Morady, F., Adomian, G., Swan, H.J.C.: Presence of widened and multiple intercalated discs in the hypertrophied heart. Circulat. Res. *27*, 391–402 (1970)
4. Maron, B.J., Ferrans, V.J.: Significance of multiple intercalated discs in hypertrophied human myocardium. Amer. J. Pathol. *73*, 81–87 (1973)

◁ Fig. 11. Irregularities of the cell surface are evident in this area of fibrosis (left ventricular myocardium of same patient as in Fig. 3C). Numerous microfibrils are present in close vicinity to the basement membrane and the surrounding collagen fibrils and portions of cytoplasm of adjacent connective tissue cells (*right*). A small, circular nexus (*arrowheads*) connects the cell on the left to a small process of another cell, the main portion of which is not seen in this section. This small area of junction is regarded as the last remnant of what must have been a much larger connection between the two cells. × 53 500

5. Adomian, G., Laks, M.M., Morady, F., Swan, H.J.C.: Significance of the multiple intercalated disc in the hypertrophied canine heart. J. mol. cell. Cardiol. *6*, 105–109 (1974)
6. Maron, B.J., Ferrans, V.J., Henry, W.L., Clark, C.E., Redwood, D.R., Roberts, W.C., Morrow, A.G., Epstein, S.E.: Differences in distribution of myocardial abnormalities in patients with obstructive and non-obstructive asymmetric septal hypertrophy (ASH): Light and electron microscopic findings. Circulation *50*, 436–446 (1974)
7. Maron, B.J., Ferrans, V.J.: Intramitochondrial glycogen deposits in hypertrophied human myocardium. J. mol. cell. Cardiol. *7*, 697–702 (1975)
8. Maron, B.J., Ferrans, V.J., Roberts, W.C.: Ultrastructural features of degenerated cardiac muscle cells in patients with cardiac hypertrophy. Amer. J. Pathol. *79*, 387–434 (1975)
9. Maron, B.J., Ferrans, V.J., Roberts, W.C.: Myocardial ultrastructure in patients with chronic aortic valve disease. Amer. J. Cardiol. *35*, 725–739 (1975)
10. Jones, M., Ferrans, V.J., Morrow, A.G., Roberts, W.C.: Ultrastructure of crista supraventricularis muscle in patients with congenital heart diseases associated with right ventricular outflow tract obstruction. Circulation *51*, 39–68 (1975)
11. Jones, M., Ferrans, V.J.: Myocardial degeneration in congenital heart disease. A comparison of morphologic findings in young and old patients with congenital heart diseases associated with muscular obstruction to right ventricular outflow. Amer. J. Cardiol. (in press)
12. Buja, L.M., Ferrans, V.J., Maron, B.J.: Intracytoplasmic junctions in cardiac muscle cells. Amer. J. Pathol. *74*, 613–648 (1974)
13. Ferrans, V.J., Thiedemann, K.-U., Maron, B.J., Jones, M., Roberts, W.C.: Spherical microparticles in human myocardium. An ultrastructural study. Lab. Invest. *35*, 349–368 (1976)
14. Maron, B.J., Ferrans, V.J.: Aggregates of tubules in human cardiac muscle cells. J. mol. cell. Cardiol. *6*, 249–264 (1974)
15. Ferrans, V.J., Jones, M., Maron, B.J., Roberts, W.C.: The nuclear membranes in hypertrophied human cardiac muscle cells. Amer. J. Pathol. *78*, 427–460 (1975)
16. Ferrans, V.J., Morrow, A.G., Roberts, W.C.: Myocardial ultrastructure in idiopathic hypertrophic subaortic stenosis. A study of operatively excised left ventricular outflow tract muscle in 14 patients. Circulation *45*, 769–792 (1972)
17. Ferrans, V.J., Massumi, R.A., Shugoll, G.E., Ali, N., Roberts, W.C.: Ultrastructural studies of myocardial biopsies in 45 patients with obstructive or congestive cardiomyopathy. In: The Cardiomyopathies. Recent Advances in Studies on Cardiac Structure and Metabolism. Bajusz, E., Rona, G., Brink, A.J., Lochner, A. (eds.), Vol. II, pp. 231–272. Baltimore: University Park Press 1973
18. Becú, L., Somerville, J., Gallo, A.: "Isolated" pulmonary valve stenosis as part of more widespread cardiovascular disease. Brit. Heart J. *38*, 472–482 (1976)
19. Thornell, L.-E., Sjöström, M., Andersson, K.-E.: The relationship between mechanical stress and myofibrillar organization in heart Purkinje fibres. J. mol. cell. Cardiol. *8*, 689–695 (1976)

11. Endomyocardial Catheter Biopsy in Heart Disease of Unknown Etiology

H. KUHN, G. BREITHARDT, H.-J. KNIERIEM, and F. LOOGEN

The technique of endomyocardial catheter biopsy (EMCB) was described as early as 1962 by Sakakibara and Konno [22]. In the following years biopsy material was studied for diagnostic reasons mostly by use of light microscopy, which revealed specific findings only in rare cases (e.g. sarcoidosis and myocarditis). Furthermore, publications about biopsies consisted primarily of case reports and information about technical problems or modifications of the original Konno bioptome [10, 12].

Systematic studies and the use of both light and electron microscopy on larger groups of patients and on different stages of heart disease with established clinical morphologic correlations have been performed only in recent years [3, 6, 10–12, 15, 16, 20; see also Chapters 6, 7 and 8]. From 1971 until January 1977 EMCB was performed in our hospital in 182 patients with various heart diseases. Of these 182, 48 with COCM were the subject of follow-up studies as part of prospective program which is reported on in detail in Chapter 22.

In this chapter a summary of the clinical and microscopic findings in all patients is presented. In addition, detailed findings in 21 patients with heart disease of unknown etiology, 10 of whom showed latent cardiomyopathy (LCM) (6 with LBBB), are reported. LBBB in 7 patients and cardiac arrhythmias in 4 were the only pathologic findings. The studies in these patients were done originally in an attempt to detect a prestage of COCM.

Patients and Methods

Clinical Diagnosis, Diagnostic Criteria and Methods

Clinical diagnosis in patients in whom biopsy was obtained for light- and electron-microscopic examination are summarized in Table 1. Classification and diagnosis of CM patients were made according to angiographic and hemodynamic data (Fig. 1) using in principle Goodwin's proposals [7, 13, 16]. Coronary heart disease, congenital and acquired valvular heart disease, arterial hypertension, and CMs of known etiology (secondary CM) were excluded in cases with primary CM. In all patients right and left heart catheterization, left ventricular cineangiograms, coronary angiography, chest x-rays, ECG, phonocardiogram, apex cardiogram, external carotid pulse tracings and laboratory tests were done and in some echocardiography was performed. Left ventricular enddiastolic volume index (LVEDVI), stroke volume index (SVI, unit = vol/m^2 surface area) and ejection fraction (EF, %) were calculated from monoplane left ventricular cineangiograms using the area length method [23].

Table 1. Clinical diagnosis of patients (n = 151) from whom biopsies were obtained appropriate for light- and/or electron-microscopic examination of myocardium.

Congestive CM (COCM supposed, carditis?)	n = 62
Latent CM	n = 20
LBBB	n = 13
Alcoholic CM	n = 12
Cardiac arrhythmia	n = 5
Hypertrophic CM	n = 6
Congenital and aquired valvular disease	n = 8
Restrictive CM (Pericarditis constric.?, endomyocardial fibrosis?)	n = 6
Post-(peri-)partum CM	n = 4
Neuromuscular disease	n = 4
Collagen disease	n = 4
Cardiocutaneous syndrome	n = 3
Endocarditis Löffler	n = 2
Acromegaly	n = 1
Postcardiotomy syndrome	n = 1

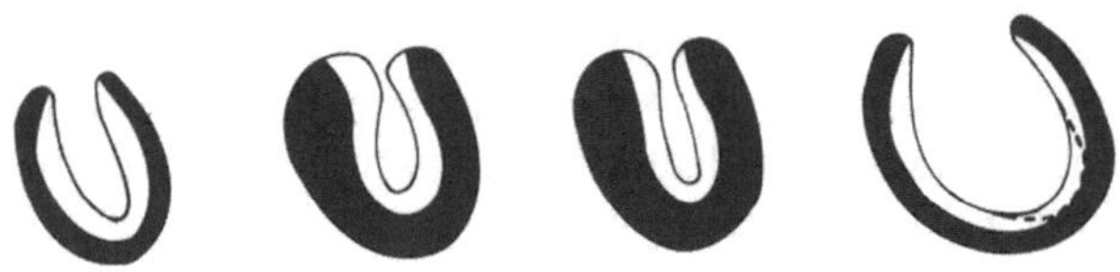

	LCM	HOCM	HNCM	COCM
EDV	N	N(↓)	N(↓)	↑
EF	N	N(↑)	N(↑)	↓
EDP	↑	↑(N)	↑(N)	↑(N)
Compliance		↓(N)	↓(N)	N(↑)
Obstruction	–	+	–	–
Wall-thickness	N	↑	↑	N ↑↓

Fig. 1. Classification of primary cardiomyopathies. The different diagnostic criteria are shown. LCM = latent cardiomyopathy; HOCM = hypertrophic obstructive cardiomyopathy; HNCM = hypertrophic nonobstructive cardiomyopathy; COCM = congestive cardiomyopathy; EDV = enddiastolic volume; EF = ejectionfraction; EDP = left ventricular enddiastolic pressure; N = normal value; arrow up = abnormal increase; arrow downward = abnormal decrease of values; () = rare findings; + = obstruction between left ventricle and aorta present at rest or after provocation

Patients With Latent Cardiomyopathy, Left-Bundle-Branch Block, and Cardiac Arrhythmias

LCM was defined by normal wall thickness (septum and free wall of left ventricle), normal LVEDVI, normal EF, and no outflow tract obstruction but with elevated LVEDP at rest or – in most cases – on exercise [16, 17]. LVEDP was estimated in patients with LCM, in patients with LBBB, and in patients with arrhythmias indirectly by measuring the mean pulmonary artery pressure (MPAP), which correlates best with LVEDP under exercise [1], using the bicycle ergometer. In patients with LBBB (without LCM) and in patients with arrhythmias (Table 2) ECG alterations were the only pathologic finding.

Table 2. Endomyocardial catheter biopsy in patients with cardiac arrhythmia.

Patient	Age (yr)	Sex.	Arrhythmias
G.U.	19	f	Atrial and ventricular p.b., S-A block
R.E.	18	f	Ventricular p.b., bidirectional tachycardia
D.M.	28	f	Atrial and ventricular p.b., atrial tachycardia
S.G.	37	m	Ventricular p.b., (couples)

In addition, to exclude pulmonary disease in patients with LCM, spirometry was performed. EMCB was taken in nearly all cases from the right ventricle by the transfemoral approach using either Konno's [22] (up to 1974) or the King's bioptome [21] (Table 3). As a rule one to three specimens were obtained.

Table 3. Number of patients in whom endomyocardial catheter biopsy (EMCB) was performed from March 1971 up to January 1977, with techniques and complications of EMCB.

Endomyocardial catheter biopsies performed		
transvenous, right ventricle		n = 166
transarterial, left ventricle		n = 16
	total	n = 182
with Konno's bioptome		n = 73
with King's bioptome		n = 109
Complications		
Severe: none		
Other: n = 4 (transient RBBB, LBBB, a-v-block II^0 and III^0)		

The myocardium was examined by light- and electron-microscopy (see Ch. 8, 22) without knowledge of the clinical data.

The morphologic findings were estimated according to their frequency, extent and severity using the following semiquantitative morphological score already applied in earlier studies [3, 10–12, 15–17] (Table 4). The following were considered to be degenerative changes: myelin figures, frequent lipofuscin granules, increased number of lipid droplets, proliferation of sarcoplasmic reticulum, lysis of myofilaments, and lysosomal changes. Alterations of mitochondria consisted of extreme variations in size, abnormally large or small mitochondria and mitochondriosis. Abnormal arrangement of myofibers, and myofibrils

Table 4. Morphologic score for semiquantitative evaluation of endomyocardial catheter biopsies.

		points
1. Degenerative changes		
	rare-slight	1
	frequent-severe	2
2. Alterations of mitochondria		
	rare	1
	frequent	2
3. Myofibrillar changes		
	rare	1
	frequent	2
4. Interstitial fibrosis		
	moderate	1
	severe	2
5. Hypertrophy	slight	1
	moderate	2
	severe	3

running in adverse directions, abnormal thickening of Z bands and irregular Z bands were considered to be myofibrillar changes. Interstitial fibrosis was evaluated from semithin sections. Myocardial hypertrophy was classified according to the size of the myofibers: slight, 15–20 μm; moderate, 21–25 μm; and severe, ⩾26 μm.

The Wilcoxon test for paired or unpaired data was used for statistical analysis.

Results

Summarizing Observations in the Total of All Patients

In the beginning biopsy was indicated to exclude myocarditis. Subsequently, biopsies were done for prognostic evaluation of patients with COCM or to detect prestage of COCM. Out of the total of 182 patients in whom biopsies were performed since 1971, samples appropriate for both light- and electron-microscopic examination were obtained in 151 cases. In 31 cases no microscopic investigation was possible, mostly because of damage to the sample. To date, light-microscopic evaluation in 151 patients and both light- and electron-microscopic evaluation in 131 patients has been completed (light- and electron-microscopic examination is incomplete in 3 patients with COCM, 10 patients with LCM, 6 patients with LBBB, and 1 patient with cardiac arrhythmia out of the groups shown in Table 1).

Abnormal findings were present in 93% of all patients examined up to now. Qualitatively, we observed a uniform ultrastructural pattern consisting of degenerative, myofibrillar, and mitochondrial alterations, hypertrophy of muscle fibers, interstitial and/or endocardial fibrosis. Degenerative changes in the form of proliferation of sarcoplasmic reticulum, lysis of myofilaments, lysosomal changes, myelin figures, frequent lipofuscin granules, and increased number of lipid droplets were observed. Alterations of mitochondria were extreme variations in size, abnormally large or small mitochondria, and mitochondriosis. No hypoxic changes of the mitochondria could be observed. Myofibrillar changes were found in the form of abnormal arrangement of myofibers and myofibrils showing different degrees of disarrangement, in some cases thickening of Z bands or irregular Z bands. No group of patients showed typical changes, e.g., there was no striking morphologic difference between the alterations in patients with COCM, hypertrophic, alcoholic, or postpartum CM and severe congenital or acquired valvular heart disease. For quantitative analysis of COCM, see Chapter 22. In only four cases were relatively specific or unusual findings observed. In one patient, in whom COCM was supposed, a diffuse myocardial storage disease of unknown etiology could be detected [10]. One patient with the clinical diagnosis of endomyocardial fibrosis showed the very unusual occurrence of specific granules in the right ventricular myocardium (Fig. 2). In another patient in whom COCM was present, changes suspect of virus-like particles could be observed. In the fourth case with neuromuscular disease extreme proliferation of sarcoplasmic reticulum was found.

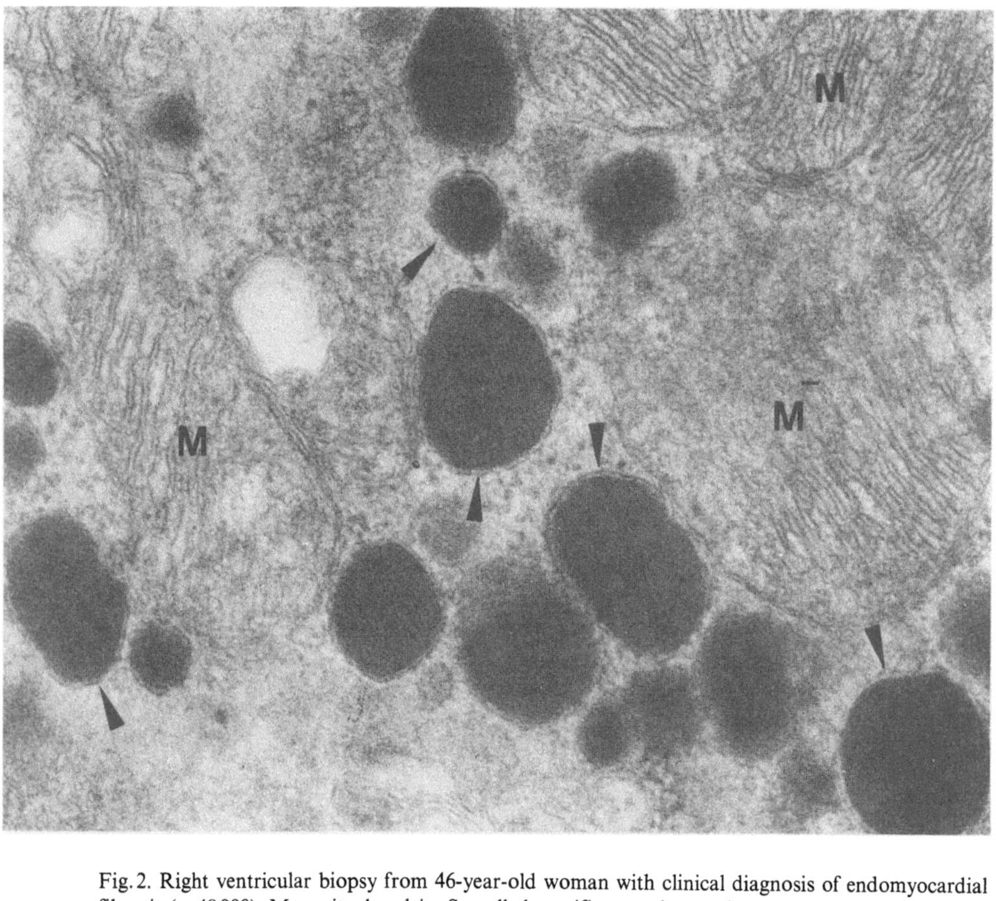

Fig. 2. Right ventricular biopsy from 46-year-old woman with clinical diagnosis of endomyocardial fibrosis (×48000). M = mitochondria. So-called specific granules can be seen (*arrowheads*)

Findings in Patients With Latent Cardiomyopathy, Left Bundle Branch Block, and Cardiac Arrhythmias

The complaints of the 20 patients with LCM were mostly uncharacteristic heart pains (70%), dyspnea (40%), weakness (25%), dizziness (10%) or irregular pulse (10%). Their mean age was 41 $\pm$ 9 years.

Hemodynamic and ventriculographic findings in patients with LCM and LBBB are shown in Figures 3 and 4. Mean pulmonary artery pressure (MPAP) on exercise in patients with LCM was the only value that was significantly higher than in normals ($P < 0.005$).

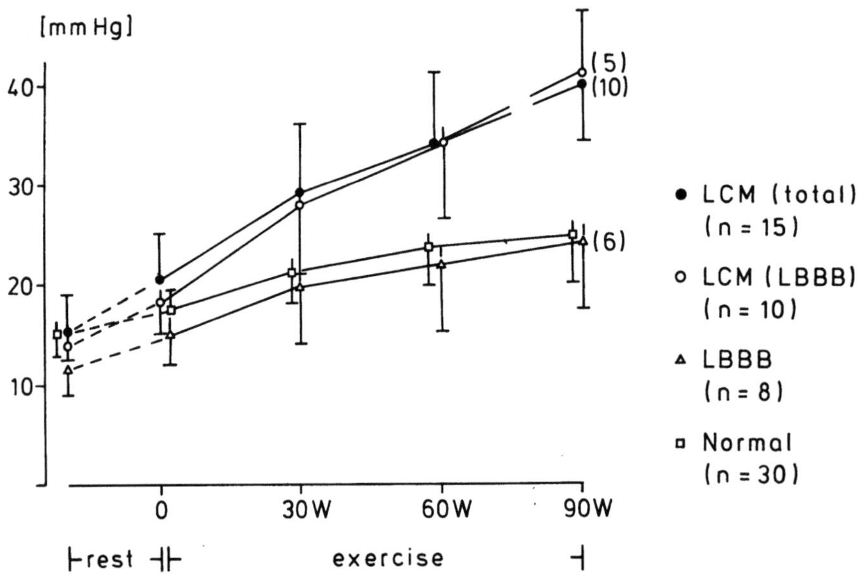

Fig. 3. Mean pulmonary artery pressure (MPAP, $\bar{x} \pm s_x$) at rest and during exercise in patients with latent cardiomyopathy (LCM), with left bundle branch block (LBBB), and in normals. Values of normals are obtained from [8]. Patients with LCM show a significantly higher increase of MPAP ($p < 0.005$). The values were obtained in the supine position, at rest with legs down (*on the left*) and on the ergometer (point 0 on the abscissa)

In addition to patients with LCM or LBBB, EMCB was performed in four patients with cardiac arrhythmias (Table 2). MPAP at rest or exercise, LVEDVI and SVI, thickness of septum and the free wall of the left ventricle, and coronary angiography were normal in these patients. In contrast to the other patients it must be noted that with the exception of patient G. U. the patients were treated for periods from several weeks to many months with various antiarrhythmic drugs such as Chinidin, aprindine, ajmaline, and/or beta-blockers.

To date light- and electron-microscopic examination of biopsy specimen has been completed in 21 patients: 10 patients with LCM, 6 showing LCM with LBBB, 4 LCM with depression of the ST-segment in the ECG; in 7 patients with LBBB and in 4 patients with arrhythmias.

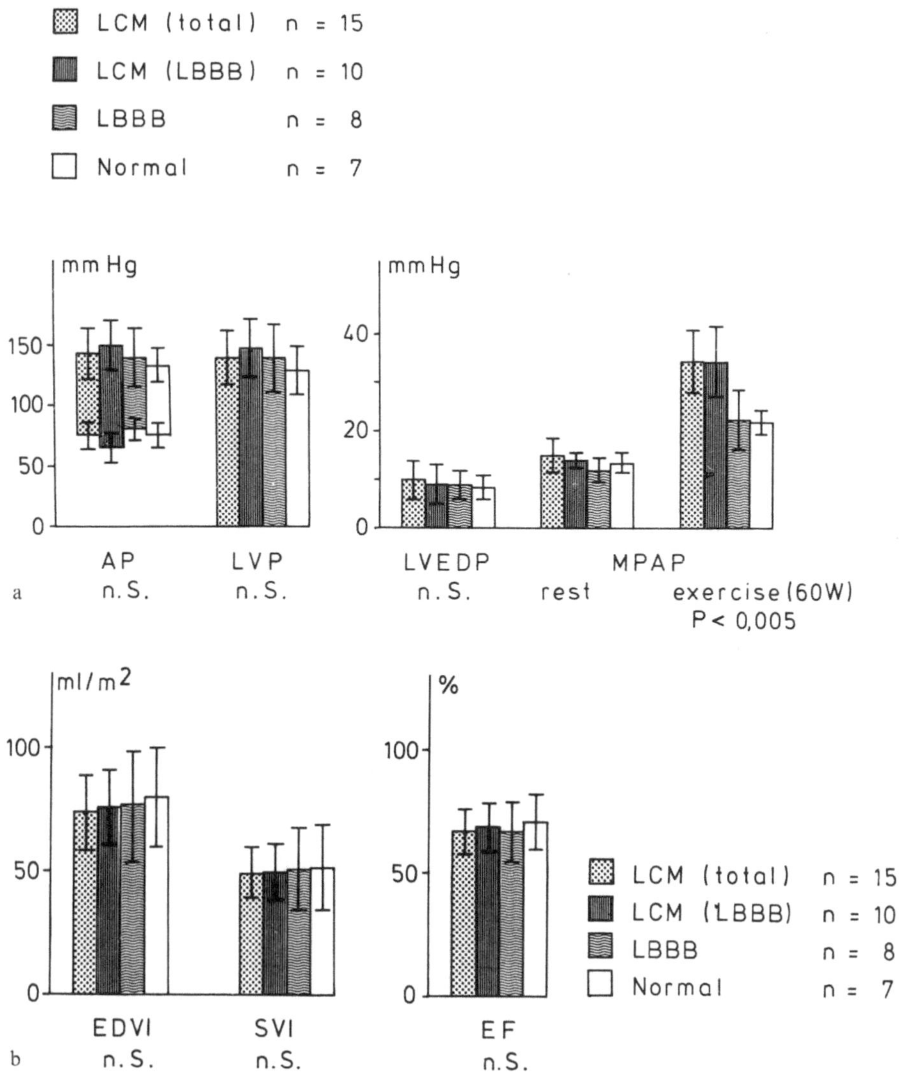

Fig. 4. In (a), aortic pressure (AP), left ventricular peak pressure (LVP), left ventricular enddiastolic pressure (LVEDP), mean pulmonary artery pressure (MPAP). In (b), enddiastolic volume index (EDVI), systolic volume index (SVI) and ejection fraction (EF) in patients with latent cardiomyopathy (LCM), with left bundle branch block (LBBB), and in normal subjects ($\bar{x} \pm s_x$). The only significant difference was found in MPAP at exercise, for example at 60 W

The results are shown in Figures 5 and 6. Electron-microscopic examples are shown in Figures 7–9. A completely normal microscopic picture was found only in one patient with LBBB. In all other patients slight or severe alterations were seen consisting of degenerative, mitochondrial and myofibrillar changes, interstitial fibrosis and/or hypertrophy. In patients with LBBB alone, myofibrillar changes were not seen. In each group all types of degenerative change occurred.

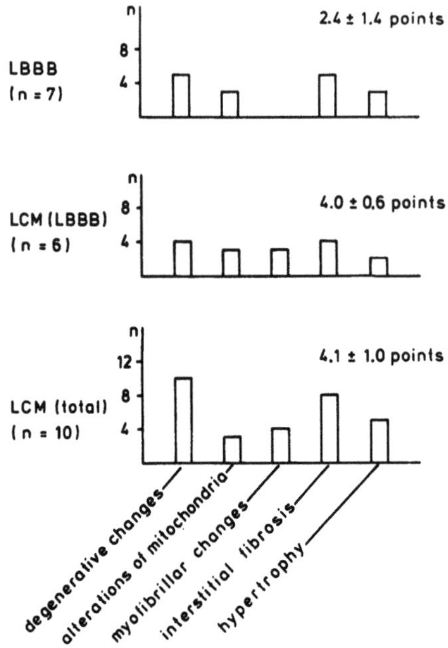

Fig. 5. Frequency (n = number of patients) of morphologic score ($\overline{x} \pm s_x$ points) in patients with latent cardiomyopathy (LCM) and left bundle branch block (LBBB)

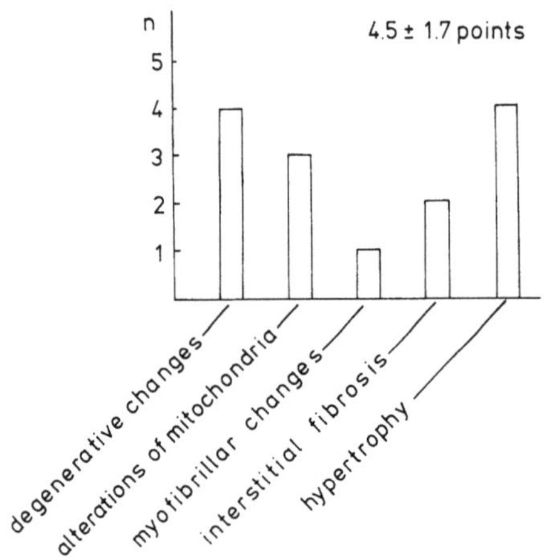

Fig. 6. Frequency (n = number of patients) of morphologic findings and morphologic score ($\overline{x} \pm s_x$ points) in patients with cardiac arrhythmia

Besides other changes, in three patients with cardiac arrhythmias, which were treated with antiarrhythmic drugs, but not in the fourth untreated patient (G. U.) a striking frequency of increased number of lipid droplets was found (Fig. 9). By semiquantitative evaluation of the biopsies 4.1 $\pm$1.0 points were calculated in patients with LCM, 4.5 $\pm$1.7 points in patients with cardiac arrhythmias and 2.4 $\pm$1.4 points in patients with LBBB.

Following clinical examination in December 1976, COCM is apparently developing in one patient with LCM and LBBB who showed severe electronmicroscopic changes.

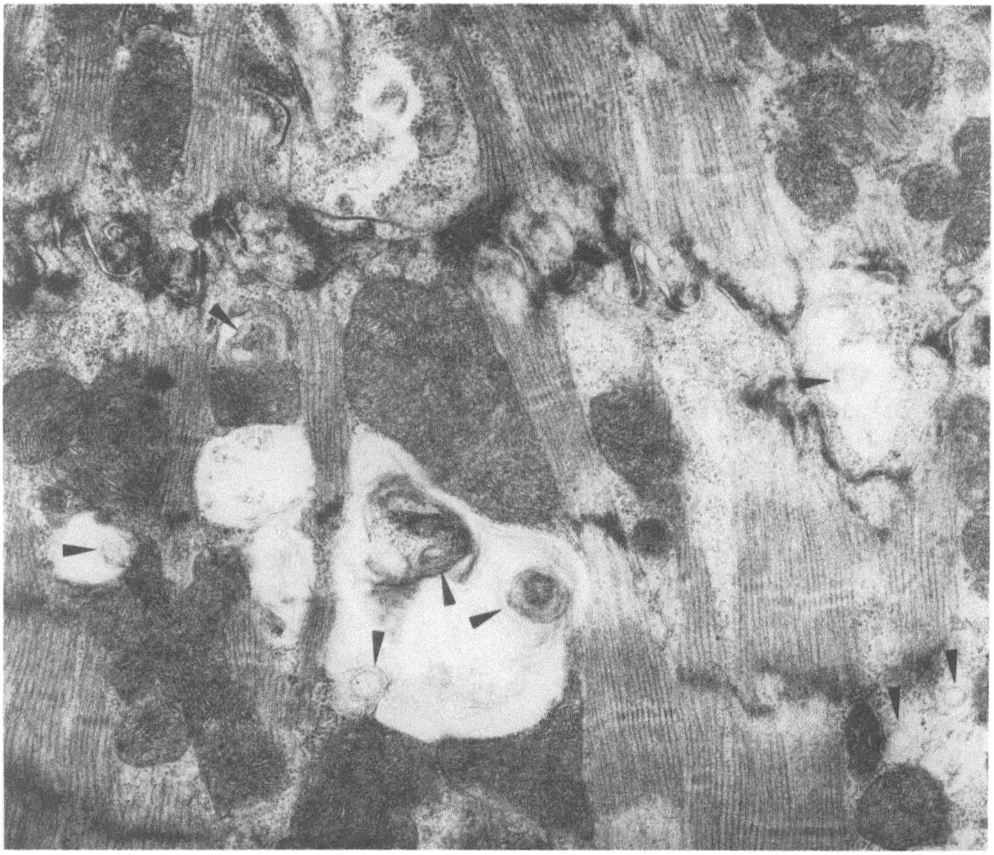

a

Fig. 7. Right ventricular biopsy from 37-year-old man with LBBB (×18000). Degenerative changes with increased number of myelin figures can be seen (*arrowheads*) (a). Myelin figures of the same patient with higher magnification (×24000) (b)

Discussion

Diagnostic Value of EMCB

Pathologic or abnormal findings of varying degree were observed in nearly all patients (93%). But although EMCB was performed in groups of patients with very different clinical diagnoses, with regard to the quality of changes the myocardium of these patients examined by both light and electron microscopy showed a homogeneous picture: the degenerative, myofibrillar, and mitochondrial alterations described above, hypertrophy of muscle fibers, interstitial fibrosis, and/or endocardial thickening. In only four patients were unusual ultrastructural findings in the right ventricle seen. These were so-called specific granules, deposits suspect of virus-like particles, extreme proliferation of sarcoplasmic reticulum and intracellular storage of unknown substance. In no case could an acute, subacute or chronic myocarditis be demonstrated.

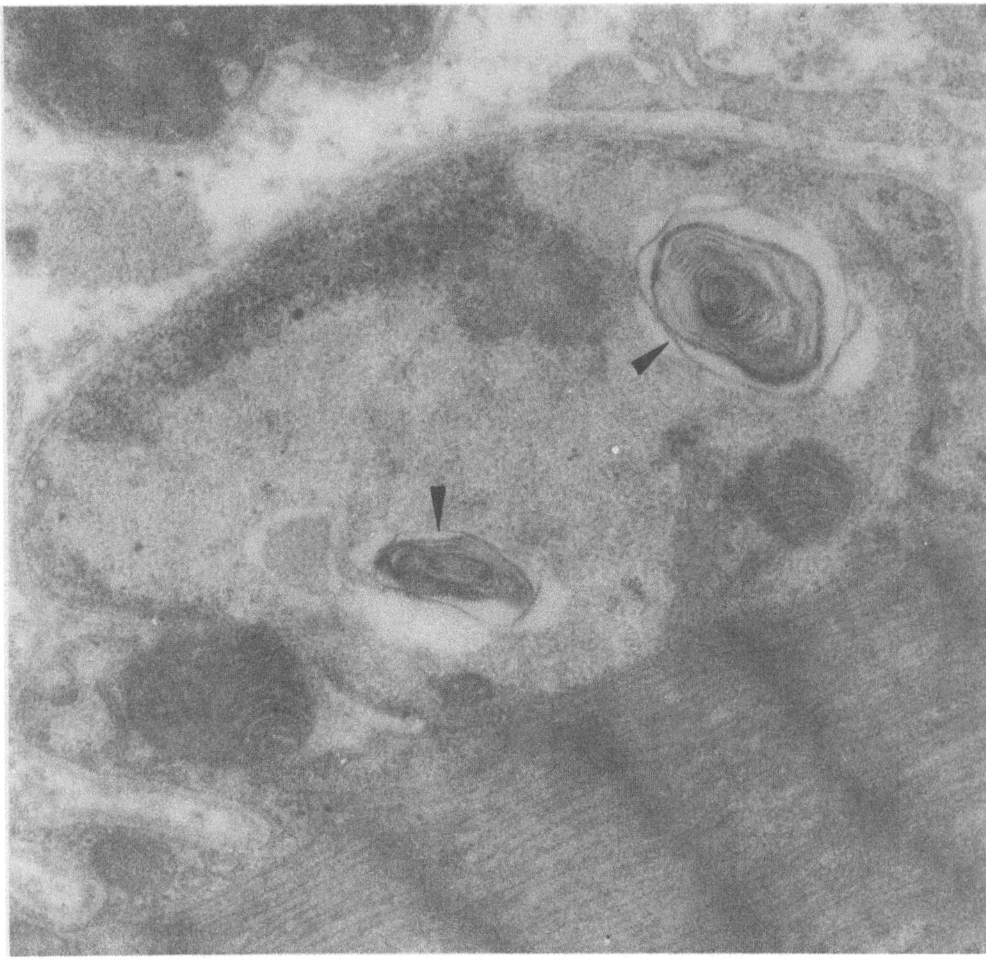

Fig. 7b. Legend see page 129

These data suggest a high sensitivity of EMCB for detecting disorders of myocardial cell structure by electron microscopy. However, there is little probability of finding specific or characteristic alterations in myocardial tissue, i.e., the high sensitivity and low specifity of EMCB, which is investigated by electron microscopy, can be assumed. Furthermore myocarditis, the exclusion of which is often the indication for EMCB, apparently does not play a causative role in heart disease of unknown etiology (Table 1).

With regard to the uncharacteristic ultrastructural picture seen in the great majority of patients, without knowledge of the clinical situation the diagnostic evaluation of biopsy or confirmation of the clinical diagnosis, as has been attempted [20], would appear to be impossible. With knowledge of the clinical data, the clinically suspected diagnosis could or could not be supported. Only rarely, e.g., in sarcoidosis where there is a specific morphologic picture, can a real diagnostic contribution by EMCB be expected.

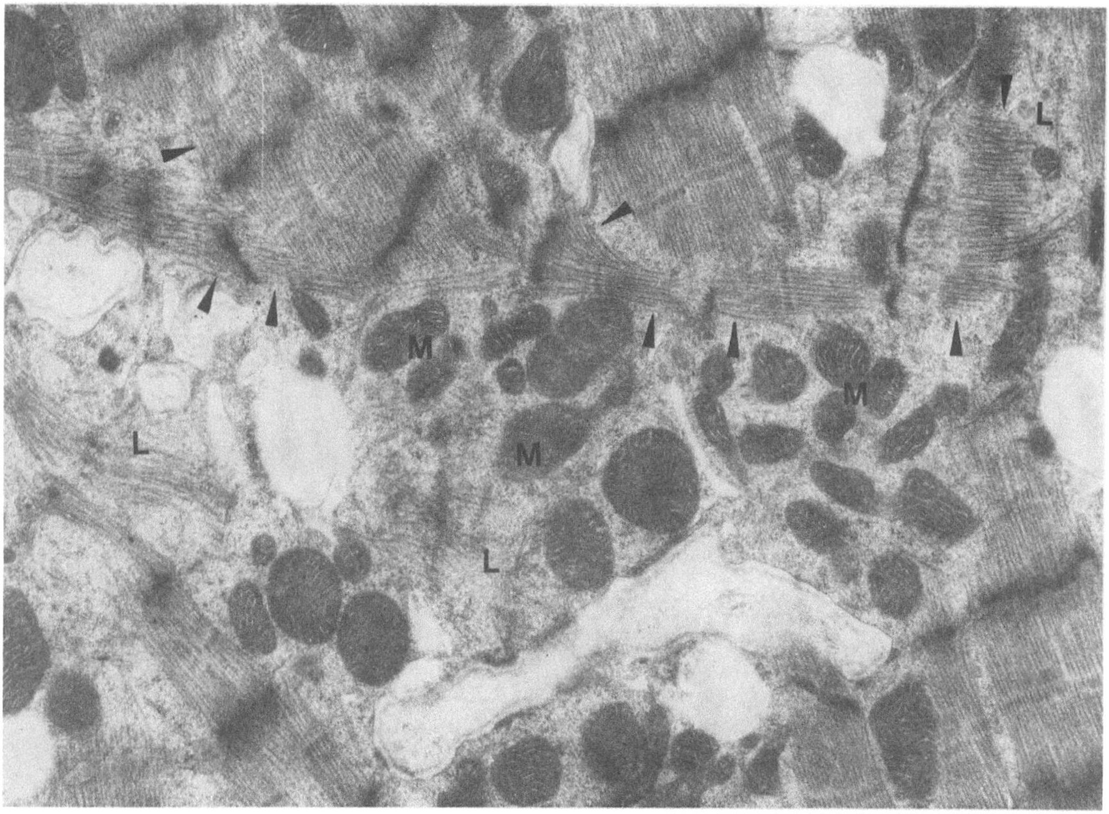

Fig. 8. Right ventricular biopsy from 39-year-old woman with latent cardiomyopathy and left bundle branch block (×16800). Disorientation of myofibrills (*arrowheads*), great variation in size of mitochondria (*M*), and lysis of myofilaments (*L*) is shown

Semiquantitative Evaluation of Endomyocardial Catheter Biopsy

To obtain a useful clinical contribution by morphologic evaluation of EMCB in a greater proportion of patients, semiquantitative evaluation of electron-microscopic criteria is proposed (Table 4). As confirmed by others [2], the prognostic value of EMCB in patients with COCM was demonstrated, i.e., a group of patients with high and low mortality rates could be clearly separated, indicating possibly two groups of patients with heart disease of different etiology [12, 16, Chapter 22].

Latent Cardiomyopathy and Left Bundle Branch Block

In order to find evidence for a prestage of COCM, by catamnestic studies of patients with COCM, the occurrence of cardiac arrhythmias or LBBB, present in many patients with COCM [14] (e.g., LBBB in 40%), could be proved as far back as 22 years before the clinical onset of COCM (Table 5) [10–12, 16]. In no

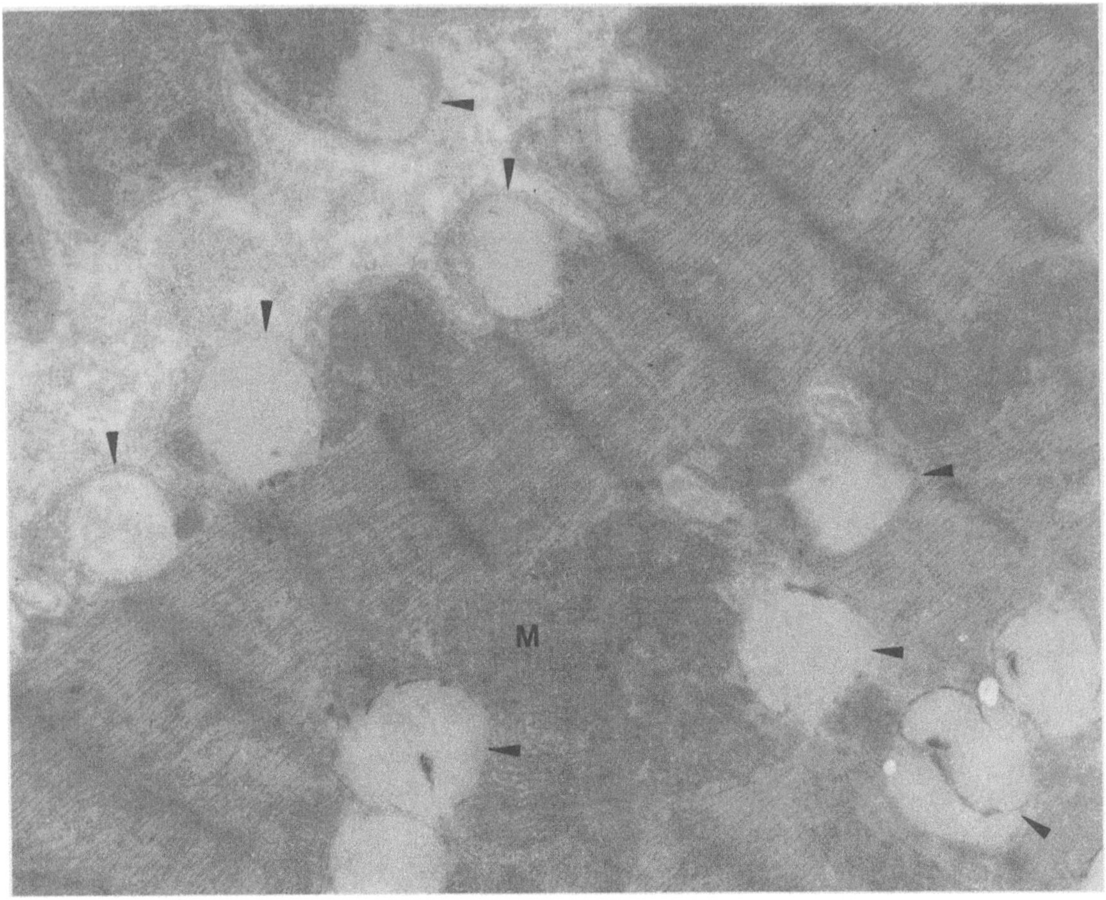

Fig. 9. Right ventricular biopsy from 28-year-old woman (D. M., see Table 2), treated with different antiarrhythmic drugs (see text). Increased number of lipid droplets (*arrowheads*) are demonstrated. M = mitochondria (×24000)

case did common LBBB develop during the course of patients who already showed COCM [14]. Because of these findings EMCB was performed in patients with possible early stages of COCM, i.e., in patients with LBBB, in patients with LCM and LBBB, and in patients with arrhythmias.
Patients with LCM mostly suffer from uncharacteristic angina pectoris similar to the early complaints of patients with COCM (Table 5). In contrast to other CMs the only pathologic finding in patients with LCM is an elevation of LVEDP. Similar hemodynamic and angiographic observations were made by Herman *et al.* [9].

The designation LCM is proposed because the elevation of LVEDP becomes in most cases evident only on exercise and because theoretically according to our catamnestic studies in COCM, the preexistence of COCM in some of these patients may be assumed. These observations are supported by prospective studies

Table 5. ECG-findings in patients with congestive cardiomyopathy (COCM) before clinical onset of disease. LBBB could be demonstrated as far back as 22 years before the beginning of COCM. In several patients X-ray of the chest was obtained or described (< 0.5), showing normal cardiothoracic ratio (CT-ratio) in the years before COCM. Duration of COCM was defined from the beginning of complaints (mostly dyspnea) up to the date of heart catheterization by which diagnosis of COCM was made. Period before COCM describes the interval from detection of abnormal ECG up to the beginning of first symptoms indicative of possible COCM. In four patients (+) cardiac complaints were transient, present many years before the clinical onset of COCM in the form of uncharacteristic heart pains or abnormal pulse (in cases of ventricular premature beats)

Patient		ECG-finding	Before COCM (years)	Cardiac complaints	CT-ratio Before COCM	After COCM	Duration of COCM (years)
H.K.	33y.	Atrial fibr.	8	–	0.475	0.590	1
W.G.	37y.	Atrial fibr.	3.5	–	0.465	0.580	3
M.P.	58y.	Ventr. p.b.	12	(+)	0.480	0.563	3
N.A.	47y.	Ventr. p.b.	13	(+)		0.540	2
P.W.	40y.	LBBB	3.5	–	(< 0.500)	0.560	6
V.F.	40y.	LBBB	13	–	0.487	0.651	2
S.W.	57y.	LBBB (intermitt.)	3	(+)	0.462	0.600	7
L.W.	47y.	LBBB	8	–		0.540	6
P.H.	53y.	LBBB	2.5	–	0.498	0.594	2.5
W.H.	49y.	LBBB	2	–	(< 0.500)	0.617	8
L.E.	49y.	LBBB	5	(+)	0.434	0.520	3
T.H.	51y.	LBBB	22	–	0.470	0.630	0.5
K.J.	48y.	LBBB (intermitt.)	14	–	0.430	0.540	2
S.G.	38y.	LBBB	9	–		0.530	2

(Framingham Heart Study) reported recently by Schneider *et al.* [24], who found that the onset of LBBB was associated in 37% with subsequent development of congestive heart failure.

EMCB revealed distinct electron-microscopic alterations of the myocardial cell not only in patients with LCM but also in patients with LBBB alone. Degenerative, mitochondrial and myofibrillar changes, interstitial fibrosis, and hypertrophy of myocardial cells were observed, i.e., changes of the same quality as those found in severe cardiac failure, (e.g. in COCM) [6, 10, 15, and Ch. 20].

The cause of myocardial changes is unclear. Inflammation is rather unlikely. No anamnestic, clinical, or light-microscopic evidence of myocarditis was found, and a higher frequency of LBBB in patients with former myocarditis is unproven. A possibility is that the electron-microscopic changes are caused by formerly severe and transient arterial hypertension. This idea is supported by the observation that slight elevation of blood pressure was present in some patients with LCM and LBBB (Fig. 4) and that some patients with COCM suffer from arterial hypertension many years before the clinical onset of COCM (authors' observations, 5, 7).

The morphologic findings obtained from right ventricular biopsies indicate a generalized myocardial disorder in patients with LCM and LBBB which apparently is not confined to the left ventricle and in the case of LBBB to the conduction system. The results are supported by His bundle recordings in the same patients (see Ch. 20) which revealed significantly longer HV-intervals in patients with LBBB than in normals, indicating a diffuse myocardial disorder in patients with LBBB. In considering the normal hemodynamic and angiographic findings in patients with LBBB, EMCB seems to be more sensitive in detecting myocardial disorder than the various invasive and noninvasive methods which have been applied.

The mean morphologic score of LCM (4.1 points) reaches the values seen in COCM [15, 16, and Ch. 22]. In addition, noteworthy is the occurrence of degenerative changes such as myelin figures, which are considered to be degenerated mitochondria. These findings are in disagreement with previous assumptions that such changes possibly characterize a late stage of cardiac failure or hypertrophy [6, 19]. The quantitative results in LCM and LBBB are supported by similar findings in COCM which also were largely independent of hemodynamic and ventriculographic changes (Ch. 8, 22). Furthermore a high morphologic score in COCM was strongly associated with rapid progression of COCM and a high mortality rate. Taking these prognostic observations in COCM into consideration, it can be speculated that the occurrence of severe or frequent electron-microscopic changes in patients with LCM or LBBB indicates subsequent COCM. These prognostic aspects need further biopsies and follow-up studies in patients with LCM. In one of our patients with LCM and LBBB showing severe electron-microscopic changes, COCM seems to be developing three years after biopsy.

A lower morphologic score (2.4 points, Fig. 6) was found in patients with LBBB than in patients with LCM (4.1 points). Nor were myofibrillar changes present. These findings can possibly be explained by an earlier stage of myocardial disorder being present in patients with LBBB who do not yet show an elevation of LVEDP or MPAP on exercise.

Today, therapy in COCM, is unsatisfactory. It seems to be necessary to find out patients with prestage of COCM which possibly could be influenced by preventive therapy, i.e., taking into consideration theoretical "risk factors" of COCM like arterial hypertension [5, 7], virus infection, alcohol, or pregnancy [7]. According to the results reported here, EMCB possibly helps to detect a prestage of COCM or "risk patients" among patients with LBBB and/or LCM, demonstrated by severe electron-microscopic alterations in myocardial tissue. Thus far a new indication for performing EMCB exists.

Patients With Cardiac Arrhythmias

As was shown in Figure 6 distinct light- and electron-microscopic changes with a high morphologic score were found in patients with cardiac arrhythmia, indicating, as in patients with LBBB or LCM, a diffuse myocardial disorder. According to our catamnestic studies in patients with COCM (Table 5), the prognostic considerations are similar to those in patients with LBBB or LCM. The etiologic considerations, however, are different. It cannot be excluded that the morphologic alterations in patients with arrhythmias were at least partly caused by the various antiarrhythmic drugs administrated, i.e., chinidine, aprindine, ajmaline, and/or beta blockers. Morphologic changes of the myocardial cell provoked by other drugs are described in the literature [4, 18]. The striking incidence of an increased number of lipid droplets, which was present in all three patients treated, and which was not present in the untreated patient, G. U., is possibly caused by the antiarrhythmic therapy. With regard to the known negative inotropic effect of these drugs, which can be seen at therapeutic dosages, a causative relationship between the hemodynamic effect and morphologic changes cannot be excluded. These findings need further investigation in larger numbers of patients.

Summary

Since 1971, EMCB has been performed in 182 patients with various cardiac diseases. No severe complications occurred. Up to now, light-microscopic examination of biopsy has been carried out in 151 patients, and both light- and electron-microscopic examination in 131 patients. In 93% of these patients abnormal morphologic findings were observed consisting of degenerative, mitochondrial, and myofibrillar alterations, hypertrophy of myocardial cells, interstitial fibrosis and/or endocardial thickening. In no case was myocarditis seen. In only four cases were uncommon changes found (myocardial storage disease, specific granules, extreme proliferation of sarcoplasmatic reticulum, virus-like particles). These data indicate high "sensitivity" but low "specifity" of electron-microscopically studied biopsies. Support of clinical diagnosis seems to be possible, but not confirmation. Light-microscopic judgment alone is mostly insufficient.

For better clinical use of EMCB, semiquantitative evaluation is proposed using a morphologic scoring system. By this means a high prognostic value in patients with COCM could be proved (see Ch. 22).

The findings in 21 patients with heart disease of unknown etiology showing only slightly impaired left ventricular function, or no impairment at all, are reported in detail. This group consisted of 10 patients with LCM, 6 of whom showed LBBB, 7 patients with LBBB without LCM; and 4 patients with cardiac arrhythmias. In order to study possible prestages of COCM, selection of these patients for biopsy was done according to catamnestic studies in COCM by which LBBB and cardiac arrhythmia could be demonstrated as far back as 22 years before clinical onset of COCM. With one exception, in all remaining 20 patients morphologic alterations were found which were qualitatively and in part quantitatively similar to those observed in advanced stages of myocardial disease, e.g., in COCM. Therefore these changes, found in right ventricular biopsies do not characterize a late stage of cardiac failure or hypertrophy as was previously assumed. Furthermore, a generalized disorder of the myocardium, not confined to the conduction system or the left ventricle, can be assumed. With regard to the follow-up studies in COCM, the combination of LCM or LBBB with severe electron-microscopic changes possibly indicates subsequent development of COCM. Thus EMCB probably helps detect prestage of COCM and leads to better prognostic differentiation in patients with LBBB.

In the biopsy of all four patients with arrhythmia, distinct morphologic alterations were found, suggesting a diffuse myocardial disease. The etiology of ultrastructural changes is unclear. But there is some evidence for antiarrhythmic drug-induced disorder of myocardial cell structure.

References

1. Bonzel, T., Schmidt, H., Sigwart, U., Mertens, H.M., Gleichmann, U.: Pulmonalarteriendrücke und linksventrikulärer enddiastolischer Druck in Ruhe und unter dynamischer Belastung. Vergleichende Untersuchungen zur Druckübertragung im kleinen Kreislauf bei simultaner Messung. Z. Kardiol. *64*, 1088 (1976)
2. Bouhour, J.B., Petitier, H., De Lajartre, A.Y., Almanzor, M., Nicolas, G., Horeau, J.: La biopsie myocardique dans les myocardiopathies congestives en apparence primitives. Arch. Mal. Cœur *69*, 485 (1976)
3. Breithardt, G., Knieriem, H.-J., Kuhn, H., Loogen, F., Gleichmann, U.: Comparison of clinical data and ultrastructural findings in myocardial biopsy of patients with cardiomyopathies. In: Kölbel, F.: Adaptability of Cardiac Muscle, Symposium of the European Section of the International Study Group for Research in Cardiac Metabolism. Prague 1974 (in press)
4. Buja, L.M., Ferrans, V.J., Roberts, W.C.: Drug-induced cardiomyopathies. Adv. Cardiol. (Basel) *13*, 330 (1974)
5. Dickinson, J., Oakley, C.M., Brockington, I.F., Goodwin, J.F., Dollery, C.T.: Debate: That congestive cardiomyopathy is really hypertensive heart disease in disguise. Seminar on cardiomyopathies. Postgrad. med. J. *48*, 777 (1972)
6. Ferrans, V.J., Massumi, R.A., Shugoll, E.J., Ali, N., Roberts, W.C.: Ultrastructural studies of myocardial biopsies in 45 patients with obstructive or congestive cardiomyopathy. In: Cardiomyopathies. Bajusz, E., Rona, G. (eds.). Munich: Urban und Schwarzenberg 1974, p. 231
7. Goodwin, J.F.: Prospects and predictions for the cardiomyopathies. Circulation *50*, 210 (1974)
8. Haerten, K., Both, A., Krelhaus, W., Loogen, F.: Die Hämodynamik des kleinen Kreislaufs bei Herzgesunden unter mehrstufiger Ergometerbelastung. Med. Welt *27*, 2386 (1976)
9. Herman, M.V., Gorlin, R., Kreulen, T.H.: Ventriculographic classification of primary myocardial disease. In: Comparative pathology of the heart. Adv. Cardiol. (Basle) *13*, 53 (1975)
10. Kuhn, H.: Die congestive Cardiomyopathie. Klinische und experimentelle Untersuchungen. Habilitationsschrift, Düsseldorf (1975)
11. Kuhn, H., Breithardt, G., Knieriem, H.-J., Seipel, L., Loogen, F.: Linksschenkelblock bei congestiver Kardiomyopathie. Z. Kardiol., Suppl. *2*, 30 (1975)
12. Kuhn, H., Breithardt, G., Knieriem, H.-J., Seipel, L., Loogen, F., Both, A., Stroobandt, R.: Die Bedeutung des Elektrokardiogramms und der endomyokardialen Katheter-Biopsie für Diagnose und Verlaufsbeobachtung der congestiven Kardiomyopathie. Verh. dtsch. Ges. Inn. Med. *81*, 211 (1975)
13. Kuhn, H., Kübler, W., Loogen, F., Gleichmann, U.: Die congestive Kardiomyopathie. 119. Tagung Rhein.-Westf. Ges. Inn. Med., Düsseldorf (1972). Med. Welt *24*, 996 (1973)
14. Kuhn, H., Breithardt, L.K., Breithardt, G., Seipel, L., Loogen, F.: Die Bedeutung des Elektrokardiogramms für Diagnose und Verlaufsbeurteilung von Patienten mit congestiver Kardiomyopathie. Z. Kardiol. *63*, 916 (1974)
15. Kuhn, H., Breithardt, G., Knieriem, H.-J., Loogen, F., Both, A., Schmidt, W.A.K., Stroobandt, R., Gleichmann, U.: Die Bedeutung der endomyokardialen Katheter-Biopsie für die Diagnostik und die Beurteilung der Prognose der congestiven Cardiomyopathie. Dtsch. med. Wschr. *100*, 717 (1975)
16. Loogen, F., Kuhn, H.: Classification and natural history of primary cardiomyopathy. International symposium on myocardial failure, Rottach-Egern, June 1976. In: Myocardial failure. G. Riecker, A. Weber, J. Goodwin (Ed.). Berlin-Heidelberg-New York: Springer-Verlag 1977, p. 232
17. Loogen, F., Kuhn, H., Neuhaus, L.K.: Störungen der Ventrikelfunktion bei Kardiomyopathien. Verh. dtsch. Ges. Kreisl.-Forsch. *42*, 63 (1976)
18. Lüllmann, H., Lüllmann-Rauch, R., Wassermann, O.: Arzneimittelinduzierte Phospholipidspeicher Krankheit. Dtsch. med. Wschr. *98*, 1616 (1973)

19. Maron, B.J., Ferrans, V.J., Roberts, W.C.: Ultrastructural features of degenerate cardiac muscle cells in patients with cardiac hypertrophy. Amer. J. Pathol. *79*, 387 (1975)
20. Olsen, E.G.J.: Diagnostic value of the endomyocardial bioptome. Lancet I, *1974*, 658
21. Richardson, P.J.: King's endomyocardial bioptome. Lancet *1974/I*, 660
22. Sakakibara, S., Konno, S.: Endomyocardial biopsy. Jap. Heart J. *3*, 537 (1962)
23. Sandler, H., Dodge, H.T.: Angiocardiographic methods for determination of left ventricular geometry and volume. In: Cardiac Mechanics: Physiological, Clinical and Mathematical Considerations. Mirsky, I., Ghista, D.N., Sandler, H. (eds.). New York-London-Sydney-Toronto: John Wiley and sons, 1974, p. 141
24. Schneider, J.F., Thomas, H.E., Kreger, B., Mc Namara, P.: Left bundle branch-block in Framingham. Circulation *53*, *54*, II/128 (1976) (Abstract)

Influence of Hypertrophy and Ischemia on Morphologic Patterns

12. Ultrastructure of Left Atrial Myocardium in Patients With Mitral Valvular Disease

K.-U. THIEDEMANN and V. J. FERRANS

Introduction

Knowledge of ultrastructural changes in diseased human ventricular myocardium has increased considerably during recent years [1–5]. However, only a few studies have been made of the ultrastructural pathology of human atria [6–17]. Although to date investigations of the fine structure of normal human atrial myocardium [15, 18, 19] have been much less detailed than have those of atrial muscle of other mammals [20–23], there is general agreement that the ultrastructure of atrial muscle cells is similar in man and a number of other mammals [20–23]. This chapter describes light-microscopic and ultrastructural findings on operatively obtained left atrial biopsies from 14 patients with mitral valvular disease.

Materials and Methods

Patients Studied

All 14 patients had valvular heart disease involving the mitral valve exclusively (8 patients) or the mitral valve as well as other valves (6 patients). Three patients had pure mitral stenosis; five had pure mitral regurgitation; and six had combined mitral stenosis and regurgitation, with predominant mitral stenosis in five patients and predominant mitral regurgitation in one patient.

Preparation of Tissues

Biopsies of the left atrial wall were taken from the area directly adjacent to the atriotomy incision and fixed in cold 3% glutaraldehyde in 0.1 *M* phosphate buffer, pH 7.2, immediately after excision. Tissues were postfixed in 1% osmium tetroxide in Millonig's phosphate buffer, dehydrated in ethanol and propylene oxide, and embedded in Maraglas [24]. Semithin sections were stained with alkaline toluidine blue for light-microscopic evaluation. Ultrathin sections were cut from selected areas, stained with alcoholic uranyl acetate and lead citrate, and viewed with a JEOL 100B electron microscope.

Results

Light-Microscopic Observations

Examination of semithin sections revealed considerable degrees of interstitial fibrosis in all biopsy specimens. Atrial muscle cells tended to be isolated from neighboring cells by fibrous tissue (Figs. 1–3). Atrial muscle cells were 10–30 μ in width and 50–160 μ in length, but small (< 4 μ in diamter) as well as very large (> 30 μ in diamter) cells often were observed.

Cells that had lost their connections to other cells frequently were spindle shaped and had irregularly invaginated ends that gradually tapered off into the interstitium (Fig. 2). Large numbers of pale-staining cells that often contained some dark-staining granular material and only a few marginally arranged myofibrils were commonly present in, or close to, areas of interstitial fibrosis. They frequently were isolated from neighboring cells by layers of fibrous tissue (Fig. 2). Ultrastructural study of these cells disclosed features of moderate to severe degeneration.

Variable degrees of degeneration of atrial muscle cells were present in all 14 patients. Severe changes were present in 10 of the 14, which indicated a relation to the presence of atrial fibrillation and of mitral regurgitation. Of the 10 patients with atrial fibrillation (8 with permanent atrial fibrillation, 2 with intermittent fibrillation), 9 showed severe degenerative changes, including 1 of the 3 patients with pure mitral stenosis, 4 of the 5 patients with pure mitral regurgitation, and 4 of the 6 patients with combined mitral stenosis and regurgitation. In contrast, severe degeneration was present in only 1 (who had pure mitral stenosis and cardiac symptoms for 27 years) of the 4 patients with normal sinus rhythm; the other 3 patients in this group (2 with pure mitral stenosis and 1 with pure mitral regurgitation) had mild to moderate degenerative changes. Severe degeneration occurred in 1 of the 3 patients with pure mitral stenosis, and in 9 of 11 patients having mitral regurgitation, either pure (4 of 5 patients) or associated with mitral stenosis (4 of 6 patients).

Electron-Microscopic Findings in Hypertrophied, Nondegenerated Cells

Muscle cells wider than 15 μ and/or longer than 100 μ were commonly present in all specimens and were considered to be hypertrophied and nondegenerated when they exhibited a qualitatively normal morphology. They had normal cellular arrangement and were connected to adjacent cells by end-to-end and side-to-side junctions. Their shape frequently was irregular. On electron-microscopic study, hypertrophied cells showed: (1) increased amounts of myofilaments and

---

Fig. 1–3. Light micrographs of $^1/_2$-μ sections, stained with alkaline toluidine blue, of tissue embedded in Maraglas. Figure 1 is from left atrium of a 22-year-old woman who had mitral valve replacement for mitral regurgitation and congestive heart failure of eight years' duration. Figures 2 and 3 are from left atrium of a 36-year-old woman who underwent triple valve replacement; her predominant lesion was mitral regurgitation ▷

Fig. 1. Atrial muscle cells, shown in cross section, exhibit great variation in size and are separated from one another by fibrous tissue. × 400

Fig. 2. Two atrial muscle cells (right) have lost all their contractile elements, have tapered ends that do not form connections with adjacent cells, and are filled with granular material (compare with Fig. 13). Cell at left shows prominent sarcolemmal invaginations. × 750

Fig. 3. Marked accumulations of Z-band material (*arrows*) are present in atrial muscle cell. Compare with Figure 4. × 750

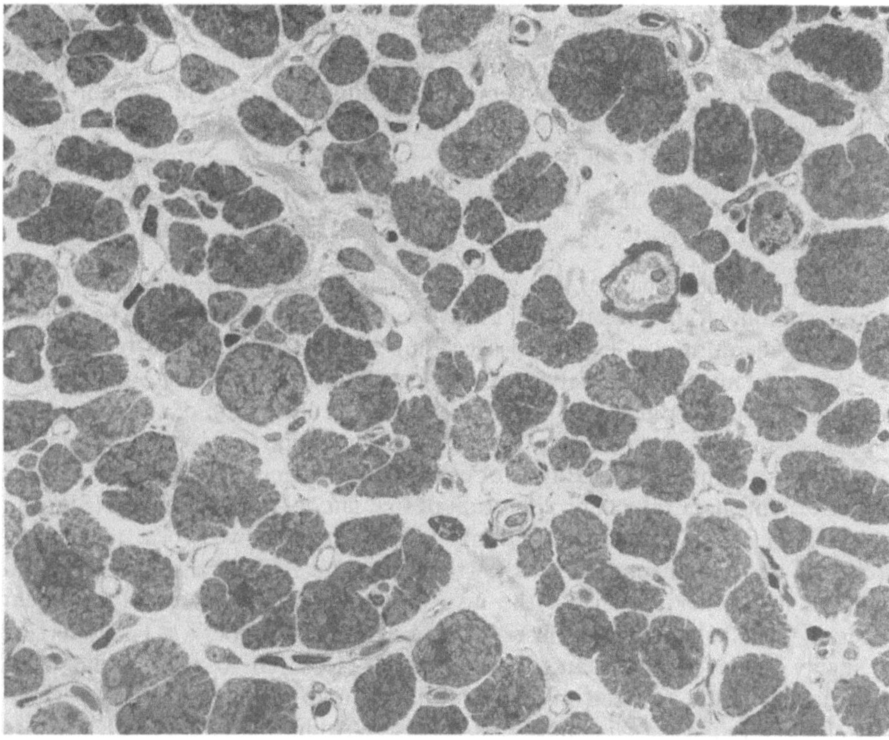

1

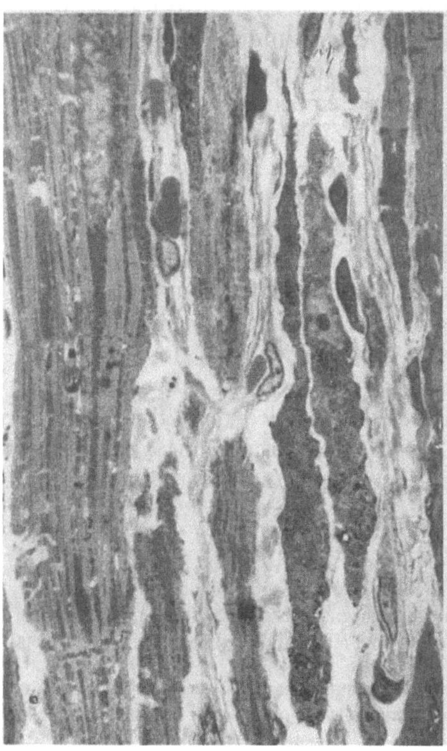

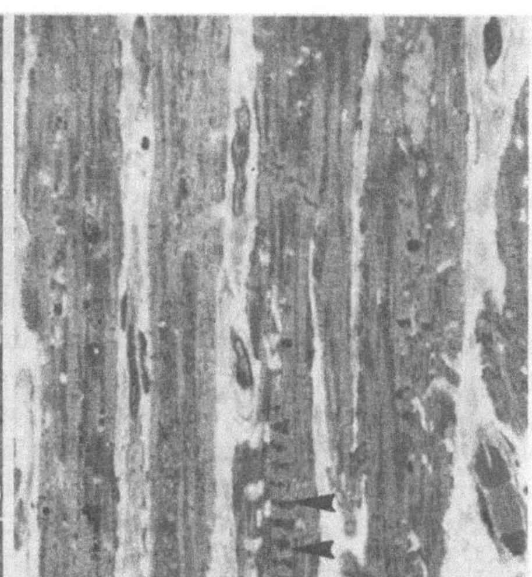

3

mitochondria; (2) increased numbers of free or membrane-bound ribosomes; (3) large and highly lobulated nuclei; (4) enlarged Golgi complexes; (5) irregularly shaped invaginations of the sarcolemma extending deep into the interior of the cells (Fig. 2); (6) focal widening and splitting of Z bands; and (7) small accumulations of Z-band-like material.

Degenerative Changes

A large spectrum of changes that were considered to be of a degenerative nature were commonly found in left atrial muscle cells from all 14 patients. The severity of the degeneration was evaluated according to the criteria of Maron *et al.* [5].

Left atrial myocytes in early stages of degeneration showed not only the basic features of hypertrophied cells, but also selective proliferation of certain cellular organelles and loss of others. The process of degeneration involved: (1) alteration of Z-band structure; (2) focal lysis of contractile elements, with preferential loss of thick filaments; (3) focal proliferation of free sarcoplasmic reticulum (SR) and (4) proliferation of extended junctional SR. Z bands showed focal thickening, splitting, and fragmentation, with irregular, elongated extension of Z-band material into other regions of the myofibrils. Two morphologically different types of Z-band changes were observed. The first of these types was characterized by highly regular arrangement of filaments that measured 70–90 Å in diameter, were connected by an electron-dense substance, and exhibited a 200-Å periodicity (Fig. 4). Extensive widening of Z bands showing this type of substructure was found frequently in several adjacent sarcomeres of single myofibrils (Fig. 3). These changes resembled those described in other studies of hypertrophied hearts [1–5, 7, 9, 25–27]. The second type of widened Z bands contained fine, short filaments that showed no periodicity and were embedded in varying amounts of an electron-dense amorphous matrix (Fig. 5). Z-band material of this latter type was present in subsarcolemmal accumulations, in elongated masses that extended over the length of several sarcomeres, and in areas of lateral connections between adjacent myofibrils. Contractile elements adjacent to altered Z bands frequently showed focal disorganization and loss of myofilaments. This loss affected myosin filaments to a larger extent than actin filaments, resulting in the presence of disproportionately higher numbers of thin filaments. Focal loss of contractile filaments was associated with proliferation of a closely knit network of branching and anastomosing tubules of free SR. This network, together with cytoskeletal filaments (100 Å in diameter), occupied myofibril-free areas of degenerated atrial muscle cells (Fig. 6). Mitochondria in these areas were either very small or absent. Specific atrial granules showed variable decreases in numbers.

Fig. 4. Accumulations of Z-band material with a highly organized substructure fill cytoplasm of atrial muscle cell from 47-year-old woman with mitral regurgitation and severe pulmonary hypertension. Note that only a few thick (myosin) filaments (*arrows*) remain in this area of the cell. × 29,800 ▷

Fig. 5. Elongated subsarcolemmal and intramyofibrillar accumulations of Z-band material associated with thin myofilaments are present in atrial muscle cell from 31-year-old woman with mitral stenosis. × 28,300

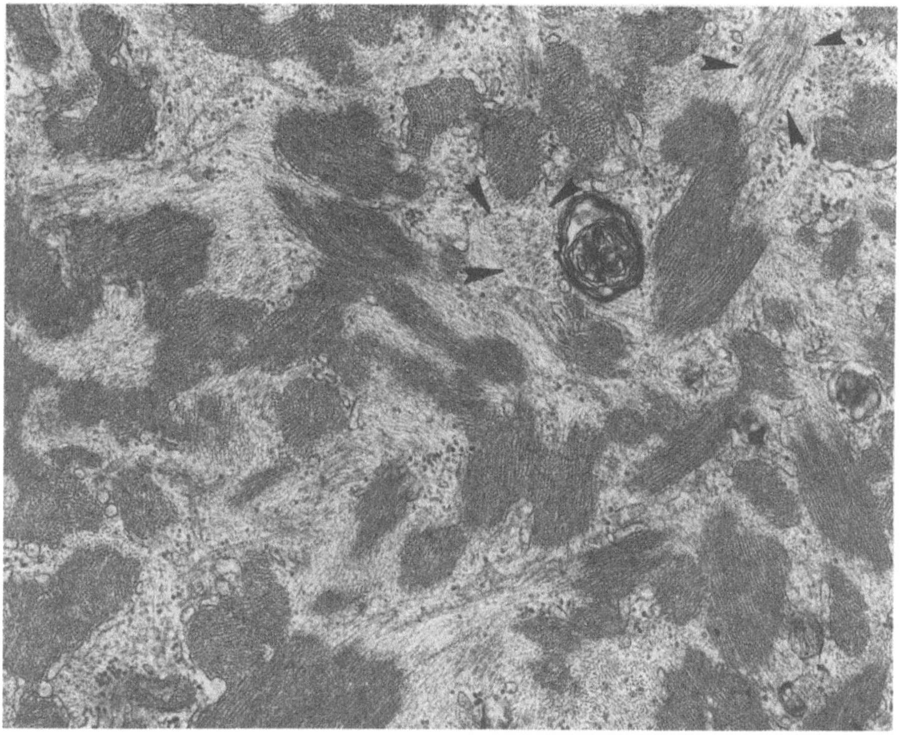

4

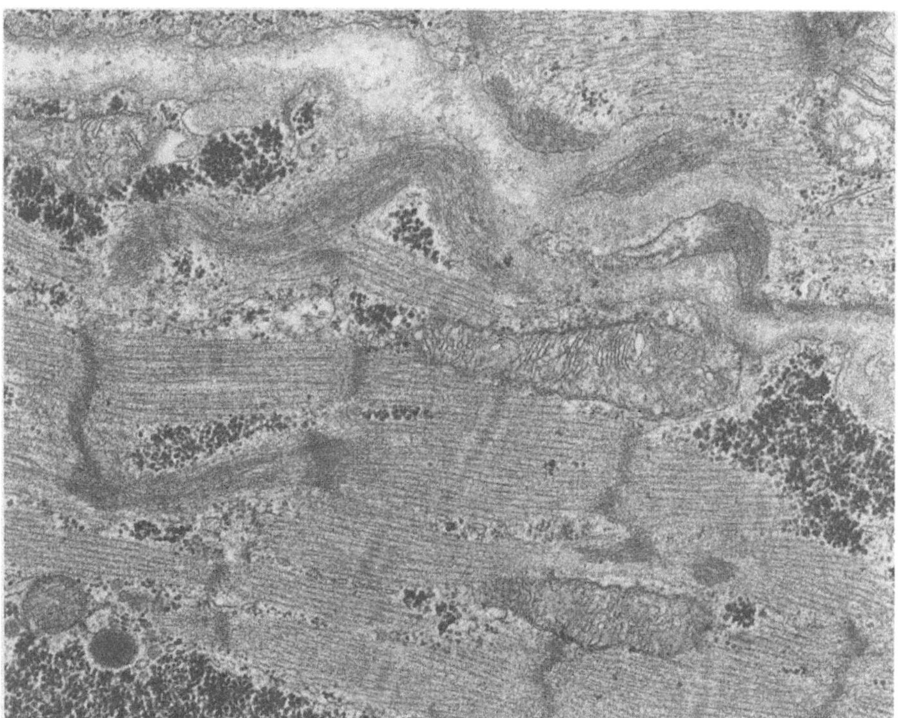

5

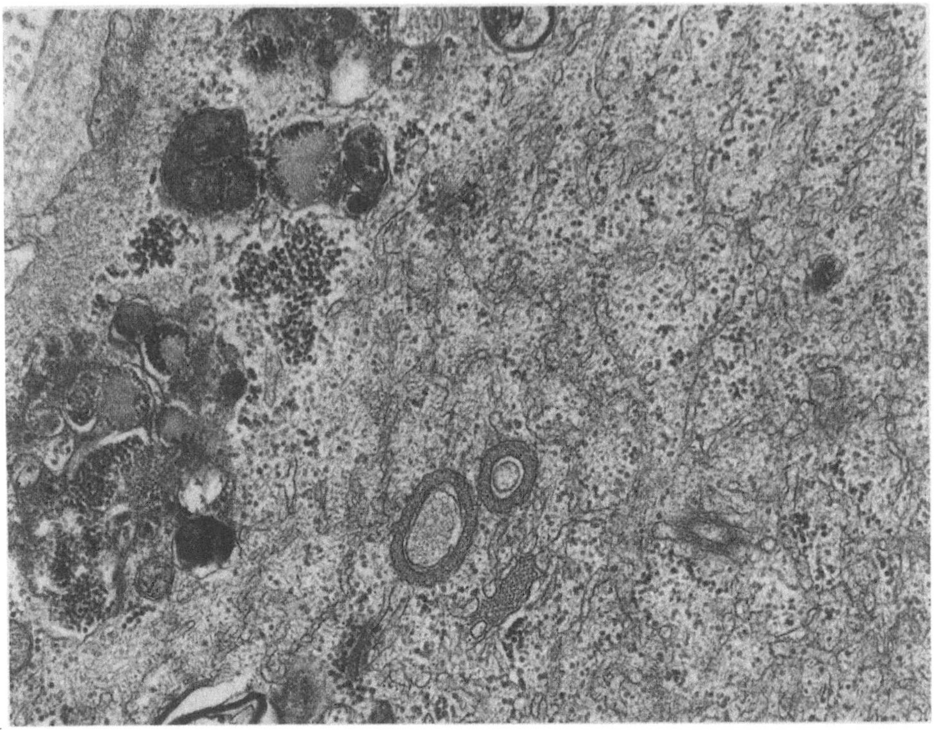

6

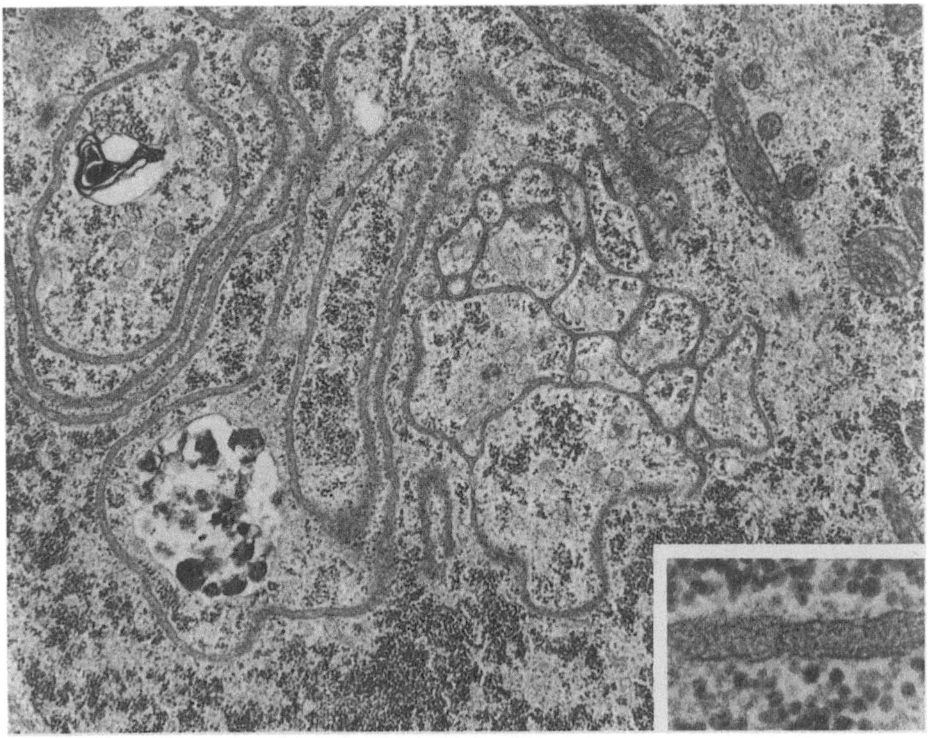

7

Proliferation of two morphologically different types of cisterns of extended junctional SR (herein designated type A and type B) was a common finding in hypertrophied and degenerated atrial myocytes of all patients [17]. Elements of extended junctional SR are morphologically similar in several respects, including their granular, electron-dense content, to cistern of junctional SR. Extended junctional SR components are continuous with those of junctional SR, but do not form special contacts with the sarcolemma [17, 28–30]. Type A cisterns were 550–650 Å wide, straight, curved, or circular, and had an uncoated outer surface and a finely granular moderately electron-dense content (Fig. 6 and 7). Type B cisterns were 220–300 Å wide, occasionally exhibited an outer coating layer, had a finely granular, moderately electron-dense content, and showed a dense central lamina (Fig. 8). Both type A and type B cisterns formed variously arranged, often very extensive complexes.

The alterations in moderately degenerated atrial muscle cells represented further progression of the degenerative process and consisted of the following additional features: (1) marked interstitial fibrosis; (2) dissociation of end-to-end and side-to-side intercellular junctions (Fig. 9); (3) isolation of cells, the ends of which tapered into the interstitial space (Fig. 10); (4) intracytoplasmic junctions in cells undergoing dissociation (Fig. 10); (5) occurrence of spherical microparticles and of small nexus-like structures in the space between sarcolemma and basement membrane and in areas of dissociating junctions (Fig. 9); (6) extensive proliferation of Z-band material; (7) streaming of Z bands and loss of regular arrangement of sarcomeres; (8) progressive loss of myofilaments and replacement by cytoskeletal filaments; (9) occurrence of hexagonally arranged tubules of free SR associated with widened Z bands (Fig. 11); (10) extensive proliferation of free SR; and (11) various mitochondrial abnormalities, including marked variations in mitochondrial size and the presence of several types of intramitochondrial inclusions.

Atrial myocytes in or adjacent to areas of severe interstitial fibrosis appeared to undergo dissociation from adjacent cells by separation of the membranes forming intercalated discs (Fig. 9). The ends of cells that were completely separated from neighboring cells formed long, shallow projections that gradually tapered into the interstitial space (Fig. 10). Spherical microparticles averaging 500 Å in diameter and composed of dense cores surrounded by single trilaminar membranes were found in the space between the sarcolemma and the basement membranes in these areas, and between the membranes of dissociating junctions. Some of these microparticles were connected by small nexus-like structures (Fig. 9).

◁ Fig. 6. Area of atrial muscle cell from 65-year-old woman with long-standing (15 years) mitral regurgitation. Only a few organized contractile elements remain (upper left). Note the masses of residual bodies, the proliferation of elements of free SR, which form a closely knit network, and two circular cisterns (type A) of extended junctional SR with dense, finely granular content. × 35,000

Fig. 7. Large, highly convoluted type A cisterns of extended junctional SR occupy large area of cytoplasm in atrial muscle cell (same patient as in Fig. 4). × 25,300. *Inset* shows high magnification view of one of the cisterns, which are filled with fine granular material and do not have an external coating or a central dense lamina. × 77,500

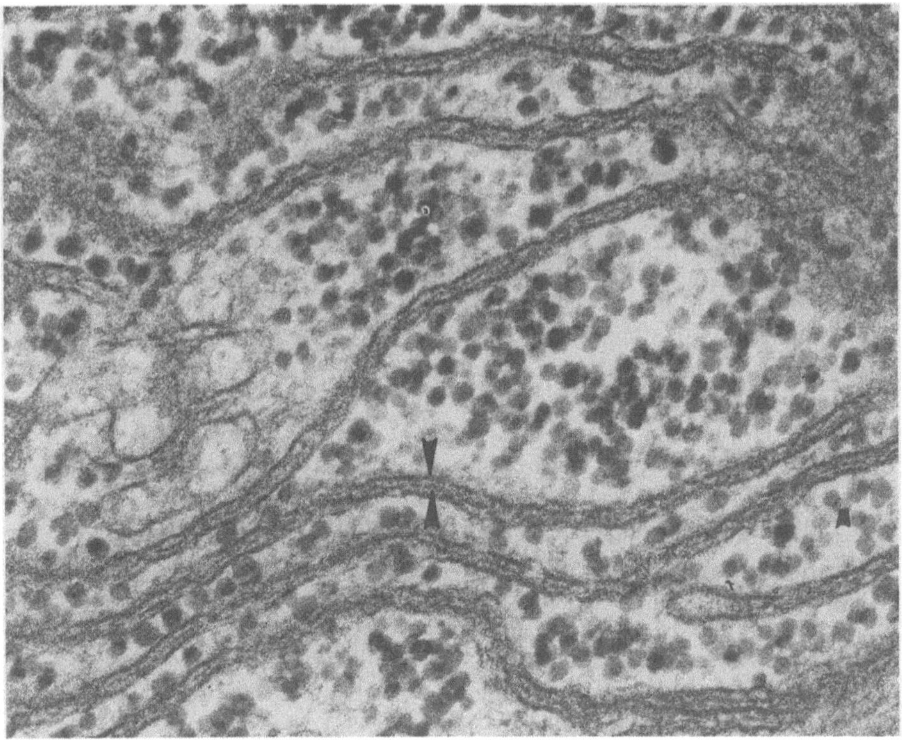

Fig. 8. High-magnification view of type B cisterns of extended junctional SR in atrial muscle cell from 49-year-old woman with mitral stenosis and regurgitation. Note the central dense lamina (*arrows*) and the outer coating. ×85,000

Severely degenerated and atrophic myocytes showed nearly complete loss of regularly arranged contractile material. They also showed proliferation or accumulation of one or more of the following cytoplasmic components, which replaced the myofibrils (Figs. 12 and 13): (1) cytoskeletal filaments, (2) tubules of free SR, (3) mitochondria, (4) glycogen granules, and (5) myelin figures and lysosomal residual bodies.

Clusters of small, atrophic, severely altered muscle cells that contained practically no cell organelles other than cytoskeletal filaments and very few tubules of free SR, masses of Z-band material, or aggregates of hexagonally arranged tubules were invariably observed in biopsies showing severe degenerative changes. These cells were connected to each other by junctions similar to those of more normal myocytes. Only by these features could they be identified as atrial myocytes.

Fig. 9. Clusters of spherical microparticles are present in space between dissociating membranes of intercellular junctions between muscle cells in left atrium of 61-year-old woman who underwent aortic and mitral valvular replacement for treatment of aortic and mitral stenosis and regurgitation. Note fragment of nexus (*arrows*) in disc space. × 44,000. *Inset* shows high magnification view of such a nexus fragment with typical substructure. × 96,500 ▷

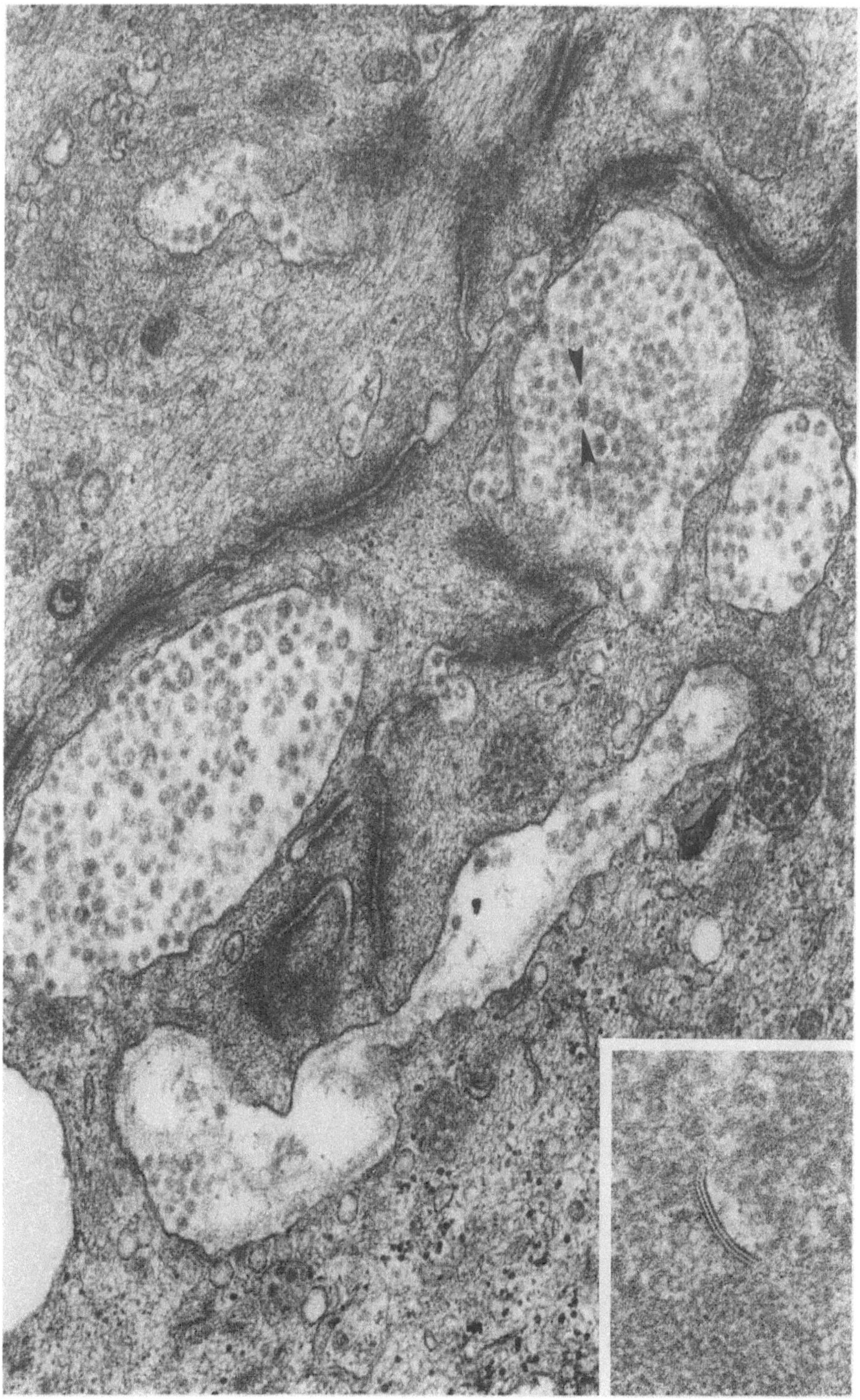

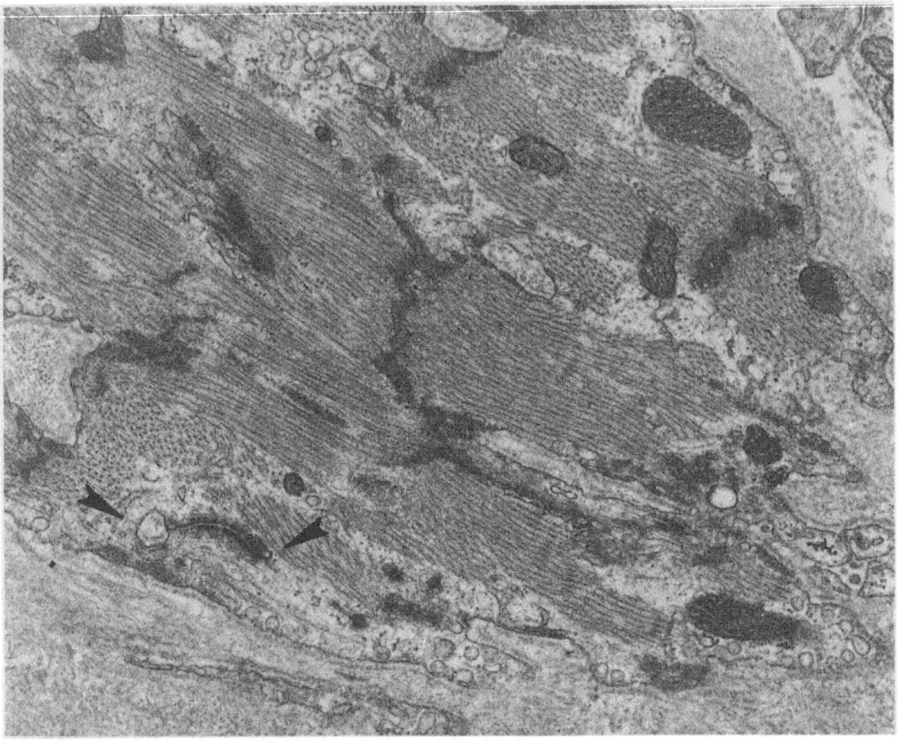

10

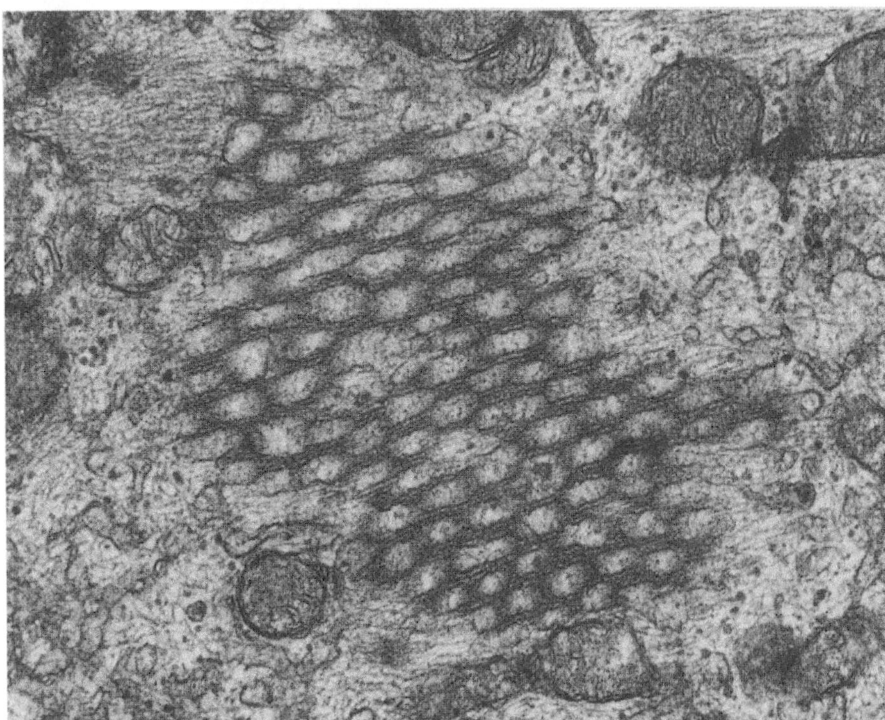

11

Severely degenerated myocytes commonly were completely isolated from other cells by fibrotic tissue, but occasionally were connected by junctional areas to only mildly or moderately degenerated cells.

Discussion

The observations described in this communication show that a large variety of changes of hypertrophy and degeneration are present in left atrial myocardium of patients undergoing operative repair of mitral valvular disease. These changes appeared similar to those in left and right ventricular myocardium of patients with hypertrophy due to various causes [1–5]. However, certain alterations were much more severe in atrial muscle of patients with mitral valvular disease.

Other alterations, such as the two types of complexes of cisterns of extended junctional SR, have not been reported in human ventricular myocardium. From our experience with a large number of myocardial biopsies, it is clearly evident that atrial muscle cells can develop degenerative changes that greatly exceed in extent and severity those that occur in ventricular muscle cells. The ultrastructural features of severely degenerated atrial muscle cells suggest that they contribute very little to contractile function since they contain little or no regularly arranged contractile material. It must be remembered, however, that the contractile function of large, dilated atria, especially of those that are chronically fibrillating, is very minimal, and that the development of comparable degenerative changes in ventricular myocardium would be incompatible with survial of the patient.

Changes in Contractile Elements

The sizes of left atrial myocytes were variable in each of the 14 patients. These variations would appear to reflect not only differences in the numbers of new sarcomeres added to individual muscle cells during hypertrophy, but also differences in the degree to which regressive changes (atrophy) occur in the late stages of cellular degeneration.

Although a number of reports (see [3, 5, 25–27] for reviews) have dealt with morphologic aspects of sarcomerogenesis in cardiac muscle cells, this process needs further elucidation. There is general agreement that Z-band material is involved in the formation of new sarcomeres. The role of extensive accumulations of Z-band-like material is less clear. Bishop and Cole [25] and Bishop [27] found masses of Z-band material in dogs in which banding of the pulmonary artery [25] or aorta [27] had led to hypertrophy and congestive heart failure, but not in

◁ Fig. 10. Atrial muscle cell (same patient as in Fig. 4) is isolated from its neighbors and shows an intracytoplasmic junction (*arrows*), accumulations of Z-band material, thickened basement membranes, and tapered ends that terminate free in the interstitium. ×24,150

Fig. 11. Aggregate of hexagonally arranged tubules of free SR associated with thin (actin) myofilaments is present in degenerated atrial muscle cell (same patient as in Fig. 6). Note large numbers of disorganized 100-Å filaments. ×50,000

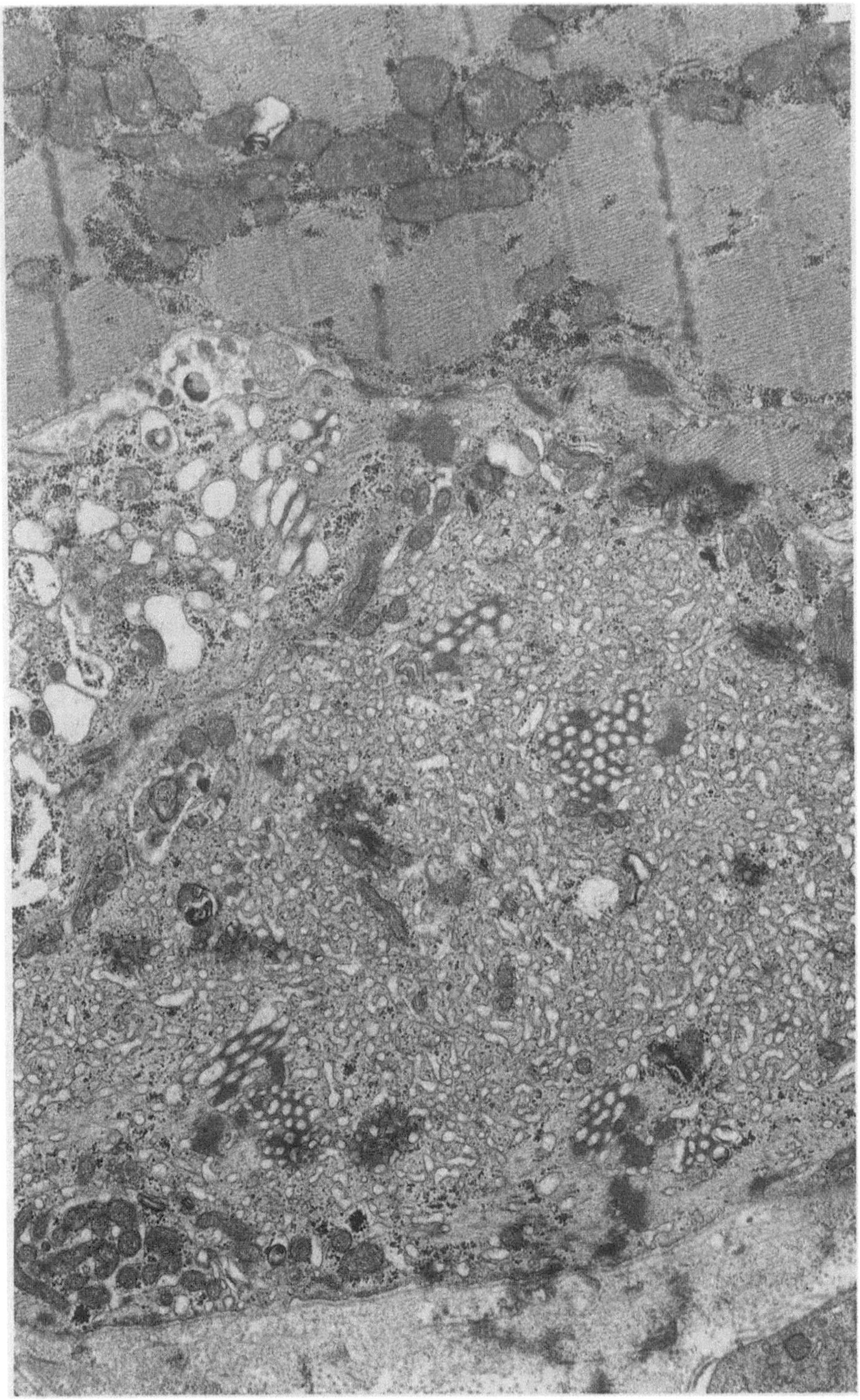

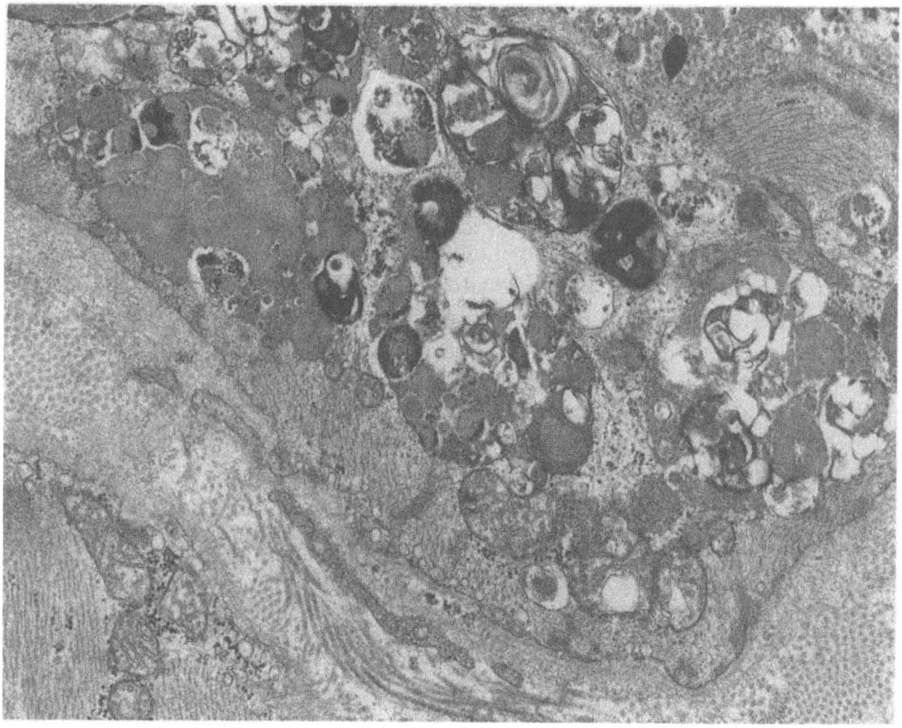

Fig. 13. Severely degenerated atrial muscle cell (same patients as in Figs. 6, 11, and 12) contains few myofibrils and mitochondria, and is filled with large, pleomorphic residual bodies. ×22,000

normal newborn dogs in which the cardiac weight was increasing at an extremely rapid rate [27]. These observations indicate that normal formation of sarcomeres need not be accompanied by formation of masses of Z-band material. We consider that the various forms of intramyofibrillar and subsarcolemmal accumulations of Z-band material observed in hypertrophied atrial muscle cells are indicative of an imbalance between the rates of synthesis of Z-band material and of other myofibrillar components. The occurrence of masses of Z-band material, particularly those having a paracrystalline substructure, which were the sites of attachment of many thin (actin) filaments not associated with thick (myosin) filaments, also suggests some form of interference with completion of sarcomerogenesis. For the preceding reasons, and because of extensive evidence derived from studies of skeletal muscle (see [5] for review), we conclude that such Z-band changes are indicative of abortive rather than of normally proceeding sarcomerogenesis.

◁ Fig. 12. View of degenerated atrial muscle cells (same patient as in Figs. 6 and 11) that have lost practically all their contractile elements and are filled with tubular aggregates and variably dilated tubules of SR. These cells are connected to a nondegenerated cell (*top*) by a side-to-side junction. ×16,500

Changes in SR

Proliferation of tubules of free SR has been reported in human atrial [10, 12, 13, 16, 17] and ventricular [3–5, 31] myocardium in various pathologic conditions. Therefore, this change is not indicative of a specific type of heart disease. Proliferation of tubules of free SR may represent an effort of the cardiac muscle cell to compensate for decreased contractile function caused by the lysis of myofibrils [17]. Accumulation of Z-band material and proliferation of tubules of free SR seem to be prerequisites for the occurrence of aggregates of hexagonally arranged tubules of SR. Such aggregates [16, 17, 31] apparently are formed by penetration of SR tubules into widened Z bands and become very regularly spaced in later stages of their development. Hexagonally arranged tubules of SR occasionally occur in human ventricular myocardium [31], but they were found in atrial myocardium of each of the patients in the present study.

Proliferation of components of SR in atrial muscle cells involved not only the tubules of free SR but also components of the extended junctional SR. These components formed two distinct types of complexes or aggregates of cisterns, which differed from one another in regard to the width of the cisterns, the presence or absence of a central dense lamina, and the separation of adjacent cisterns by layers of glycogen granules. We regard the formation of both of these types of cysternal complexes as extreme forms of overdevelopment of extended junctional SR in atrial muscle [17].

Interstitial Fibrosis and Cellular Dissociation

Atrial biopsies from all patients exhibited interstitial fibrosis of a severity seldom found in ventricular myocardium with hypertrophy of any cause. Atrial cells undergoing dissociation from each other were most frequently found in fibrotic areas. Separation of adjacent cells would impair not only their electric coupling but also the tension development that normally is exerted upon a given cell by the contraction of adjacent cells. As is well known from studies of denervation atrophy of skeletal muscle, both kinds of abnormalities can cause muscle cells to undergo degeneration and atrophy. Separation appears to start with dilatation of unspecialized regions of intercalated discs and side-to-side junctions, finally leading to complete dissociation of all junctional components. The affected areas of specialized components of intercellular junctions undergo a remodeling process that has characteristic morphologic manifestations. Intracytoplasmic junctions [32] are believed to be areas that presumably were involved in the formation of junctions between two different cells but now form junctions between two apposed areas of one given cell. The occurrence of spherical microparticles at the periphery of dissociating cells also is related to the remodeling of cell surfaces, particularly those of intercellular junctions [33].

Cellular degeneration was found more frequently in patients with mitral regurgitation than in patients with mitral stenosis. Degeneration also was more frequent in patients with atrial fibrillation than in patients with normal sinus rhythm. Although they need to be confirmed by studying a larger group of patients, these findings suggest: 1. that the atria (as do the ventricles) tolerate pressure overloading better than volume overloading, and 2. that the presence of chronic atrial fibrillation in patients with mitral valvular disease correlates well with the occurrence of severe degeneration of atrial muscle cells.

Summary

Light and electron-microscopic observations of left atrial biopsies of 14 patients undergoing operative repair of mitral valvular disease are described. In fibrotic areas, present in all biopsies, the muscle cells were frequently isolated from each other and exhibited degenerative changes of variable severity. These changes consisted of lysis of myofibrils, with preferential loss of myosin filaments; proliferation of Z-band material; increased content of cytoskeletal (100-Å diameter) filaments; proliferation of elements of sarcoplasmic reticulum (SR), with formation of aggregates of hexagonally arranged tubules of free SR and of large complexes of cisterns of extended junctional SR; dissociation of intercellular junctions, with formation of spherical microparticles and intracytoplasmic junctions; and accumulation of lysosomal degradation products. These changes were believed to indicate the end stages of hypertrophy of atrial muscle cells.

References

1. Ferrans, V.J., Massumi, R.A., Shugoll, G.I., Ali, N., Roberts, W.C.: Ultrastructural studies of myocardial biopsies in 45 patients with obstructive or congestive cardiomyopathy. In: Recent Advances in Studies on Cardiac Structure and Metabolism, Vol. II, The Cardiomyopathies. Bajusz, E., Rona, G., Brink, A.J., Lochner, A. (eds.). Baltimore: University Park Press 1973, pp. 231–272
2. Maron, B.J., Ferrans, V.J., Jones, M.: The spectrum of degenerative changes in hypertrophied human cardiac muscle cells: an ultrastructural study. In: Recent Advances in Studies on Cardiac Structure and Metabolism, Vol. VIII, The Cardiac Sarcoplasm. Roy, P.-E., Harris, P. (eds.). Baltimore: University Park Press 1975, pp. 447–466
3. Jones, M., Ferrans, V.J., Morrow, A.G., Roberts, W.C.: Ultrastructure of crista supraventricularis muscle in patients with congenital heart diseases associated with right ventricular outflow tract obstruction. Circulation *51*, 39–67 (1975)
4. Maron, B.J., Ferrans, V.J., Roberts, W.C.: Myocardial ultrastructure in patients with chronic aortic valvular disease. Amer. J. Cardiol. *35*, 725–739 (1975)
5. Maron, B.J., Ferrans, V.J., Roberts, W.C.: Ultrastructural features of degenerated cardiac muscle cells in patients with cardiac hypertrophy. Amer. J. Pathol. *79*, 387–434 (1975)
6. Ben-Ishay, Z., Davies, A.M., Laufer, A.: Fibrogenesis in the human myocardium: an electron microscopic study. Exp. mol. Pathol. *8*, 358–369 (1968)
7. Côté, G., Mohiuddin, S.M., Roy, P.-E.: Occurrence of Z-band widening in human atrial cells. Exp. mol. Pathol. *13*, 307–318 (1970)
8. Laufer, A., Garces, C.J., Ron, N., Friedman, I., Borman, J.B.: Morphological and immunological studies in valvular heart surgery. Pathol. Microbiol. *36*, 230–242 (1970)
9. Roy, P.-E., Morin, P.J.: Variations of the Z band in human auricular appendages. Lab. Invest. *25*, 422–426 (1971)
10. Roy, P.-E., Dorais, J., Morin, P.J.: Les foyers de nécrose intracellulaire focale dans le muscle cardiaque humain. Ann. anat. Pathol. (Paris) *17*, 39–51 (1972)
11. Roy, P.-E., Morin, P.J.: Dilatations of transverse tubules and of the intercalated disc in human cardiac muscle. J. mol. cell. Cardiol. *4*, 337–343 (1972)
12. Fenoglio, J.J., Wagner, B.M.: Studies in rheumatic fever. VI. Ultrastructure of chronic rheumatic heart disease. Amer. J. Pathol. *73*, 623–640 (1973)

13. Legato, M.J., Bull, M.B., Ferrer, M.I.: Atrial ultrastructure in patients with fixed intraatrial block. Chest *65*, 252–261 (1974)
14. Tomisawa, M., Onouchi, Z., Goto, M., Nakata, K., Kusunoki, T., Asazuma, S., Watanabe, T., Hashimoto, I.: Congenital left atrial enlargement. A case report with special reference to myocardial fine structure. Jap. Circulat. J. *39*, 417–424 (1975)
15. Stein, A.A., Thibodeau, F., Stranahan, A.: Electron microscopic studies of human myocardium. J. Amer. med. Ass. (Chicago) *182*, 537–540 (1962)
16. Mitsui, H., Kawamura, K., Ishizawa, K., Ohmae, M., Kawai, C.: "Tubular aggregates" in human atrial myocardial cells. J. clin. electron. Microsc. *8*, 311–312 (1975)
17. Thiedemann, K.-U., Ferrans, V.J.: Ultrastructure of sarcoplasmic reticulum in atrial myocardium of patients with mitral valvular disease. Amer. J. Pathol. *83*, 1–38 (1976)
18. Lannigan, R.A., Zaki, S.A.: Ultrastructure of the normal atrial endocardium. Brit. Heart J. *28*, 785–795 (1966)
19. Lannigan, R.A., Zaki, S.A.: Ultrastructure of the myocardium of the atrial appendage. Brit. Heart J. *28*, 796–807 (1966)
20. McNutt, N.S., Fawcett, D.W.: The ultrastructure of the cat myocardium. II. Atrial muscle. J. Cell Biol. *43*, 46–67 (1969)
21. Jamieson, J.D., Palade, G.E.: Specific granules in atrial muscle cells. J. Cell Biol. *23*, 151–172 (1964)
22. Bencosme, S.A., Berger, J.M.: Specific granules in mammalian and non-mammalian cardiocytes. In: Methods and Achievements in Experimental Pathology, Vol. V. Bajusz, E., Jasmin, G. (eds.). Basle: Karger 1971, pp. 173–213
23. Berger, J.M., Rona, G.: Function and fine structural heterogeneity of atrial cardiocytes. In: Methods and Achievements in Experimental Pathology, Vol. V. Bajusz, E., Jasmin, G. (eds.). Basle: Karger 1971, pp. 540–590
24. Freeman, J., Spurlock, B.: A new epoxy embedment for electron microscopy. J. Cell Biol. *13*, 437–443 (1962)
25. Bishop, S.P., Cole, C.R.: Ultrastructural changes in the canine myocardium with right ventricular hypertrophy and congestive heart failure. Lab. Invest. *20*, 219–229 (1969)
26. Legato, M.J.: Sarcomerogenesis in human myocardium. J. mol. cell. Cardiol. *1*, 425–437 (1970)
27. Bishop, S.P.: Effect of aortic stenosis on myocardial cell growth, hyperplasia, and ultrastructure in neonatal dogs. In: Recent Advances in Studies on Cardiac Structure and Metabolism, Vol. III, Myocardial Metabolism. Dhalla, N.S. (ed.). Baltimore: University Park Press 1973, pp. 637–656
28. Jewett, P.H., Sommer, J.R., Johnson, E.A.: Cardiac muscle. Its ultrastructure in the finch and hummingbird with special reference to the sarcoplasmic reticulum. J. Cell Biol. *49*, 50–65 (1971)
29. Jewett, P.H., Leonard, S.D., Sommer, J.R.: Chicken cardiac muscle. Its exclusive extended junctional sarcoplasmic reticulum and sarcoplasmic reticulum fenestration. J. Cell Biol. *56*, 595–609 (1973)
30. Sommer, J.R., Jewett, P.H.: Cardiac muscle: A comparative ultrastructural, anatomical view. In: Cardiac Hypertrophy. Alpert, N.R. (ed.). New York: Academic Press 1971, pp. 89–106
31. Maron, B.J., Ferrans, V.J.: Aggregates of tubules in human cardiac muscle cells. J. mol. cell. Cardiol. *6*, 249–264 (1974)
32. Buja, L.M., Ferrans, V.J., Maron, B.J.: Intracytoplasmic junctions in cardiac muscle cells. Amer. J. Pathol. *74*, 613–647 (1974)
33. Ferrans, V.J., Thiedemann, K.-U., Maron, B.J., Jones, M., Roberts, W.C.: Spherical microparticles in human myocardium. An ultrastructural study. Lab. Invest. *35*, 349–368 (1976)

13. Hypertrophic and Degenerative Changes of the Myocardium and the Influence of Ischemia During Cardiac Surgery

JUTTA SCHAPER, F. SCHWARZ, and F. HEHRLEIN

Introduction

In a previous study [3] ultrastructural changes occurring in human myocardial tissue during ischemia and during reperfusion after ischemia were investigated in order to evaluate the tolerable duration of induced cardiac arrest during open-heart surgery. It was concluded that 45 min of ischemia resulted in a moderate degree of myocardial damage and a relatively fast recovery of the tissue structure during reperfusion of the heart. However, tolerance to ischemia as indicated by ultrastructural changes was not the same in all patients.

In our study [3] human hearts with aortic valve defects showed hypertrophy and in most cases the hypertrophied myocardium exhibited degenerative changes of subcellular structures. We therefore tried to determine to what extent the degree of hypertrophy influenced the tolerance to ischemia during cardiac surgery.

Material and Methods

In 15 patients with aortic valve disease (stenosis or insufficiency or a combination of both, see Table 1) left ventricular catheterization including ventriculography were carried out. From the hemodynamic data, EF was used as an indicator of left ventricular function. The angiographically determined muscle mass (g/m^2 body surface) served as a measure of the degree of hypertrophy. Replacement of the diseased aortic valve was carried out under total cardiopulmonary bypass. Cardiac standstill was induced by injection of a precooled (4 °C) potassium-free solution containing procain, magnesium aspartate, and sorbitol [1] which was injected directly into the aortic root at 2 ml/kg body weight after aortic cross clamping. After replacement of the valve, coronary perfusion was reestablished, resulting in spontaneous rhythmic activity of the heart. For ultrastructural investigations, three needle biopsies were taken from the anterior wall of the left ventricle. The first tissue sample was removed before induction of cardiac arrest and served as control for the quality of histologic fixation. The second biopsy was taken at the end of cardiac standstill, which was after an ischemic period of 45 min in all patients. Before closure of the pericardium and after coronary perfusion had been reestablished for at least 20 min, the third biopsy was removed. All tissue samples were immediately fixed in cold 3% glutaraldehyde buffered in 0.1 *M* cacodylate and embedded in Epon. Semithin sections were stained with toluidine blue. By means of light microscopy, areas free of artifacts were chosen

Table 1. Fifteen patients with aortic valve defects were ranged according to their angiographically determined muscle mass, which stands for the degree of cardiac hypertrophy. Cardiac function, as indicated by EF, declines with increasing muscle mass.

Patient	Age (yr.)	Diagnosis	Mm	EF	CM changes[a]	Ischemic injury score[a]
Group A: Muscle mass (< 200 g/m^2)						
H.E.	26	A.I.	141	62	1	1
S.E.	67	A.S.	163	84	1	1
D.G.	19	A.I.	184	63	1	1
G.K.	35	A.I.	190	61	1	2
B.R.	51	A.I. + A.S.	200	60	1	1
P.M.	45	A.S.	200	57	2	1
	Mean value		180	64		
Group B: Muscle mass (> 250 g/m^2)						
V.L.	62	A.I. + A.S.	258	54	2	2
N.H.	57	A.S.	260	61	2	2
E.E.	51	A.I.	275	61	1	2
S.A.	32	A.I. + A.S.	285	58	2	2
A.D.	36	A.I. + A.S.	296	25	1	2
K.H.	21	A.I. + A.S.	306	63	1	1
B.R.	41	A.S.	334	43	2	2
B.R.	46	A.I. + A.S.	345	34	1	2
G.G.	37	A.I.	583	18	2	2
	Mean value		329	46		

[a] Scoring system for ultrastructural observations: Scores from 0–3 were employed. 0 = no changes; 1 = slight; 2 = moderate; 3 = severe changes. The same gradings were used in the evaluation of both degenerative alterations and the degree of ischemic injury

for the preparation of ultrathin sections. After staining with uranyl acetate and lead citrate the sections were viewed with a Philips EM 300 electron microscope.

Qualitative Evaluation of the Myocardial Ultrastructure

Fixation of the myocardial tissue was optimal in the control samples. The mitochondria exhibited a dense matrix, small intercristal dark granules, and undamaged cristae. The sarcomeres were regularly arranged, glycogen was present, and the T system and sarcoplasmic reticulum were not dilated. The nucleus showed normal density and normal distribution of chromatin (Fig. 1).

Many cells, however, showed degenerative changes. Both terms, degenerative and CM changes, are used interchangeably in this study. These changes consisted of:

1. Unusually large nuclei exhibiting invaginations of the nuclear membrane, irregular distribution of chromatin, and the occurrence of tubular structures (Figs. 2 and 3)
2. Loss of myofibrils and accumulation of Z-band material (Fig. 4)
3. Accumulation of large amounts of mitochondria exhibiting variable shape and size (Fig. 5)

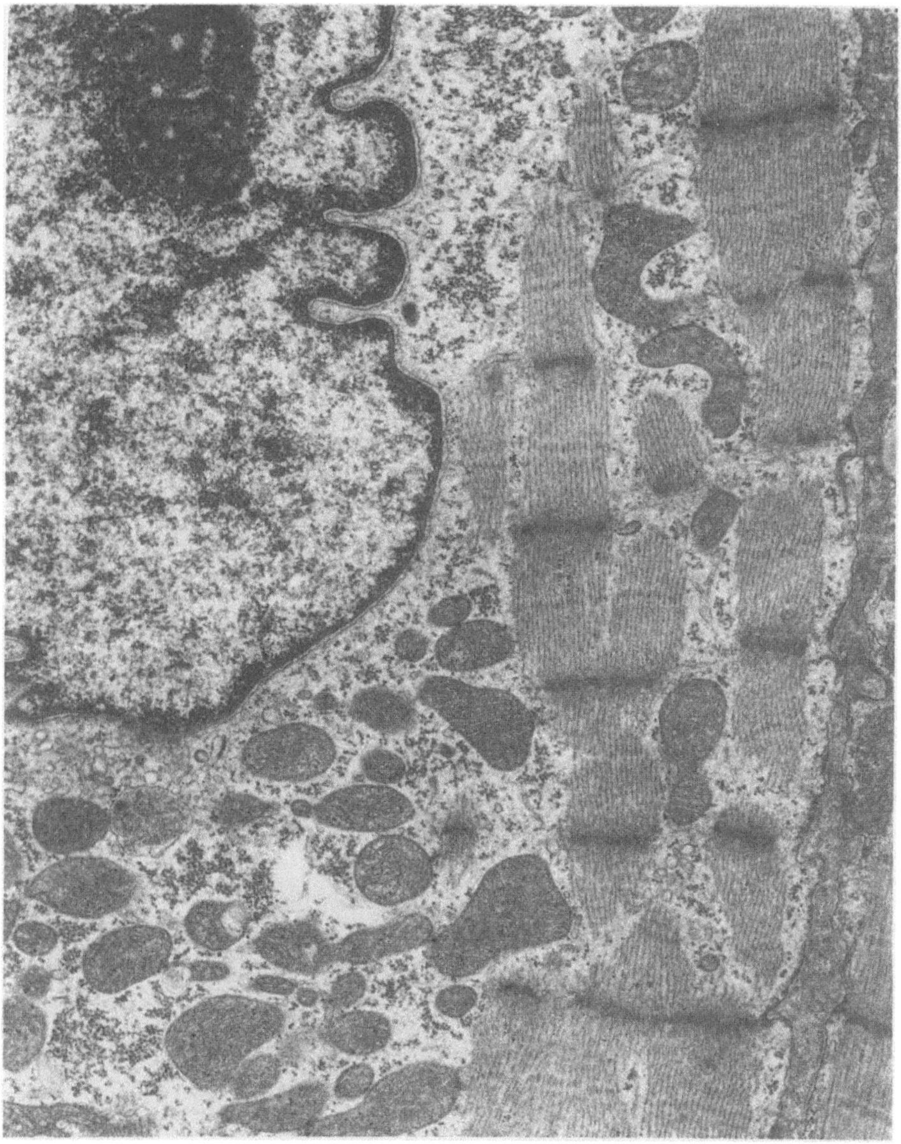

Fig. 1. Normal human myocardium. The nucleus shows normal distribution of chromatin. The mitochondria possess a dense matrix, regular cristae, and normal small dense granules. Glycogen is present. The sarcomeres have been cut tangentially. ×13800

4. Occurrence of large cytoplasmic areas devoid of contractile material, but filled with glycogen, ribosomes, and sometimes, increased amounts of sarcoplasmic reticulum (Fig. 6)
5. Presence of proliferative fibroblasts, macrophages, mast cells, and increased amounts of collagen fibers in the interstitial space

2

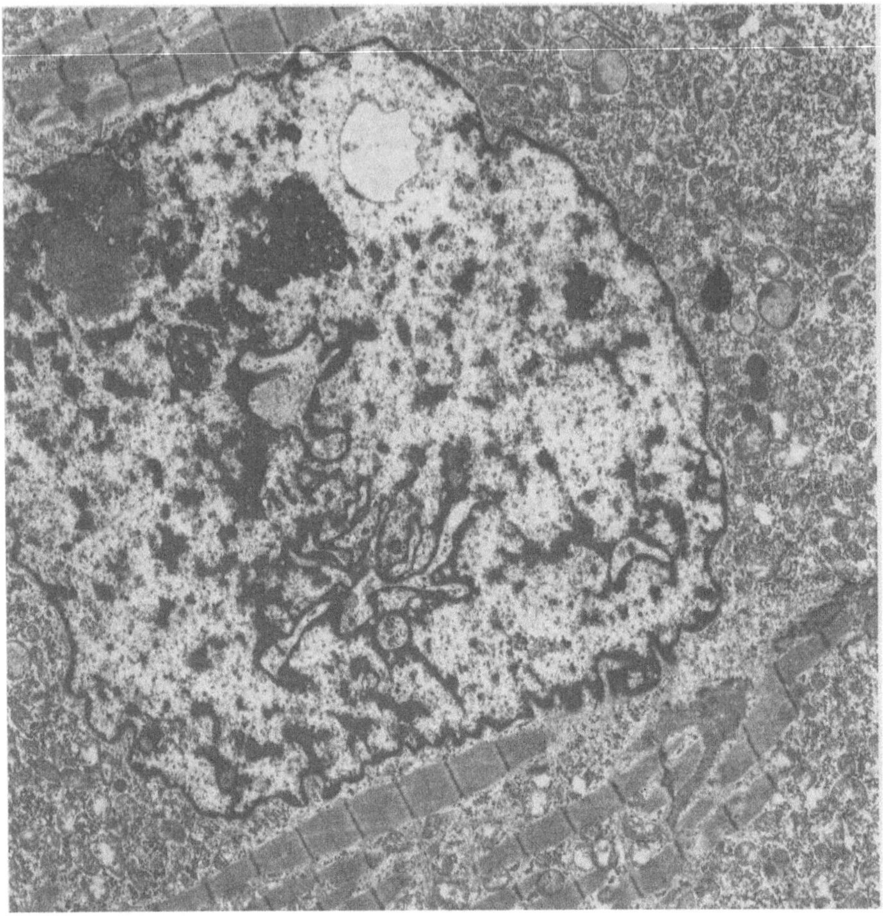

3

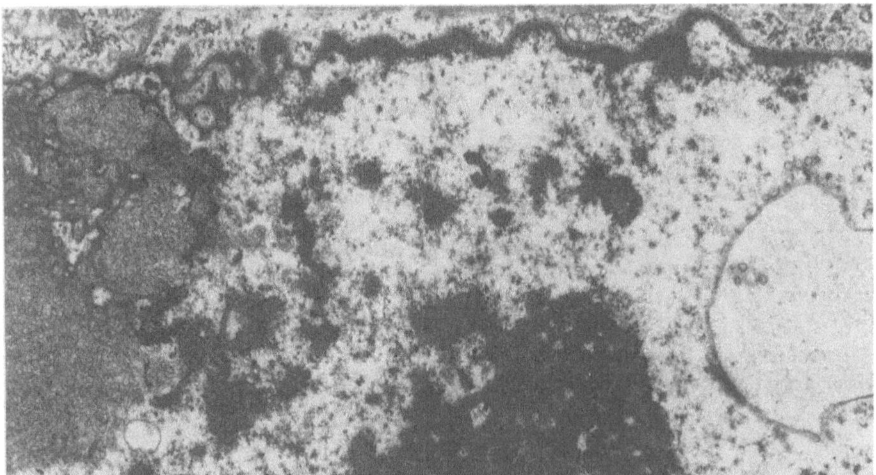

Fig. 2. Nucleus showing abnormal distribution of chromatin, numerous invaginations of the nuclear membrane, a vacuole, and tubular structures. ×9900

Fig. 3. High magnification of part of the nucleus shown in Figure 2. ×60000

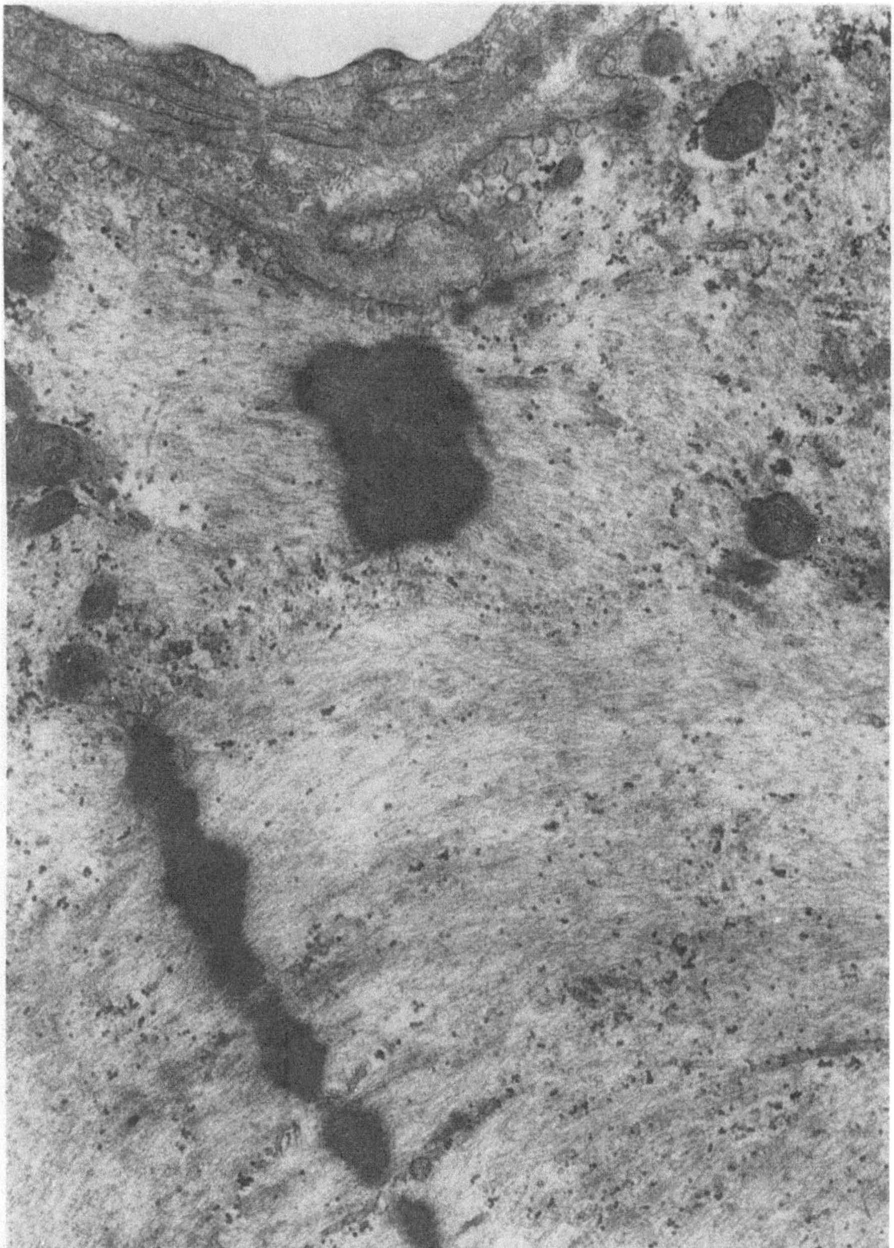

Fig. 4. Part of a myocardial cell exhibiting loss of regular contractile units. Accumulation of Z-band material and numerous fine myofibrils. × 24600

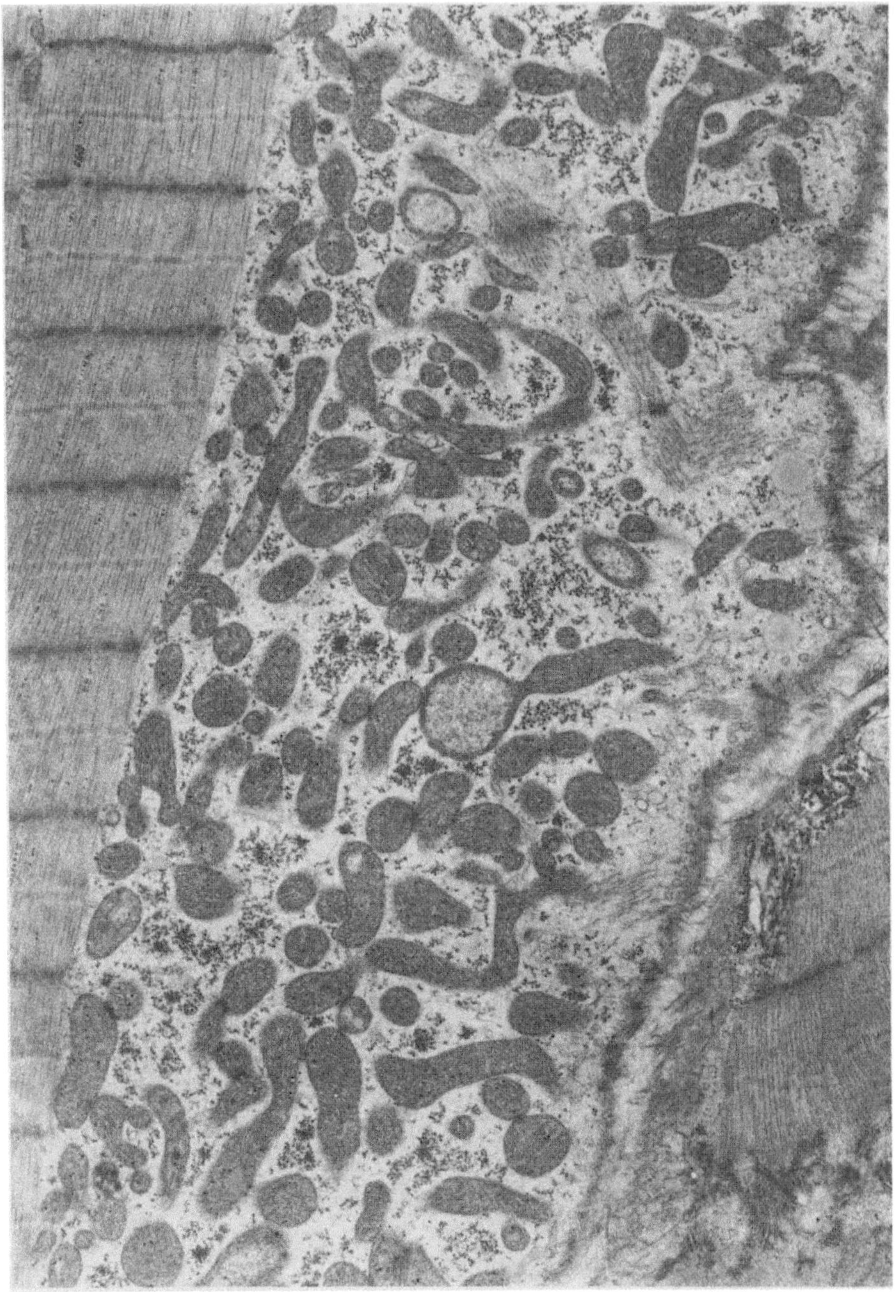

Fig. 5. Accumulation of mitochondria showing great variations in size and shape. × 13800

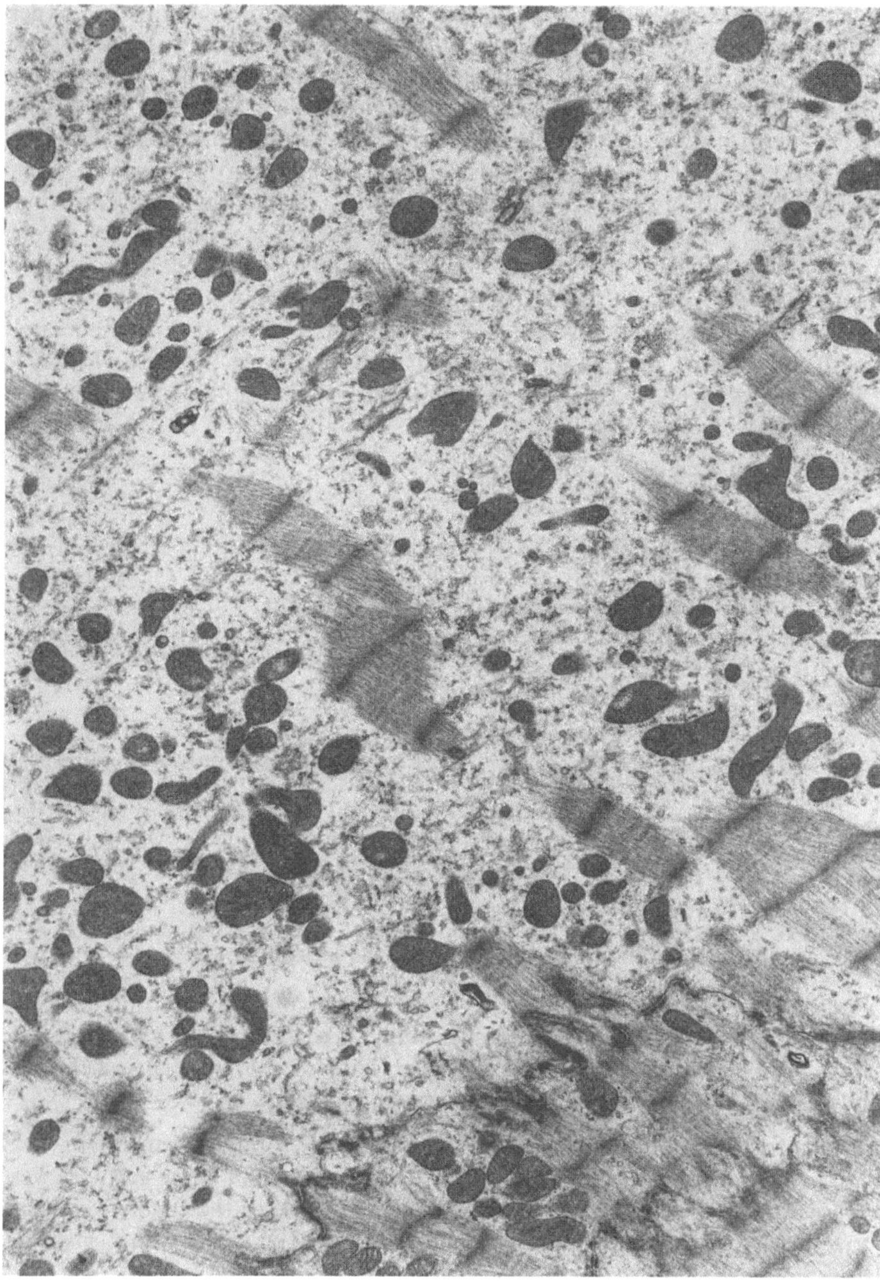

Fig. 6. Loss of contractile elements in a myocardial cell. The cytoplasm contains mitochondria, ribosomes and glycogen, T tubules and SR. ×9900

These degenerative changes were less severe than those described in hypertrophic idiopathic CM [2] or in the atria of patients with mitral valve defects [4]. The severity and frequency of ultrastructural abnormalities did not correlate with the type of aortic valve defect, as shown in Table 1.

The degenerative alterations were graded in a semiquantitative manner using a scoring system (see Table 1 for data and explanation). It was evident that in the first group of patients with a muscle mass smaller than 200 g/m^2 body surface, only slight degenerative changes were present, whereas in the second group with a much larger muscle mass both slight and moderate changes occurred. The relationship between the degree of cardiac hypertrophy and the presence of degenerative changes is shown in Figure 7. It was evident that in moderately hypertrophic hearts only slight degenerative changes were present, whereas in hearts with a severely increased muscle mass both slight and moderate degenerative changes were observed.

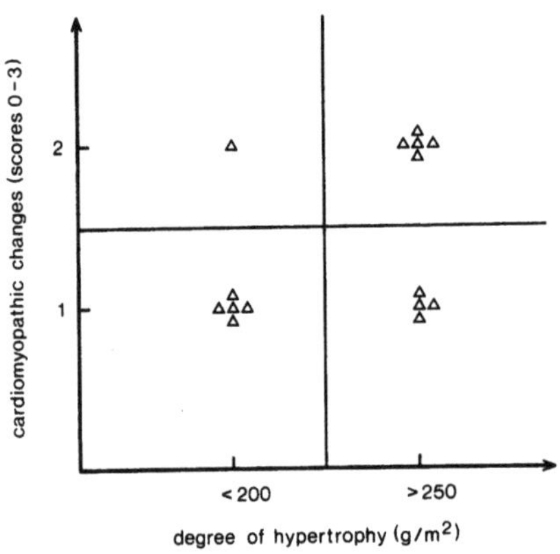

Fig. 7. In moderately hypertrophic hearts slight degenerative changes (*score 1*) are present. In hearts with severe hypertrophy (muscle mass > 250 g/m^2 body surface) slight or moderate degenerative changes were observed (*score 1 or 2*)

Tolerance to Ischemia in Human Hypertrophic Myocardium

Despite the fact that all patients had a cardiac arrest of 45 min during total cardiopulmonary bypass, the second tissue sample taken at the end of the ischemic period exhibited different degrees of ischemic injury. Myocardial ischemic injury was also evaluated using a scoring system [3] (Table 1).

a) In the first group of patients with moderate hypertrophy ischemic injury was of a slight degree (Table 1), i.e., the mitochondrial small dense granules were absent, the matric was less electron dense, and some of the cristae were fragmented or dissolved (Fig. 8). The nucleus showed slight swelling; glycogen was present; all other cell organelles were inconspicuous.

Fig. 8. Slight ischemic damage of the mitochondria after 45 min cardiac arrest. Cristae are replaced by gray flocculent material, and the normal dense granules are absent. The matrix is more electron lucent than in undamaged mitochondria. Glycogen is present. ×9900 ▷

Fig. 9. Moderate ischemic damage of the mitochondria after 45 min of cardiac arrest. Cristae are fragmented; the matrix is light. Normal dense granules are absent. Glycogen is absent. ×9900

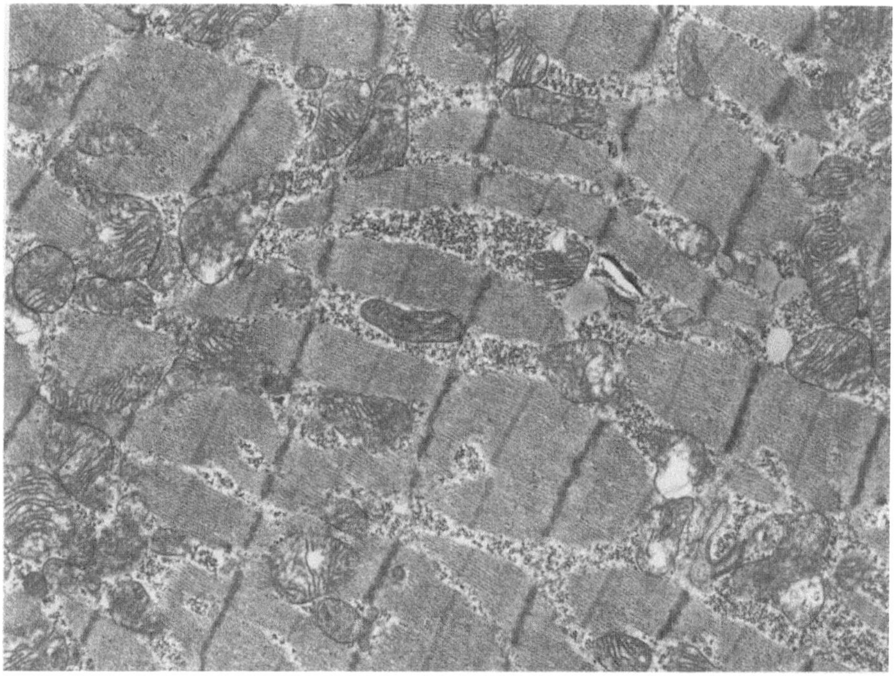

8

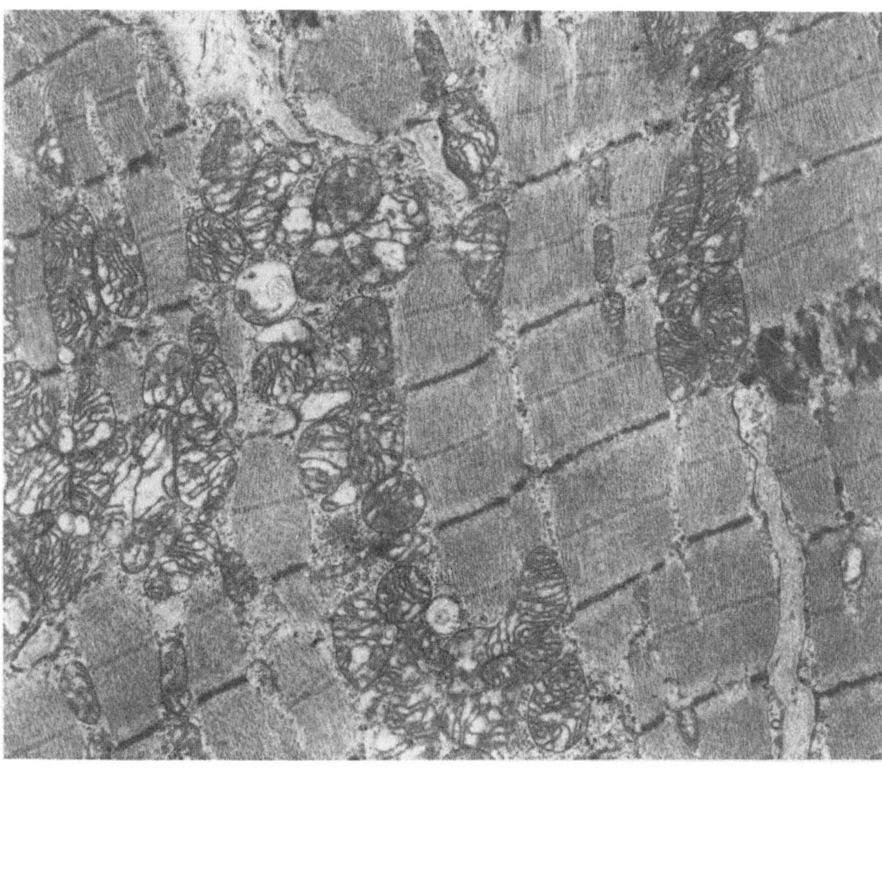

9

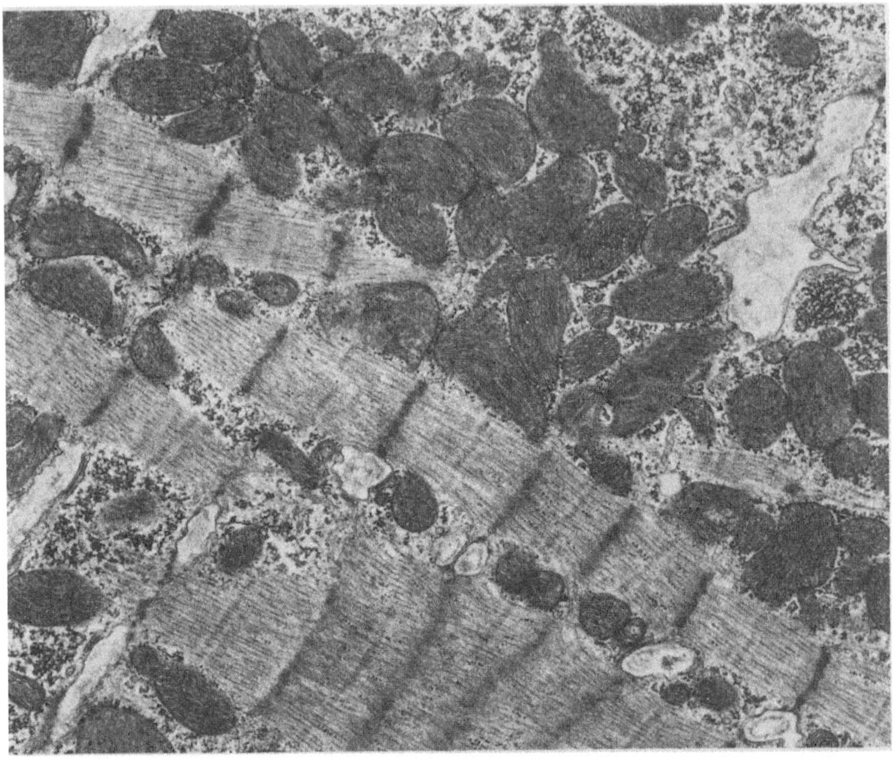
10

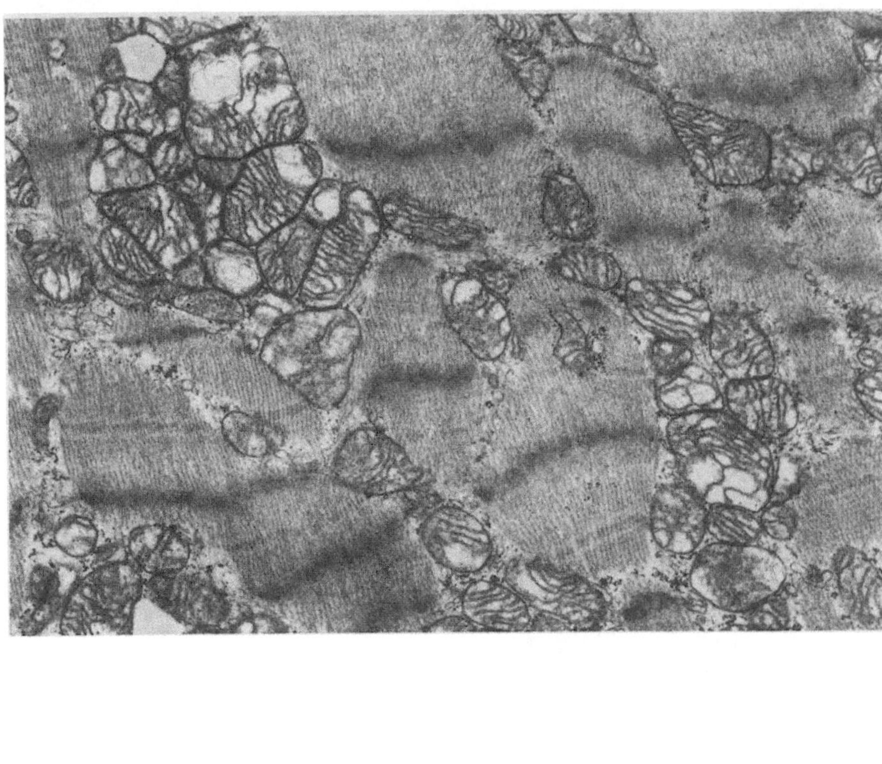
11

b) In the second group of patients ischemic injury was more pronounced: The dark mitochondrial granules were absent, the matrix was much more electron lucent, and many cristae were broken. The nuclei showed a greater degree of swelling with margination of the chromatin, but glycogen was still present and other cell components remained unchanged. Intracellular edema was absent (Fig. 9).

The tissue samples taken during coronary reperfusion of the heart showed quick recovery in the first group (Fig. 10) and a retarded but still rather good structural recovery in the second group (Fig. 11). Plotting of the scores for degenerative changes against the scores for ischemic injury (Fig. 12) showed that

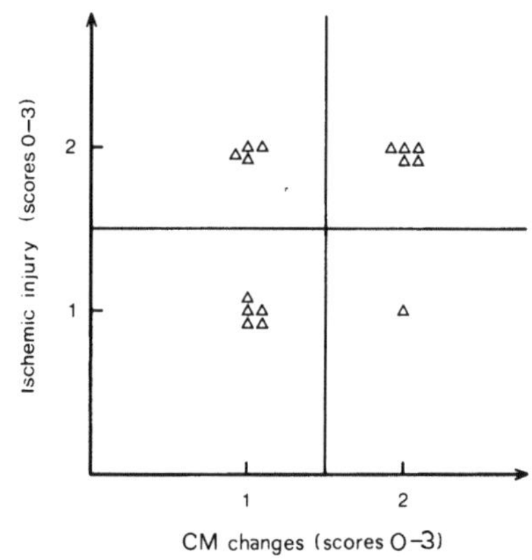

Fig. 12. In the presence of slight CM changes (*score 1*), ischemic injury is slight or moderate (*score 1 or 2*), but when moderate CM changes prevail ischemic injury is moderate (*score 2*)

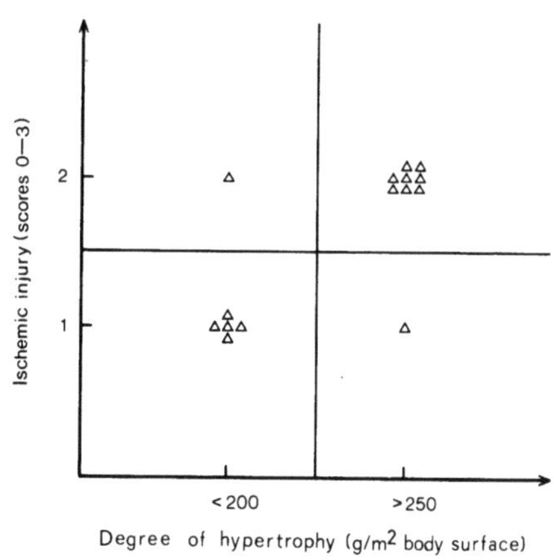

Fig. 13. Ischemic injury is slight (*score 1*) after 45 min of cardiac arrest in moderately hypertrophic hearts, but it is moderate (*score 2*) in severely hypertrophic hearts. The tolerance to ischemia during cardiac surgery decreases in severe hypertrophy

◁ Fig. 10. Mitochondria after 45 min of ischemia and 20 min of reperfusion. Normal dense granules are present, and the matrix is more electron dense than in Figure 8. × 13 800

Fig. 11. Mitochondria after 45 min of ischemia and 20 min of reperfusion. Only a few normal dense granules are present, and the number of intact cristae has somewhat increased. The matrix, however, is still more electron lucent than normal, and the gray flocculent substance is still present. A small amount of glycogen is present. × 13 800

in the presence of slight degenerative changes ischemic injury was slight or moderate, whereas in the presence of moderate degenerative changes ischemic injury of moderate degree prevailed. In moderate hypertrophy the tolerance to ischemia was better than in severely hypertrophic hearts (Fig. 13). Degenerative changes were more frequent and more severe in markedly hypertrophic hearts than in hearts with a moderately increased muscle mass. The findings of this study indicate that the tolerance to ischemia during induced cardiac arrest in heart surgery decreases with increasing hypertrophy of the heart when accompanied by degenerative subcellular changes. These findings are relevant and, it is hoped, will be helpful in finding the ideal stage at which a patient suffering from aortic valve disease should undergo surgical correction of the defect.

References

1. Kirsch, U., Rodewald, G., Kalmar, P.: Induced ischemic arrest. Clinical experience with cardioplegia in open-heart surgery. J. Thor. Cardiovasc. Surgery *63*, 121–130 (1972)
2. Maron, B., Ferrans, N.J., Jones, M.: The spectrum of degenerative changes in hypertrophied human cardiac muscle cells: An ultrastructural study. In: Recent Advances in Studies on Cardiac Structure and Metabolism. Baltimore: University Park Press 1975, Vol. III, pp. 447–466
3. Schaper, J., Hehrlein, F., Schlepper, M., Thiedemann, K.-U.: Ultrastructural alterations during ischemia and reperfusion in human hearts during cardiac surgery. J. Mol. Cell. Cardiol. *9* (1977)
4. Thiedemann, K.-U., Ferrans, V.J.: Ultrastructure of sarcoplasmic reticulum in atrial myocardium of patients with mitral valvular disease. Amer. J. Pathol. *83*, 1–24 (1976)

Ventricular Function and Angiography in Cardiomyopathies

14. Ventricular Function at Rest and During Exercise in Patients With Cardiomyopathy

W.-D. Bussmann, W. Schmidt, G. Kober, and M. Kaltenbach

In patients with diseased myocardium, ventricular function is an important factor in clinical outcome and prognosis. The capacity for exercise in patients depends on the overall ventricular contraction reserve. Many investigators have described the function of the left ventricle at rest [13, 18]. Studies of left ventricular contraction and contractility reserve during exercise, however, are rare [17, 6]. In this chapter three main aspects of ventricular function are discussed:

1. The relationship of size and volume between left and right ventricle in CM
2. Contractility and relaxation reserve in different types of CM
3. Regional contraction patterns of the left ventricle at rest and during stress (leg raising, exercise).

Relationship Between Right and Left Ventricular Volumes

It is generally accepted that CM is a diffuse disease of the whole myocardium. To verify this finding Guldner *et al.* investigated volumes of both ventricles in 40 patients with CM [10]. Volumes were determined using the biplane cine-angiographic technique and Simpson's rule [11]. It was found that enddiastolic volumes of both ventricles were equally large (Fig. 1). However, in one-third of the patients studied, left ventricular volumes were twice as large as right ventricular volumes (in Fig. 1 on the right side of the 45° axis). On the left side of the 45° axis only two patients had an excessive enlargement of the right ventricle with normal left ventricular size (Fig. 1).

These results indicate disproportionate enlargements of either the left or right ventricle. Thus, the whole heart is not evenly involved in all cases. In many patients local and regional differences caused by the disease must be anticipated, as indicated by the disproportionate increase in volume of the right or left ventricle.

Ventricular Function at Rest and During Exercise: Contractility and Relaxation Reserve in Different Types of Cardiomyopathy

The overall left ventricular function at rest and during exercise can be evaluated by measurements of left ventricular pressure, using catheters with a manometer at the tip [1]. The indices derived during isovolumic contraction and relaxation provide information on the overall contractile properties of the left ventricle. By this method regional information cannot be obtained, but the overall and

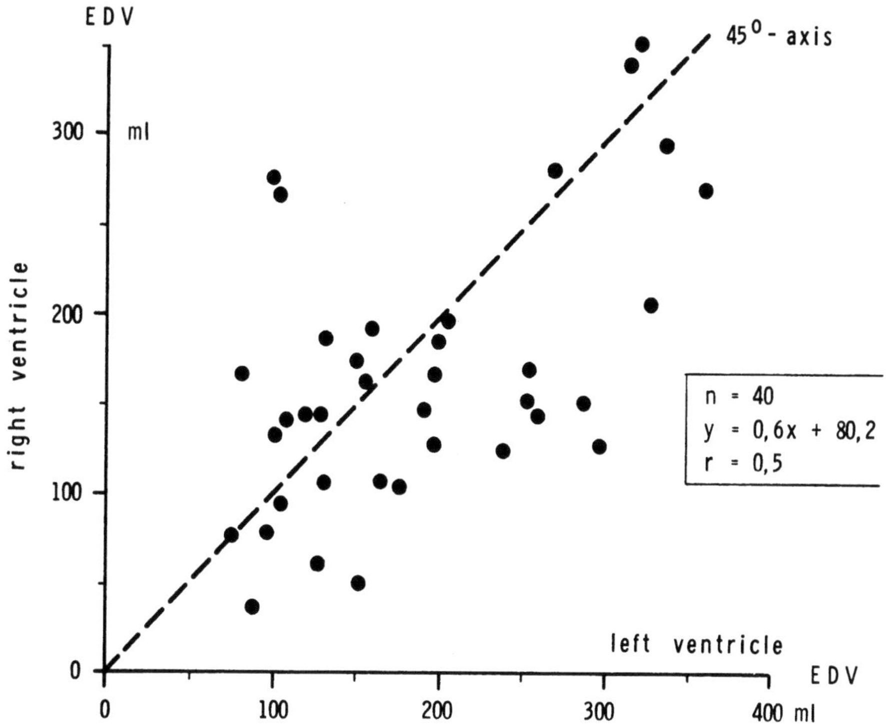

Fig. 1. Right and left ventricular volumes in 14 CM patients. EDV of both ventricles were equally large in the majority of cases. In one-third, left ventricular volume was twice as large as right ventricular volume. Two patients had enlargement of the right ventricle with normal left ventricular size

resultant left ventricular function can be determined. The latter parameters must be correlated with the basic hemodynamic data, such as left ventricular systolic and enddiastolic pressure during exercise.

Methods

Twenty-two patients were studied: in 7 with a hypertrophic CM without obstruction, diagnosis was based on a wall thickness of more than 13 mm and muscle masses above 250 ml/1.73 m^2. In 5 patients with HOCM the left ventricle had the typical angiographic configuration, muscle mass was increased and pressure gradient present at rest or upon provocation. Ten patients with COCM had a dilated left ventricle with reduced ejection fraction. Left ventricular contraction was regionally and/or locally impaired.

Physical exercise was performed on the bicycle ergometer with a work-load of 100 W, and left ventricular pressure was measured using Millar catheters with a manometer at the tip [6].

Left ventricular systolic (LVP) and enddiastolic pressure (LVEDP), maximal rate of left ventricular pressure rise ($LV dP/dt_{max}$), and maximal rate of pressure decrease during relaxation ($LV dP/dt_{min}$) were measured. Peak measured velocity of contractile elements (V_{pm} = dP/dt divided by the absolute value of P : dP/dt/P) was continuously computed by an analog device [2]. Angiographic parameters were derived from biplane left ventricular cine-angiograms at rest, i.e. endsystolic (ESV) and enddiastolic volume (EDV), ejection fraction (EF) and mean circumferential fiber shortening (mean V_{cf}).

Changes in contractility during exercise were related to changes in enddiastolic pressure. Thus, the Frank-Starling mechanism can be studied with regard to contractile state.

Results

Compared to normal controls most CM patients had decreased contractile and relaxation reserve. The 13 control patients had normal contractility of the left ventricle at rest and during exercise. The changes in contractile reserve ($\Delta dP/dt_{max}$) are plotted against changes in left ventricular enddiastolic pressure (ΔLVEDP, Fig. 2). In all cases, dP/dt_{max} increased at least 1800 mm Hg/s or more, without a simultaneous increase of enddiastolic pressure of more than 4 mm Hg. These limits are marked on Figure 2. The increase of dP/dt/P ($= V_{pm}$) was found to be at least 22 mm Hg/s, and of dP/dt_{min}, it was 1000 mm Hg/s [4]. Thus, patients with normal left ventricles had a marked increase in left ventricular contractile and relaxation properties without changes in left ventricular enddiastolic pressure.

As shown in Figure 3, only seven CM patients had a normal contractility without an increase in enddiastolic pressure. In two HOCM patients left ventricular pressure increased by more than 4 mm Hg. Almost all patients with normal contractile reserve had hypertrophic CM, indicated by increases in wall thickness.

Contractile reserve is reduced (< 1800 mm Hg/s) without increases in left ventricular enddiastolic pressure, this was classified as grade 1. All patients of grade 1 had congestive type of CM.

The other patients were classified as grade 2 and had an increase of enddiastolic pressure from 4 to over 15 mm Hg. This group included patients with severe congestive and hypertrophic CM.

Further increases in enddiastolic pressure were found in patients of grade 3 with a hypertrophic or hypertrophic-obstructive type of disease.

In five patients with asymmetric septal hypertrophy contractility reserve was large in three and low in two. In the latter two patients – despite excessive increases in enddiastolic pressure – the contractile reserve remained normal.

The maximal rate of decrease of left ventricular pressure ($\Delta dP/dt_{min}$) increased during exercise only in one of these five patients to more than 1000 mm Hg/s (Fig. 4). All other patients had a reduced reserve during relaxation. In one case, $\Delta dP/dt_{min}$ even decreased. Thus, in patients with a hypertrophic-obstructive disease, relaxation seems to be more impaired than contractile reserve. This has recently been confirmed in a larger number of patients.

A typical example is shown in Figure 5: a 34-year-old patient with a left ventricular wall thickness of 20 mm had an increase of left ventricular enddiastolic pressure to 30 mm Hg during exercise without sufficient increase of

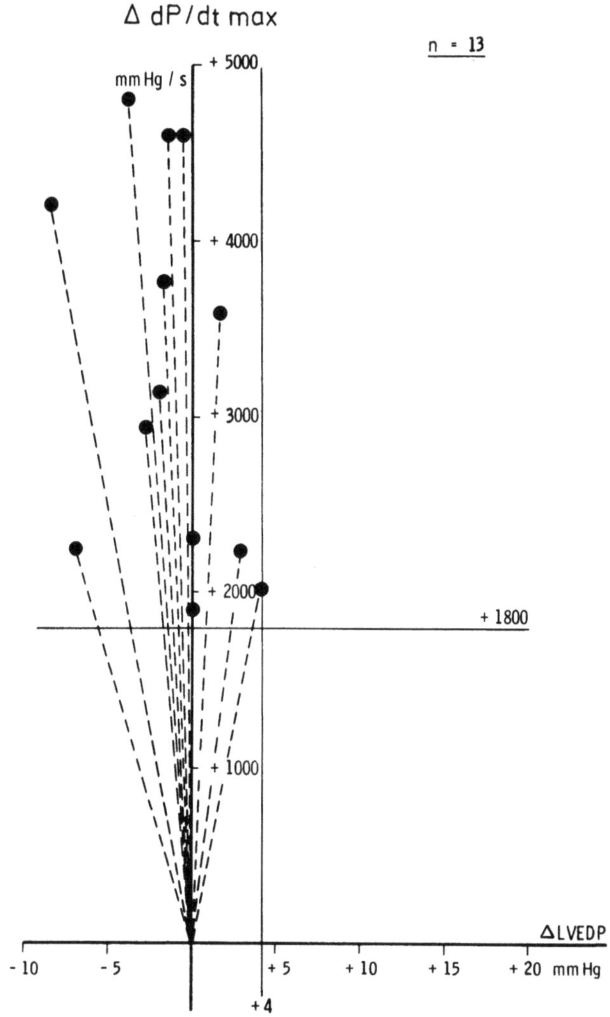

Fig. 2. Exercise in patients with normal left ventricle. $\Delta dP/dt_{max}$ increased at least 1800 mm Hg/s or more, without increase of enddiastolic pressure (ΔLVEDP) of more than 4 mm Hg

$dP/dt_{max, min}$ and dP/dt/P. The same results were found upon administration of orciprenalin.

Conclusions

1. In COCM contractility and relaxation decreased to the same extent. In patients with hypertrophic and hypertrophic-obstructive disease the relaxation reserve decreased more than the contractile function. The cause of the decreased relaxation may be due to an inhibition of diastolic filling [9].
2. Contractility and enddiastolic pressure were found to be normal during stress in patients with a *hypertrophic type* of CM (Fig. 6). In these cases the history

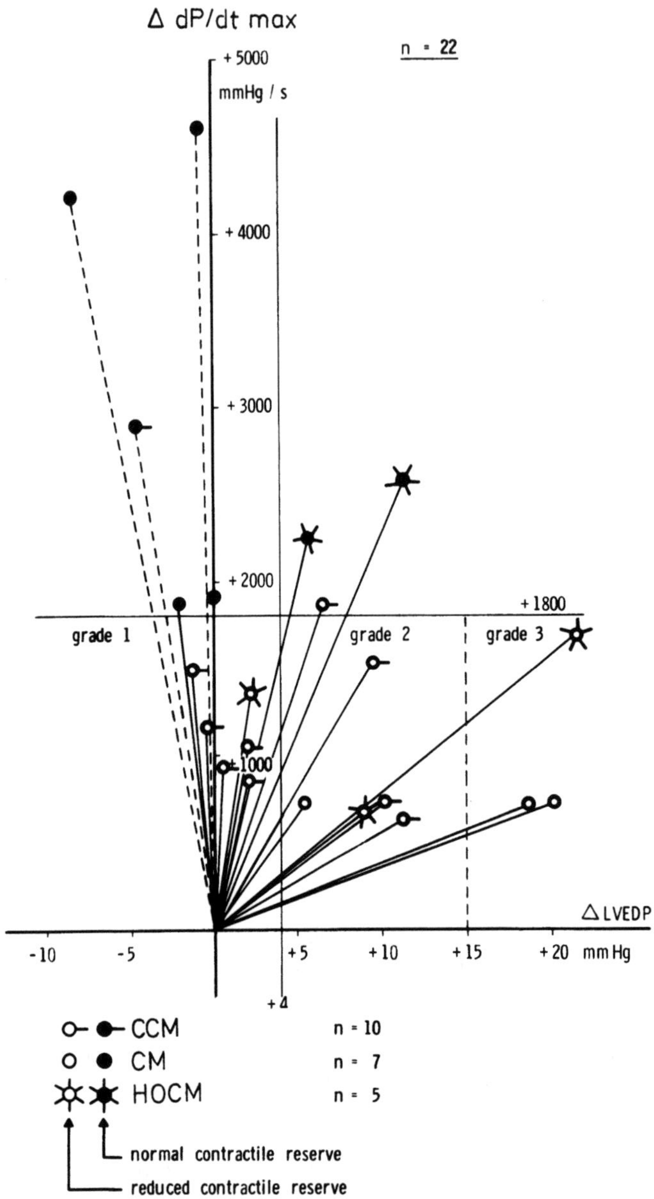

Fig. 3. Normal (*filled symbols*) and reduced (*open symbols*) contractile reserve ($\Delta\, dP/dt_{max}$) in CM patients. Patients with congestive type had reduced contractility only (*grade 1*, *left*, *lower quadrant*). Patients with severe congestive or hypertrophic CM had reduced contractile reserve and an increase of LVEDP of between 4 and 15 mm Hg (*grade 2*). Those with hypertrophic or hypertrophic-obstructive type had increase of ΔLVEDP above +15 mm Hg (*grade 3*, *right*, *lower quadrant*). In 5 patients with asymmetrical septal hypertrophy (*stars*) contractility was normal in 2 and abnormal in 3

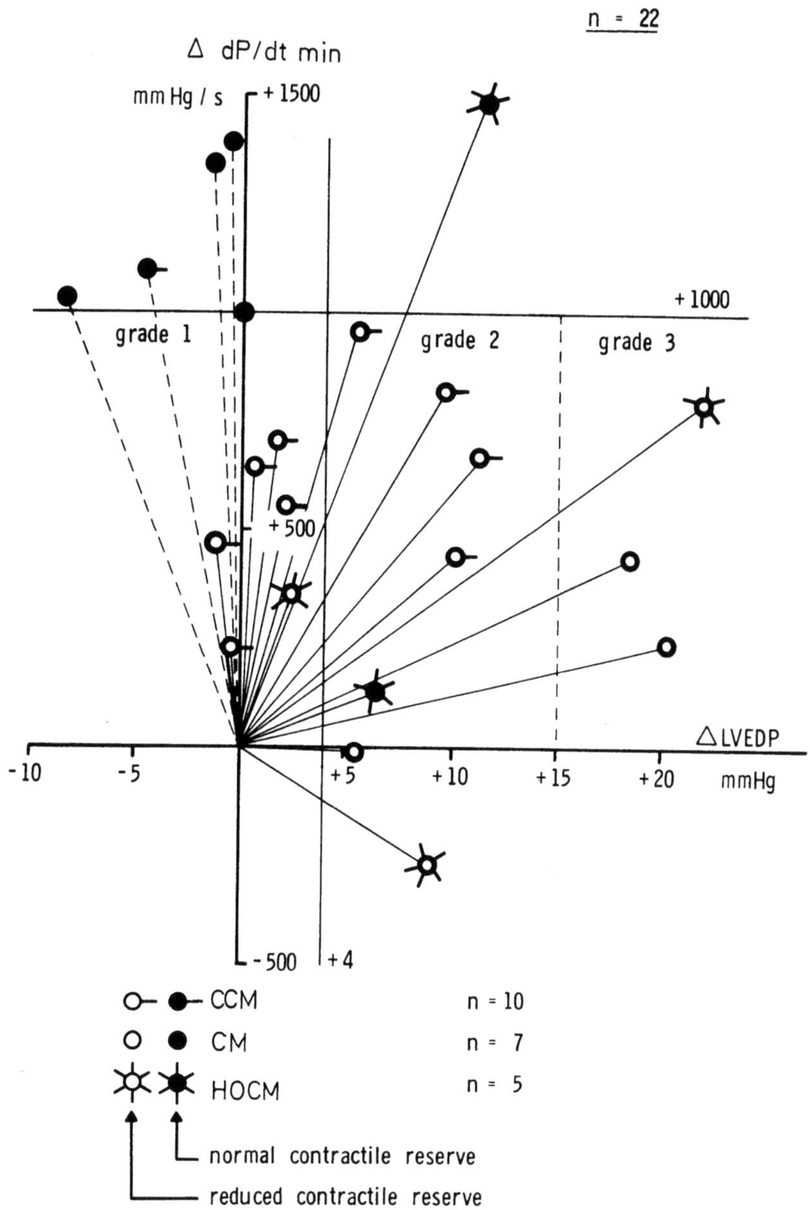

Fig. 4. Changes of maximal rate of decrease in LVP ($\Delta dP/dt_{min}$) plotted versus changes in EDP (ΔLVEDP). Reduced relaxation reserve in patients with congestive type (*grade 1*). Increase of LVEDP in patients with severe congestive or hypertrophic CM (*grades 2 and 3*). In patients with hypertrophic and hypertrophic-obstructive disease, the relaxation reserve decreased more than the contractile reserve (see Fig. 2)

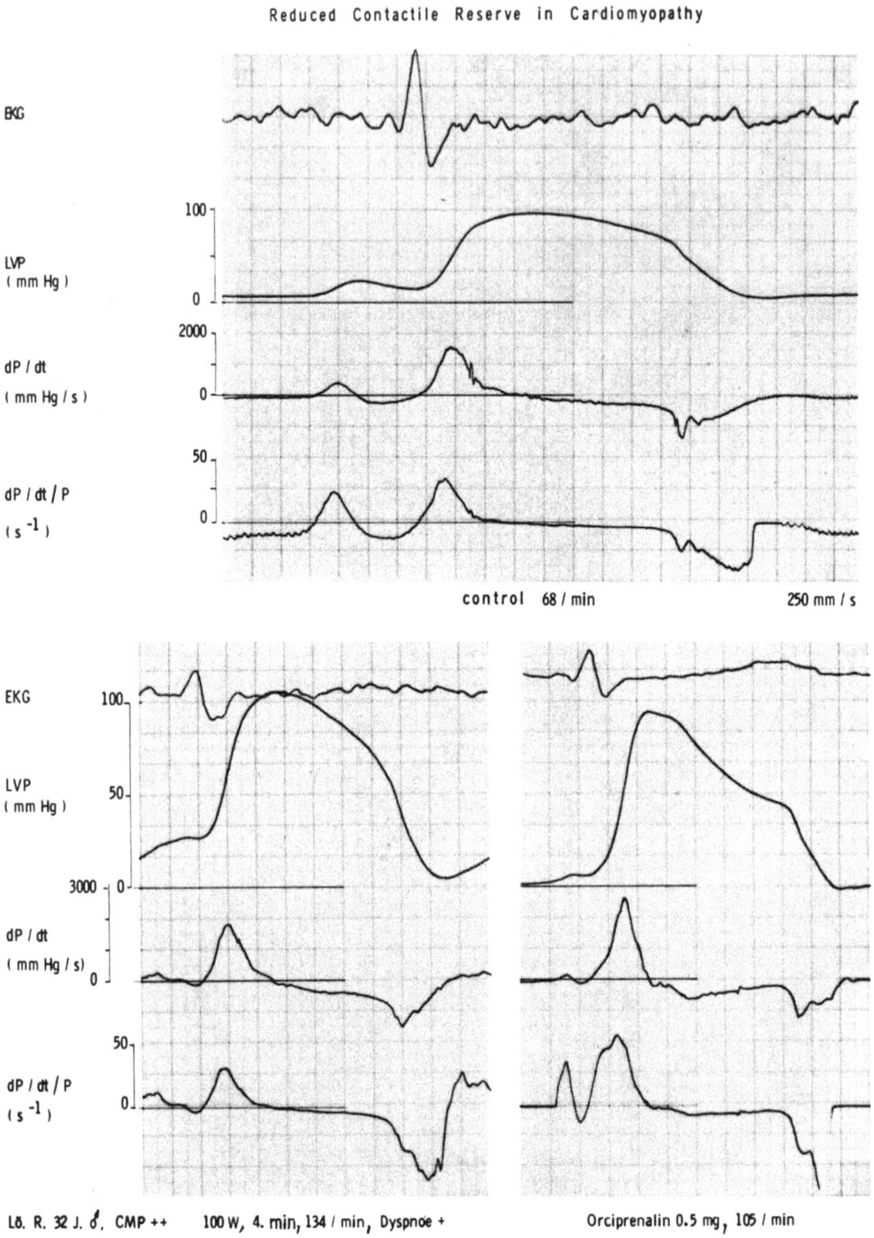

Fig. 5. Typical example of a 32-year-old patient with a left ventricular wall thickness of 20 mm. Increase of LVEDP to 30 mm Hg during exercise. Reduced contractile and relaxation reserve during exercise or administration of orciprenalin

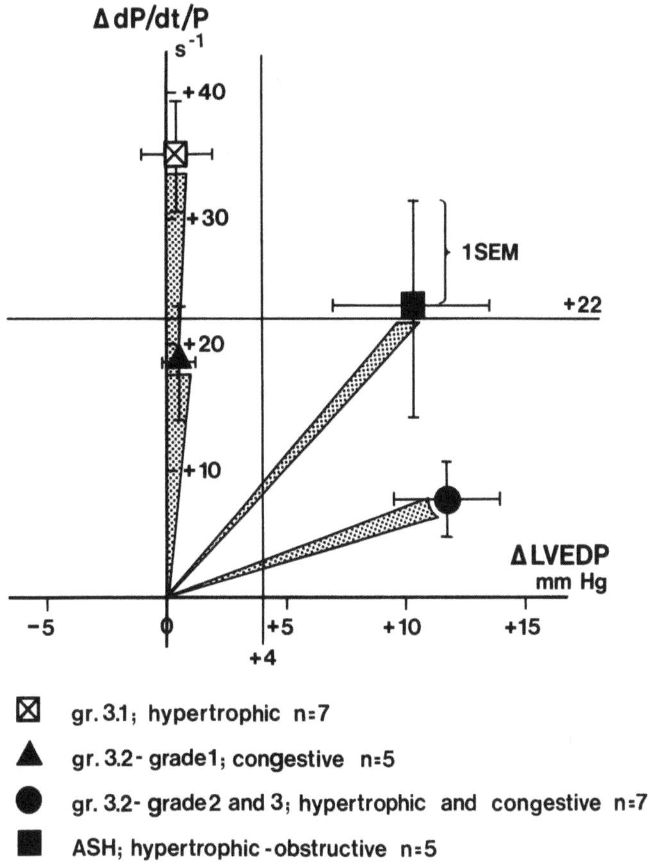

Fig. 6. Contractile reserve in different types of CM. Normal contractility and normal EDP during exercise in patients with hypertrophic type (mild degree, [*gr.* = *group*] *gr. 3.1*). Reduced contractility reserve with normal EDP in patients with mild congestive type (*gr. 3.2, grade 1*). No major increase in contractility and excessive increase of EDP in patients with severe hypertrophic or severe congestive CM (*gr. 3.2*, grade 2 and 3). Nearly normal contractile patterns in patients with asymmetrical septal hypertrophy (ASH)

of disease was short, ventricular volumes at rest were normal, and patients had no complaints during exercise.

3. Patients with a mild *congestive type* of CM were found to have a reduced contractility reserve with normal enddiastolic pressures during stress (Fig. 6).
4. Patients with *severe hypertrophic* CM and patients with a severe type of *congestive* disease were incorporated into one group. All patients demonstrated the same impaired left ventricular function during stress (Fig. 6). Enddiastolic pressure increased between 4 and over 15 mm Hg without a major increase in contractility.
5. Patients with a *hypertrophic-obstructive* disease of the myocardium formed one group, presenting with greater increases in enddiastolic pressure and nearly normal contractile patterns (closed quadrant in Fig. 6, ASH).

Thus, ventricular function in patients with CM depends upon the type of disease, history and duration of illness, and upon the amount of muscle. With increasing severity of disease, contractility is the first parameter to be impaired with a simultaneous increase in enddiastolic pressure. These particular findings are comparable to changes caused by other cardiac diseases [5, 7]. If during stress contractility is decreased due to myocardial or mechanical factors, the Frank-Starling mechanism is triggered and the work of the heart is accomplished by means of an increase in enddiastolic pressure.

Discussion of Methods

The validity of isovolumic contractility indices has been questioned recently [12]. These parameters depend upon different hemodynamic variables. dP/dt_{max} proved to be less dependent upon pre- and afterload than did other indices [15]. V_{pm} is dependent upon preload to a large extent [14]. These restrictions mainly apply when measurements taken at rest were compared. dP/dt_{max} increases threefold during exercise in patients with normal contractile reserve (Fig. 2). Thus, only a small error results from the limitations of these parameters when obtained during exercise.

Regional Left Ventricular Function at Rest and Under Stress in Patients With Cardiomyopathy

Isovolumic studies of left ventricular contractility are applicable for determination of overall ventricular function. More detailed information can be gained from regional parameters during the ejection phase.

It was mentioned above that in CMs a disparity exists between the size of the right and left ventricle. From this one may conclude that the disease not only involves the total myocardium diffusely but may also cause various regional impairments. Thus, the purpose of this part of the study was to investigate regional functional disturbances of the left ventricle at rest and during exercise, and whether or not regional contraction patterns differ in the various stages of the disease.

Methods

Thirteen patients, 8 with congestive and 5 with hypertrophic CMs were investigated by introducing a Millar-tip-angiographic catheter into the left ventricle and subsequent injection of contrast medium at rest, after leg raising and within 30 s after exercise on a bicycle ergometer. Between each left ventricular angiogram a period of 10–15 min elasped, which reportedly is adequate to restore hemodynamic changes [8]. One-plane left ventricular angiograms in the right anterior oblique position (40°) were analyzed by the hemiaxis method [3]. The velocity of circumferential fiber shortening was calculated at the basal, middle, and apical horizontal axes of the left ventricle, and the mean of all three was calculated (mean V_{cf}). Hemiaxes were numbered from m1 to m3 at the anterior and from m4 to m6 at the diaphragmatic wall.

Ventricular volumes were calculated similarly by the area-length method with an automatic device (Volumat, Siemens AG) [11]. The simultaneously registered pressure values and contractility indices were calculated in the same manner as in part 1.

Patients were divided into three groups according to the severity of clinical findings and hemodynamics at rest, i.e., mild, moderate or severe CM.

Results

In patients classified as mild, mean V_{cf} increased after leg raising and exercise (Fig. 7). On the other hand, mean V_{cf} decreased after leg raising in patients with moderate and severe disease. Ventricular function deteriorated during exercise in patients classified as severe.

In the group classified as moderate, exercise led to an increase of mean V_{cf} only slightly above values at rest.

The mean values in Figure 8 show that in mild disease, mean V_{cf} increased significantly during leg raising and physical exercise. In patients with moderate *and* severe CM, a significant decrease occurred during leg raising. During exercise the increase of mean V_{cf} was markedly reduced as compared to the mild group.

Mean V_{cf} is, like dP/dt_{max} or V_{pm}, a measurement that reflects the overall function of the left ventricle. More detailed information can be obtained by quantitative analysis of the ventriculograms. The original ventriculograms at

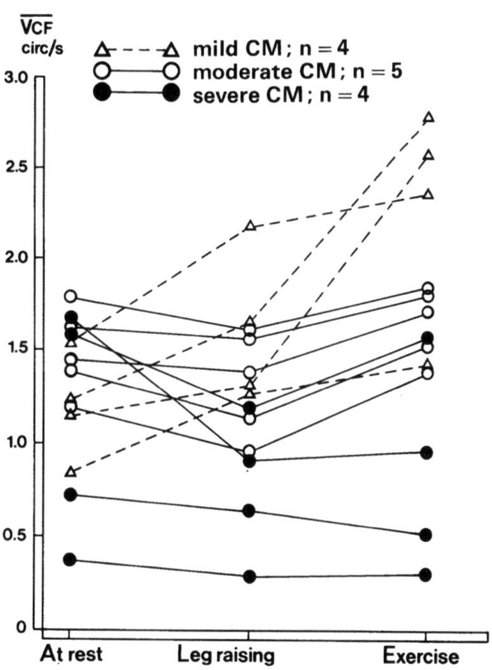

Fig. 7. Increase of mean circumferential fiber shortening ($\overline{V_{cf}}$) during leg raising and exercise in patients with mild cardiomyopathy (CM). Decrease of mean V_{cf} after leg raising in patients classified as moderate and severe CMP. Deterioration during exercise in patients with severe disease

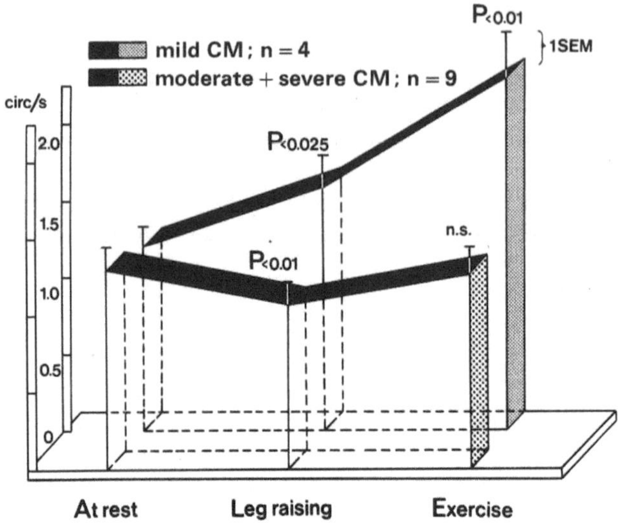

Fig. 8. Increase of mean V_{cf} during leg raising and exercise in mild CM. Decrease of mean V_{cf} during leg raising in the group with moderate and severe CM. During exercise the increase of mean V_{cf} was markedly reduced as compared to the mild group

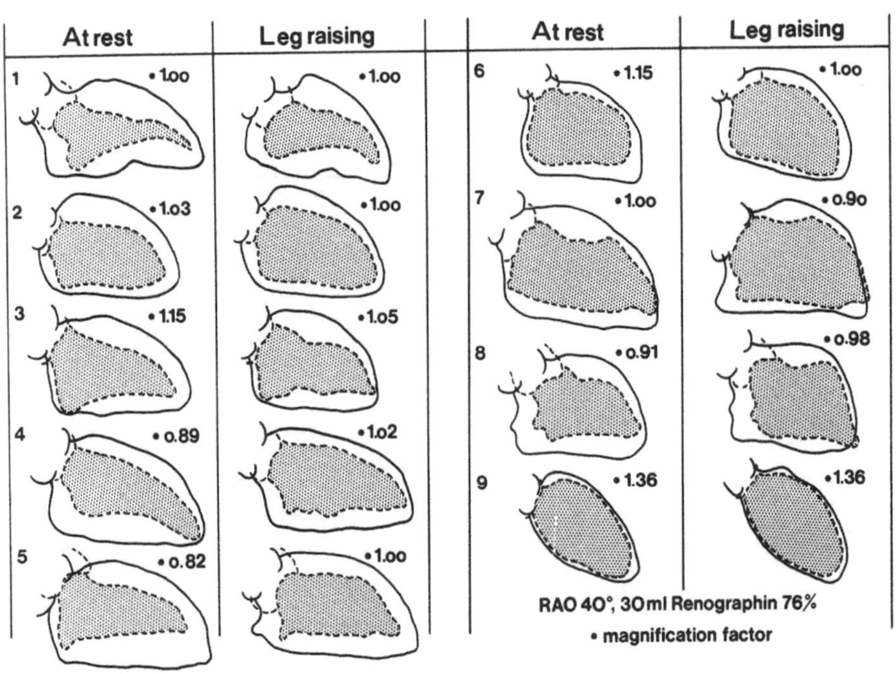

Fig. 9. Asynergy after leg raising in patients classified as moderate (1–5) and severe (6–9). Regional wall motion disturbances in the anterior and apical part of the left ventricle

rest and after leg raising are shown in Figure 9. Patient numbers 1 to 5 were in the moderate and 6 to 9 in the severe group. The qualitative evaluation indicates that regional function disturbances are most probably localized in the anterior wall and in the apical part of the left ventricle. As is apparent from most angiograms, the remaining parts of the ventricle are also involved, but to a lesser degree.

The velocity in the middle anterior hemiaxis (Vm2) decreased significantly during leg raising from 1.41 $\pm$0.53 to 1.09 $\pm$0.20 ($\pm$1 SD) s^{-1}. Significant changes were also found in the apical proportion (Vm3) but not in the other parts of the ventricle (Vm5 and Vm6).

The velocity of the middle anterior hemiaxis (Vm2) is plotted in Figure 10. In the group with mild CM, Vm2 increased after leg raising and during exercise, as in patients with normal left ventricular function. In moderate disease the contraction velocity of the segment m2 was significantly reduced during leg raising; during exercise the increase was only small. A deterioration of regional function was particularly evident in the group with severe disease. Contraction velocity of the region m2 was merely reduced during leg raising and a further decrease was observed during exercise.

The same changes in regional motion found during leg raising became apparent in patients 6 to 9 (Fig. 11) comparing ventriculograms at rest and during exercise. In patients with severe CM, ventricular function deteriorated during exercise. In these patients the velocity in the middle anterior hemiaxis decreased significantly from 1.17 $\pm$0.74 to 0.74 $\pm$0.45 s^{-1} ($P < 0.05$). In patients with moderate disease (patients 1–5, Fig. 11) ventricular function improved only slightly and insufficiently.

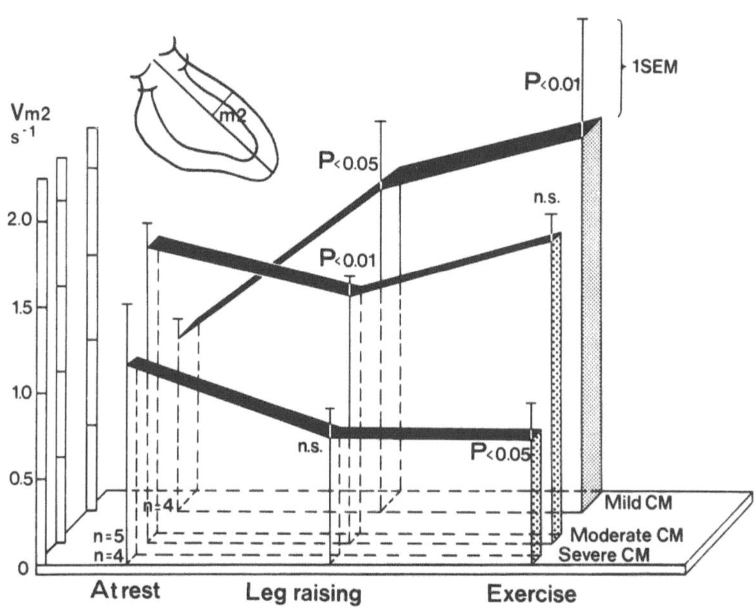

Fig. 10. Velocity of middle anterior hemiaxis (Vm2) increased in mild and decreased in moderate and severe CM during leg raising. No change of Vm2 during exercise in patients with severe CM

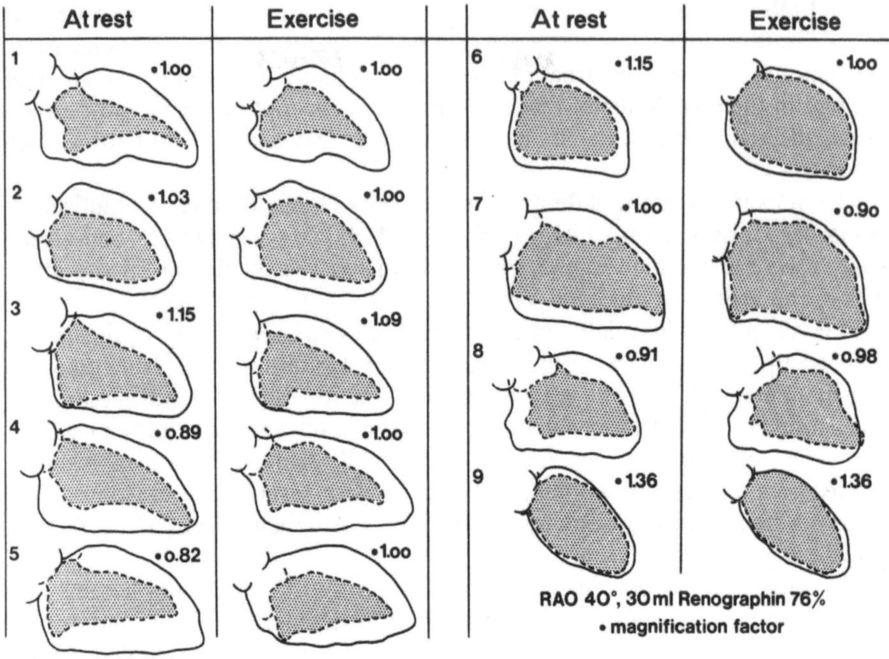

Fig. 11. Ventriculograms at rest and during exercise in patients with moderate (1–5) and severe (6–9) cardiomyopathy (CM). No major changes in patients classified as moderate, but hypo- or akinesis especially in the anterior and apical wall in patients classified as severe

Further Hemodynamic Findings

Leg Raising

The hemodynamic variables of the patients with mild, moderate *and* severe CM are illustrated in Figure 12.

In patients with mild disease, mean V_{cf} increased significantly. LVEDP increased from 18.6 ±4.9 to 27.2 ±10.8 mm Hg ($P < 0.10$), but EDV did not change markedly. ESV decreased from 49 ±25 to 38 ±30 ml/1,73 m^2 ($P < 0.10$).

In patients with moderate *and* severe disease the significant decrease in mean V_{cf} and V_{pm} was accompanied by a highly significant increase of LVEDP (from 18.8 ±7.0 to 30.5 ±6.8 mm Hg, $P < 0.0005$). EDV increased only slightly and not significantly, whereas ESV increased significantly from 84 ±52 to 102 ±59 ml/1.73 m^2 BSA.

Exercise

Comparing data of the resting and exercise period, patients had significant increases in heart rate and left ventricular systolic pressure. In patients with mild disease, mean V_{cf} increased significantly, LVEDP increased without changes in EDV, and ESV decreased. In patients with moderate and severe disease, mean V_{cf} did not change during exercise (Fig. 13). LVEDP increased from

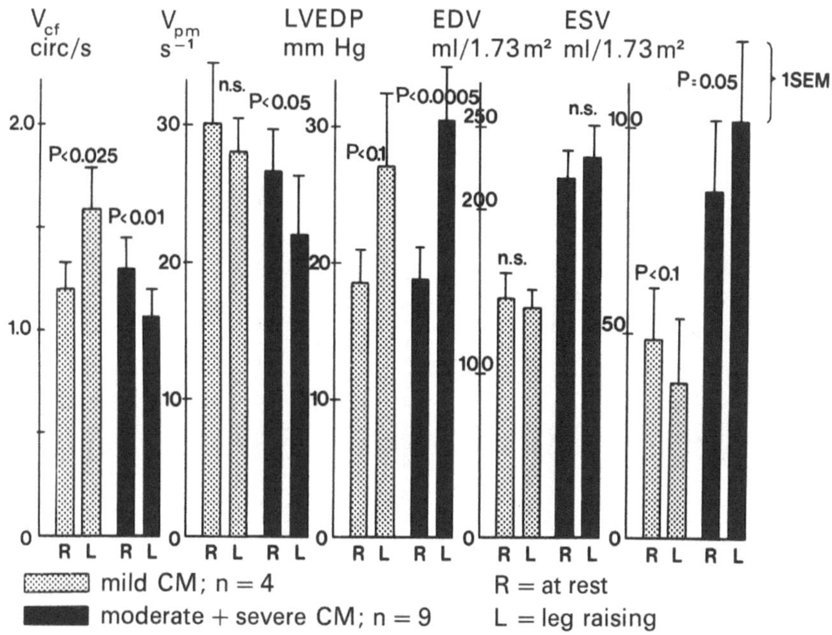

Fig. 12. Leg raising in mild CM: increase of mean V_{cf} and LVEDP, no change in enddiastolic volume (EDV) and decrease of endsystolic volume (ESV). In patients with moderate and severe cardiomyopathy mean V_{cf} and V_{pm} decreased significantly, LVEDP and ESV increased. No changes in EDV

18.8 ±7.0 to 28.5 ±12.4 mm Hg, again without major changes in enddiastolic volume. ESV tended to increase.

Conclusions

The following conclusions may be drawn:

1. Hemodynamic changes during stress (volume load, exercise) depend on the severity of the disease.
2. In patients with mild CM, contraction and contractility parameters (mean V_{cf}, V_{pm}) may increase nearly as much as in patients with normal left ventricular function.
3. In severely ill patients, ventricular function during leg raising and during exercise deteriorated, whereas in moderately ill patients—despite a slight improvement during exercise—contraction reserve was reduced.
4. Regional function of the left ventricle during stress was mainly impaired in the anterior and apical portion of the left ventricle. In most cases, however, other segments in the posterior and diaphragmatic wall were also involved.

Discussion

The question arises why patients with CM develop regional wall motion disturbances during stress testing. Two explanations are possible:

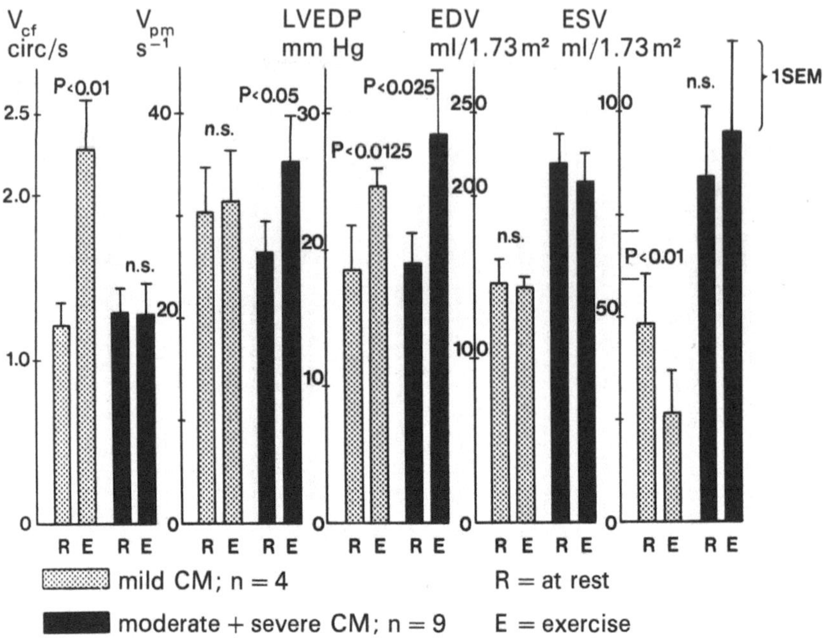

Fig. 13. Significant increase in mean V_{cf} and LVEDP in mild CM. In the moderate and severe group, mean V_{cf} did not change and LVEDP increased markedly. Endsystolic volume (ESV) tended to increase. No change in enddiastolic volume (EDV)

1. In patients with coronary artery disease hypokinesis or akinesis regularly occurs in poststenotic segments during ischemia [3]. In patients with CM, hypokinesis is less pronounced during stress and involves the ventricle regionally as well as diffusely. Relative coronary insufficiency may be considered and a decrease of endocardial blood flow through an increase of EDP – an effect of the extracoronary component of the coronary resistance [16]. As reported by Olsen, histologic changes in small vessels could not be demonstrated. Ferrans stated that in 20%–40% of the patients with CMs changes in the small vessels were observed. However, it is still unlikely that the morphologically verified narrowing of small vessels leads to functional disturbances and a reduced blood flow.
2. The other interpretation seems more likely: during exercise the contractile activity of the muscle fibers may be decreased due to fibrotic areas surrounding normal myocardial tissue. Therefore the well-functioning fibers may be overloaded, which in turn leads to an overall decrease in left ventricular contractile properties.

References

1. Bussmann, W.-D.: Kontraktilitätsreserve des linken Ventrikels unter körperlicher und pharmakologischer Belastung bei verschiedenen Herzerkrankungen. Habilitationsschrift, Frankfurt (1974)
2. Bussmann, W.-D., Jooß, B., Kaltenbach, M.: Recheneinheit zur Bestimmung der größten gemessenen Verkürzungsgeschwindigkeit der kontraktilen Elemente. Z. Kardiol. *64*, 289 (1975)
3. Bussmann, W.-D., Thaler, R., Kober, G., Hopf, R., Kaltenbach, M.: Angiographie des linken Ventrikels nach Volumenbelastung und körperlicher Arbeit bei koronarer Herzkrankheit. Z. Kardiol. *65*, 693 (1976)
4. Bussmann, W.-D., Heeger, J., Kaltenbach, M.: Kontraktilitäts- und Relaxationsreserve des linken Ventrikels. I. Normaler linker Ventrikel. Z. Kardiol. (1977) (in press)
5. Bussmann, W.-D., Heeger, J., Kaltenbach, M.: II. Kontraktilitäts- und Relaxationsreserve des linken Ventrikels bei Patienten mit rheumatischen Vitien. Z. Kardiol. (1977) (in press)
6. Bussmann, W.-D., Heeger, J., Kaltenbach, M.: III. Kontraktilitäts- und Relaxationsreserve des linken Ventrikels bei Patienten mit Myokardiopathie. Z. Kardiol. (1977) (in press)
7. Bussmann, W.-D., Heeger, J., Kaltenbach, M.: IV. Kontraktilitäts- und Relaxationsreserve des linken Ventrikels bei Patienten mit koronarer Herzkrankheit. Z. Kardiol. (1977) (in press)
8. Erbel, R., Neuhaus, K.L., Spiller, P., Benn, M., Kreuzer, H.: Beeinflussung der systolischen und diastolischen Ventrikelfunktion durch Kontrastmittelinjektion in den linken Ventrikel. Z. Kardiol. *65*, 305 (1976)
9. Goodwin, J.F.: Prospects and predictions for the cardiomyopathies. Circulation *50*, 210 (1974)
10. Guldner, N., Kober, G., Schäfer, G., Bussmann, W.-D., Hopf, R., Kaltenbach, M.: Volumenparameter des linken und rechten Ventrikels bei Kardiomyopathien. Z. Kardiol. (1977) (in press)
11. Kaltenbach, M., Schulz, W.: Kineangiographische Bestimmung von Ventrikelvolumina mit Rechnerhilfe. Dtsch. med. Wschr. *100*, 590 (1975)
12. Kreuzer, H., Neuhaus, K.L.: Invasive Untersuchungsmethoden zur Erfassung einer gestörten Kontraktilität. Verh. dtsch. Ges. Kreisl.-Forsch. *42*, 31 (1976)
13. Mathes, P., Delius, W., Sebening, H., Wirtzfeld, A., Blömer, H.: Das regionale Kontraktionsverhalten der linken Herzkammer bei kongestiver Kardiomyopathie. Dtsch. med. Wschr. *101*, 995 (1976)
14. Mehmel, H.C., Krayenbuehl, H.P., Wirz, P.: Isovolumic contraction dynamics in man according to two different muscle models. J. appl. Physiol. *33*, 409 (1972)
15. Morgenstern, C., Goebel, H., Lochner, W.: Die Beurteilung der Kontraktilität des Herzens. Dtsch. med. Wschr. *97*, 1563 (1972)
16. Raff, W.K., Kosche, F., Lochner, W.: Extravascular coronary resistance and its relation to microcirculation. Amer. J. Cardiol. *29*, 598 (1972)
17. Roskamm, H., Blümchen, G., Fiebig, H., Schnellbacher, K., Wink, K., Pabst, K., Schollmeyer, P., Lösel, E., Weidemann, H., Reindell, H.: Hämodynamik und Kontraktilitätsreserve bei Myokardiopathien. Dtsch. med. Wschr. *97*, 1681 (1972)
18. Weiss, M.B., Ellis, K., Sciacca, R.R., Johnson, L.L., Schmidt, D.H., Cannon, P.J.: Myocardial blood flow in congestive and hypertrophic cardiomyopathy. Circulation *54*, 484 (1976)

15. Disorders of Left Ventricular Performance in Congestive and Hypertrophic Obstructive Cardiomyopathy

P. SPILLER, C. BRENNER, K. L. NEUHAUS, and G. SAUER

While the histologic features of COCM and HOCM are well defined, the effects of the morphologic disorders on cardiac dynamics are not yet clear [3, 8–10, 13]. Whether ventricular function in HOCM is disturbed mainly during systole or during diastole is still controversial [5, 12]. In COCM, the data in the literature about diastolic compliance are especially contradictory [6, 11].

Therefore, the purpose of this investigation was to characterize the nature and degree of ventricular and myocardial dysfunction in patients with HOCM and COCM.

Methods

Seven patients with normal left ventricular function, 10 patients with HOCM, and 10 patients with COCM were studied. No patient had arterial hypertension or coronary arterial disease. Four patients with HOCM had mild or moderate, and two patients with COCM had mild mitral regurgitation. All patients with CM had symptoms of left ventricular failure (class II–IV, N.Y.H.A.).

Biplane cineventriculograms (100 or 150 frames/s) of the left ventricle were performed. Ventricular pressure was measured simultaneously by a catheter tip manometer. Frame-by-frame analysis of the cineventriculograms during one sinus beat yielded following parameters: left ventricular systolic (PLV) and enddiastolic pressure (PLVED), enddiastolic wall thickness (W), ratio of end-diastolic diameter to wall thickness (D/W), enddiastolic equatorial wall stress (σ_{ED}) (using the formula of Wong and Rautaharju [14]), enddiastolic (EDVI) and endsystolic (ESVI) volume (using the biplane area–length method of Dodge *et al.* [2]), stroke volume (SVI), cardiac index (CI) as the product of SVI and heart rate, peak rate of left ventricular pressure rise (dp/dt_{max}), dp/dt_{max} divided by the instantaneous pressure [$(dp/dt_{max})/IP$], and the mean velocity of circumferential fiber shortening (V_{CF}) in the basal (B), equatorial (D), and apical (A) region of the ventricle. Left ventricular and myocardial compliance were assessed by assuming an exponential function of pressure versus volume and stress versus fiber length during diastolic pressure rise [1]. According to this function, the constant ratio $(dP/dV)/P = \ln P/V$ is directly related to left ventricular compliance, the ratio $\frac{d\sigma}{dl}/\text{length} = \ln\sigma/\text{length}$ to myocardial compliance. The slopes (a) of the linear functions $\ln P$ versus volume (a_v) and $\ln\sigma$ versus length (a_m), respectively, were used as indices of ventricular and myocardial distensibility (Fig. 1). Because of the geometric abnormalities, myocardial stress in HOCM

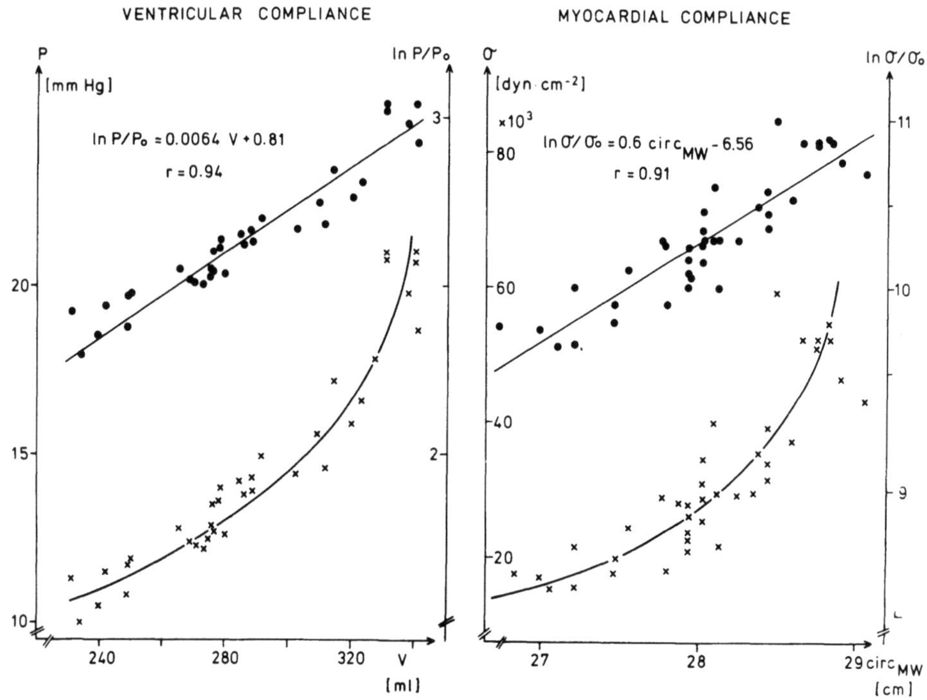

Fig. 1. Example of the determination of ventricular and myocardial compliance. Assuming the pressure volume relationship and the stress-fiber length relationship during diastole to be exponential (*below, crosses*) the constant ratios $(dP/dV)/P = \ln P/V$ and $(d\sigma/dl)/\text{length} = \ln \sigma/\text{length}$ (*above*) were directly related to ventricular and myocardial compliance, respectively. The slopes of the two linear functions were used as indices of ventricular (a_v) and myocardial (a_m) distensibility

was calculated only for the posterior free wall (Fig. 2). In three cases (two of HOCM, one of COCM) the relation between diastolic pressure and volume or stress and fiber length was not exponential; therefore no indices of compliance were calculated.

Results

On the average, external left ventricular work in patients with COCM and HOCM was quite similar to that of patients with normal left ventricular function (Fig. 3). Systolic pressures of the ventricles with HOCM were higher in the apical and normal in the subaortic region. Stroke volume and cardiac index were in the upper range of normal or slightly above the normal range. In four cases this might be due to a moderate mitral regurgitation, which led to an overestimation of stroke volume by ventriculography. Ventricles with COCM had a normal stroke volume and cardiac index. The mean value of cardiac index (4.6 $\pm$0.6 liter $\min^{-1}$ m^{-2}) was surprisingly high, even in the presence of mitral regurgitation in two patients.

2

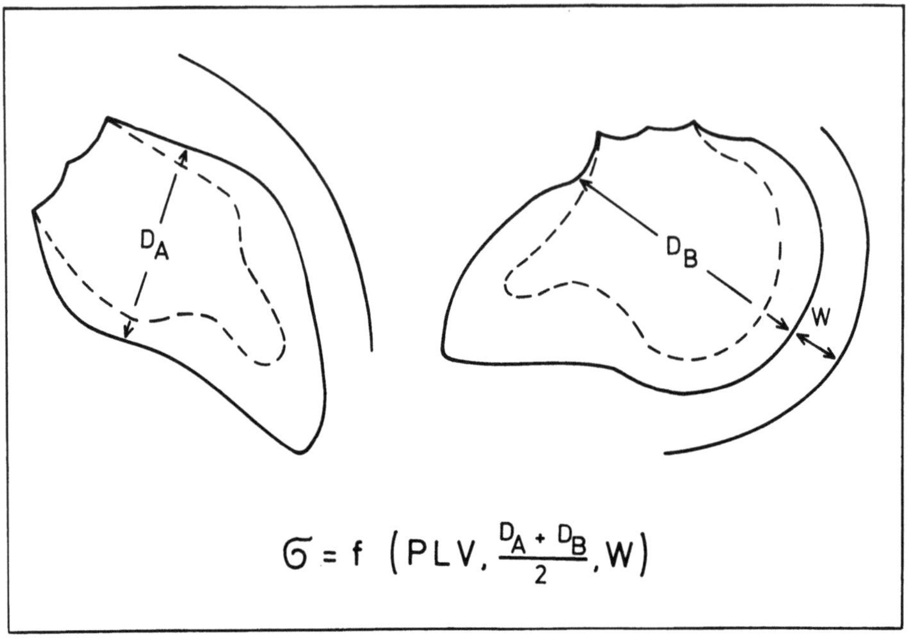

D_A
D_B
W
σ = f (PLV, (D_A + D_B)/2, W)

3

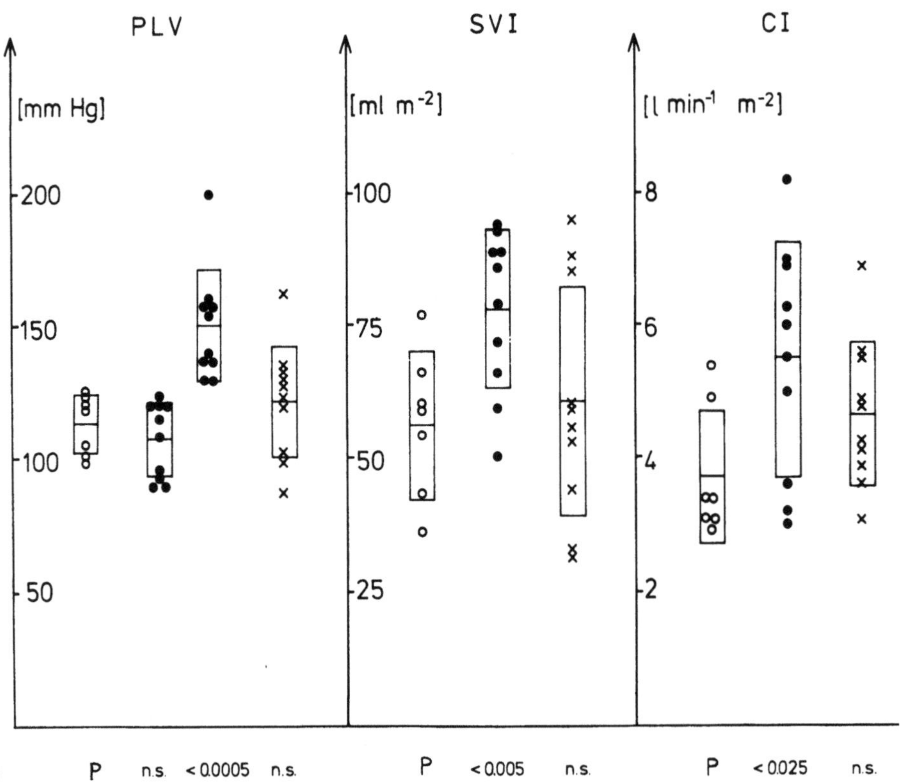

PLV
[mm Hg]
200
150
100
50
SVI
[ml m-2]
100
75
50
25
CI
[l min-1 m-2]
8
6
4
2
P n.s. < 0.0005 n.s.
P < 0.005 n.s.
P < 0.025 n.s.

Figure 4 summarizes the parameters of left ventricular pump function. EDV, ESV, and EF were normal in patients with HOCM. In patients with COCM, EDVI and ESVI were increased, and the EF considerably diminished ($34.5 \pm 16.1\%$). LVEDP was significantly elevated in both groups.

The parameters of myocardial function (Fig. 5) were in the normal range in patients with HOCM. In COCM, on the average, peak rate of left ventricular pressure rise, $(dp/dt_{max})/IP$, and the mean value of V_{CF} in three regions of each ventricle ($\overline{V_{CF}}$) were considerably reduced.

Regional diameter changes are depicted in Figure 6. With one exception, normal ventricles had an almost identical pattern of V_{CF}. In HOCM there were important variations between the different ventricular regions. In four cases, V_{CF} was abnormally high, probably because of a moderate mitral regurgitation. In nine patients with COCM, V_{CF} was reduced. Only a few had moderate regional V_{CF} differences.

Six of nine ventricles with COCM had a normal ventricular and myocardial compliance (Fig. 7). Most patients with HOCM showed a significantly reduced ventricular distensibility (high a_v values). A moderately decreased myocardial distensibility was found in three cases (high a_m values). Only one patient had a normal myocardial and ventricular compliance.

Myocardial hypertrophy was found in HOCM and COCM in all cases (Fig. 8). The mean value of enddiastolic wall thickness was 1.35 cm in HOCM and 1.17 cm in COCM, as compared to 0.94 cm in normal ventricles. On the average, the ratio of enddiastolic diameter to wall thickness was 4.42 in HOCM, 6.71 in COCM, and 6.08 in normal ventricles. Enddiastolic stress was considerably elevated in COCM ($47\,500 \pm 17\,400$ dyn cm^{-2}), as compared to normal ventricles ($20\,500 \pm 11\,800$ dyn cm^{-2}). On the average, in HOCM enddiastolic stress of the free posterior wall was increased also.

Discussion

In our CM patients (HOCM and COCM) LV pressure-volume-work was normal. In HOCM these results were similar to those published in the literature. In COCM, however, some investigators had reported a reduced cardiac output [5, 6, 8]. Although the explanation was not clear, this discrepancy might be partially due to different stages of the disease in the patients investigated or to an overestimation of stroke volume by angiocardiography. Regarding the possible errors, it must be considered that all determinations of ventricular

---

◁ Fig. 2. Scheme of the geometric data used for the determination of myocardial stress in HOCM. Myocardial stress of the posterior wall was calculated as a function of left ventricular pressure (LVP), the mean value of the ventricular diameters in two projections (D_A, D_B), and the thickness of the posterior wall (W)

Fig. 3. Systolic left ventricular pressure (LVP), stroke volume index (SVI), and cardiac index (CI) in patients with normal left ventricular function (○) and in patients with HOCM (●) and COCM (×). The two series of values in HOCM characterized systolic LVP in the subaortic (*left*) and in the apical (*right*) region. Bars indicate the mean value ± standard deviation

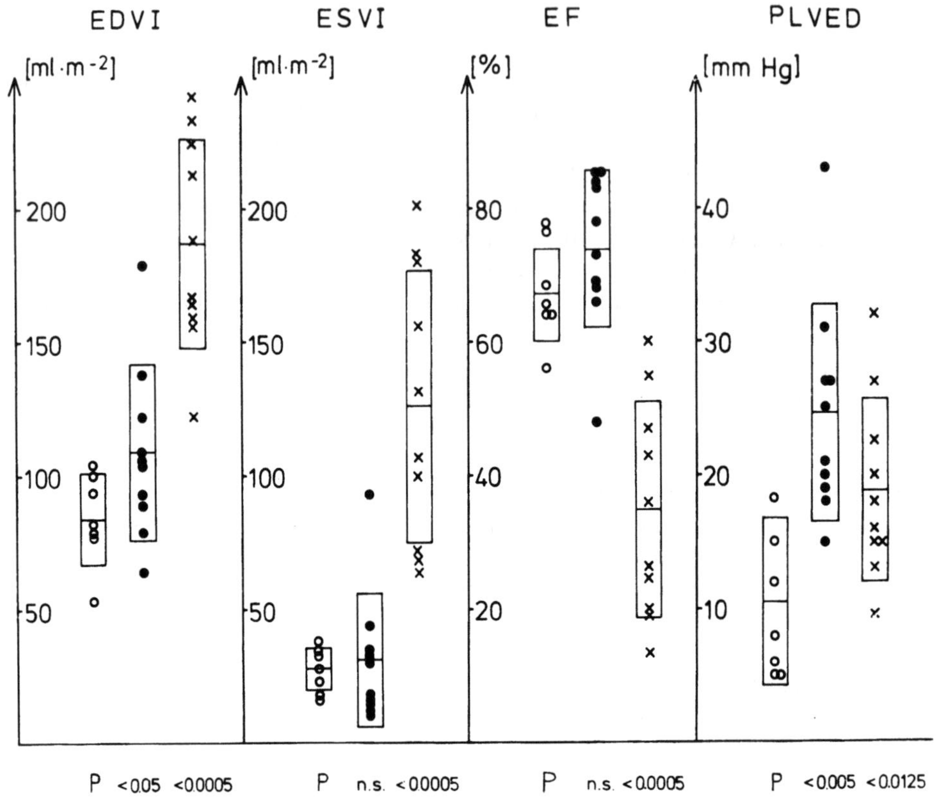

Fig. 4. EDVI, ESVI, EF, and LVEDP in patients with normal left ventricular function (○) and in patients with HOCM (●) and COCM (×). On the average, the parameters of pump function were normal in HOCM and considerably reduced in COCM. LVEDP was elevated in both groups. Bars indicate the mean value ± standard deviation

volume in vivo were approximations only. Compared to other methods, the values from biplane X-ray ventriculography seemed to be the best possible estimations of the real volume [7].

In HOCM, no essential disorder of systolic ventricular and myocardial function could be demonstrated at rest. The elevated EDP and the normal EDV, however, indicated a dysfunction during diastole. In COCM, on the contrary, a normal stroke volume was ejected by a considerably enlarged ventricle. The reduction of systolic myocardial performance in all cases was at least compensated in part by an increase in myocardial preload. In HOCM, the elevated EDP might indicate an increased preload; it might also be due to a reduction of ventricular distensibility. The increased stiffness of these ventricles in some cases could be related to a reduced myocardial distensibility; in others it could be caused by the increased wall thickness and geometric abnormalities.

The rather normal distensibility of ventricles with COCM, to a certain degree, contrasted with the conclusions of Mathes and Just [11] who had reported a reduced ventricular compliance in COCM. To explain this discrepancy, methodic

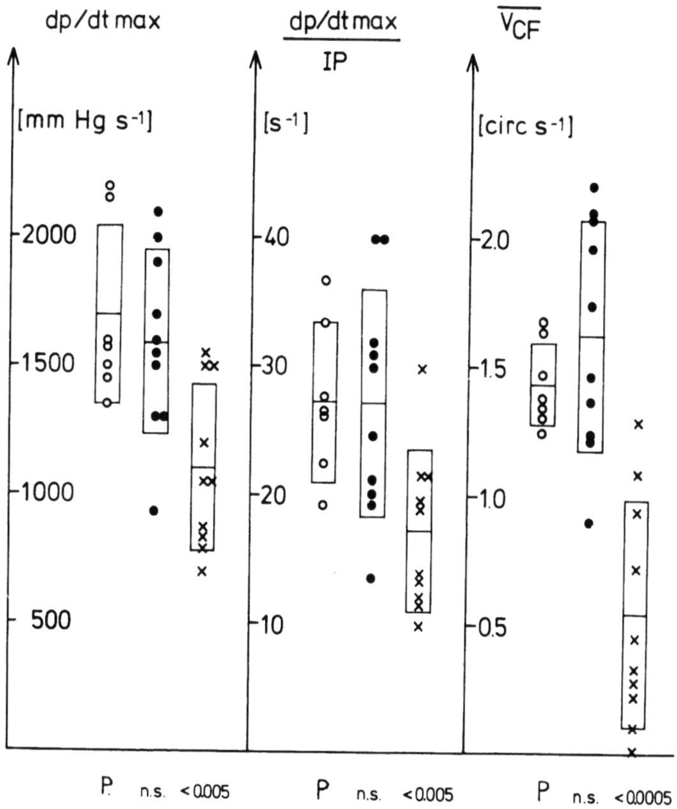

Fig. 5. Peak rate of LVP rise (dp/dt_{max}), dp/dt_{max} divided by the instantaneous pressure [$(dp/dt_{max})/IP$] and the mean value of V_{CF} in the three regions B, D, A of each ventricle ($\overline{V_{CF}}$) in patients with normal left ventricular function (○) and in patients with HOCM (●) and COCM (×). On the average, parameters of myocardial function were normal in HOCM and significantly reduced in COCM. Bars indicate the mean value ± standard deviation

differences and a different stage of the disease must be considered. The latter explanation had been supported by the results of Gotsman *et al.* [6]. They had found in a larger group of patients with COCM a reduced, a normal, or even an increased distensibility of the myocardium.

In COCM the high enddiastolic wall stress indicated an increased myocardial preload, because myocardial and ventricular compliance were nearly normal. In HOCM, on the contrary, the elevated enddiastolic stresses in most cases could be explained by two mechanisms, the decrease in myocardial compliance and the increase in myocardial preload. In our study it could not be estimated in which proportion these two factors had affected the enddiastolic stress.

Left ventricular hypertrophy was evident from the increased wall thickness in HOCM and COCM as well as from calculations of left ventricular muscle mass. In HOCM, the mean value of the ratio of enddiastolic diameter to wall thickness (D/W) was distincly lower (4.4 ±1.2), in COCM, D/W, on the average, was higher (6.7 ±1.0) than the normal value (6.1 ±0.8). In HOCM this result

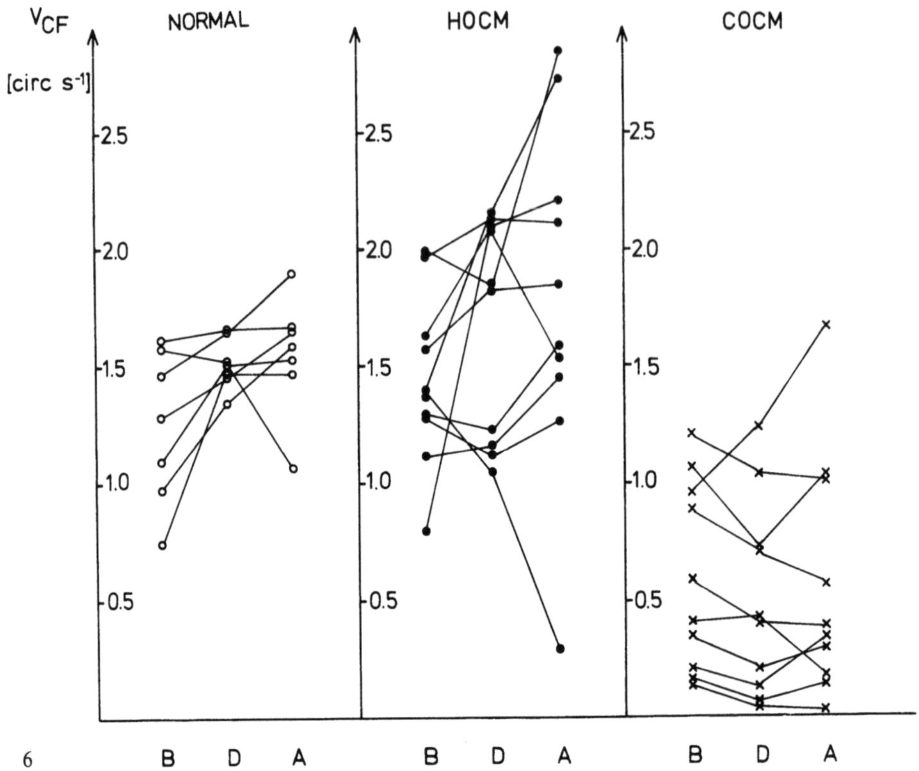

V_{CF}
[circ s-1]
NORMAL
HOCM
COCM
2.5
2.0
1.5
1.0
0.5
B D A
B D A
B D A

6

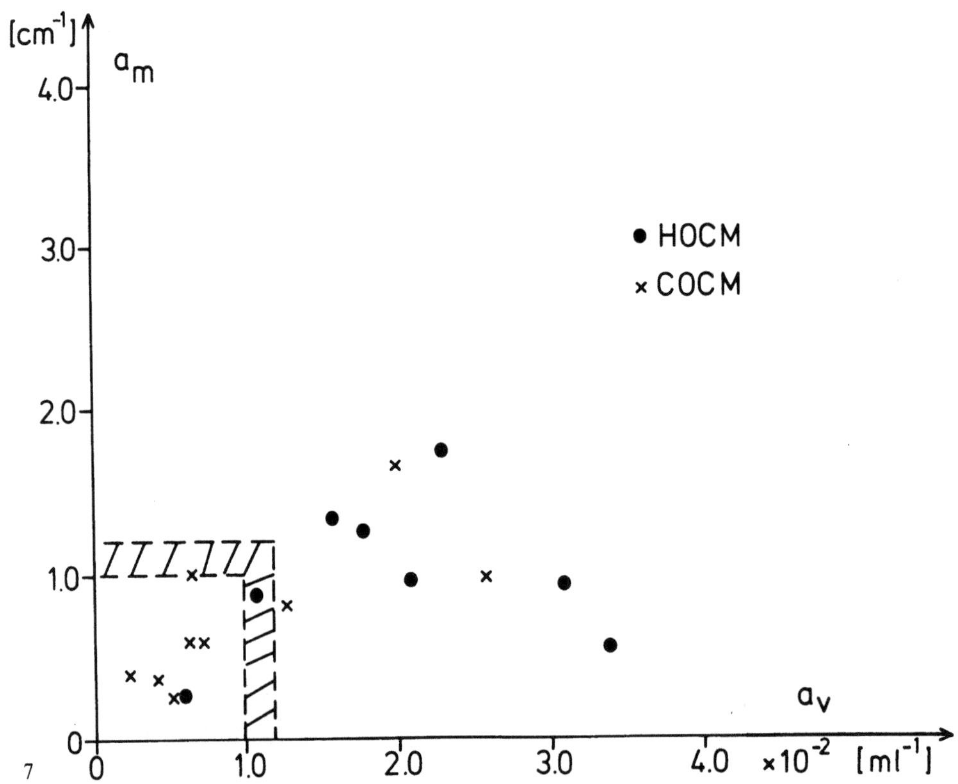

[cm-1]
a_m
4.0
3.0
2.0
1.0
0
● HOCM
× COCM
a_v
0
1.0
2.0
3.0
4.0
×10-2 [ml-1]

7

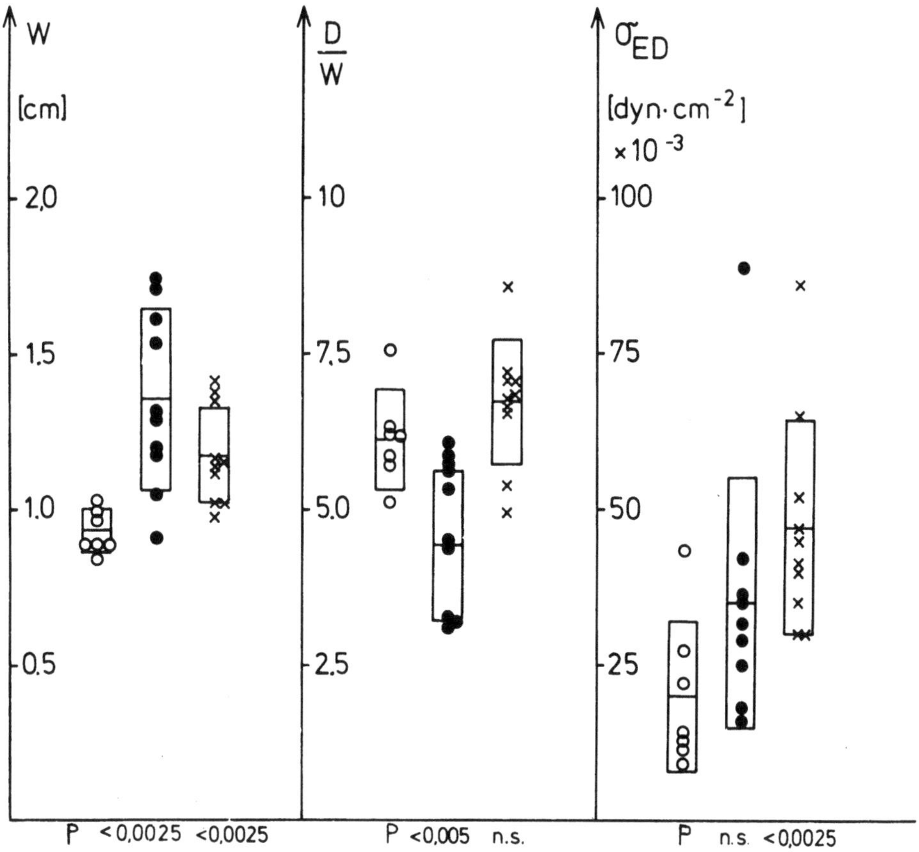

Fig. 8. Wall thickness (W), ratio of enddiastolic diameter and wall thickness (D/W) and enddiastolic wall stress (σ_{ED}) in patients with normal left ventricular function (○) and in patients with HOCM (●) and COCM (×)

represented the "concentric hypertrophy" of the ventricles. In COCM the high ratio D/W might represent the "hypertrophy, inappropriate to the degree of dilatation," postulated by Goodwin and Oakley [4, 5]. The authors suggested that in COCM, in contrast to other dilated ventricles, the usual adaptation by hypertrophy might be diminished.

Figure 9 shows the relationship of D/W (an index of left ventricular hypertrophy) to EDV for ventricles with pressure or volume overload. The values for HOCM fell below the normal range; those for COCM were at the upper

---

◁ Fig. 6. Regional V_{CF} in patients with normal ventricular function (○) and patients with HOCM (●) and COCM (×). There were great differences in the basal (B), equatorial (D), and apical (A) regions of the ventricle in HOCM. In COCM, V_{CF} was considerably reduced in all regions with one exception

Fig. 7. Left ventricular and myocardial compliance in patients with HOCM (●) and COCM (×). Limits of upper normal range are indicated by *cross-hatched area*

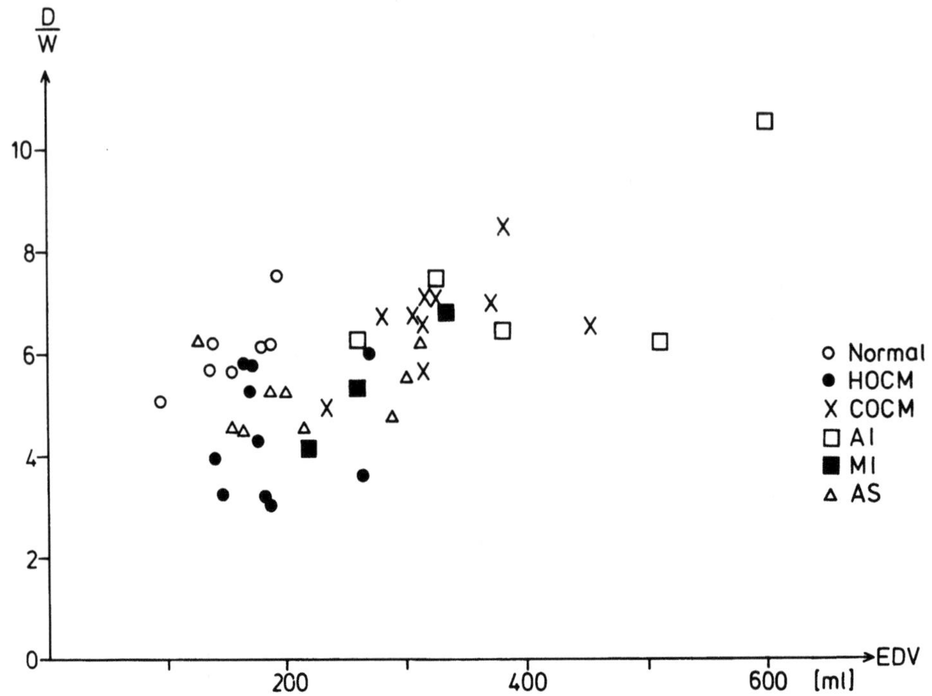

Fig. 9. Correlation of the ratio of enddiastolic diameter and wall thickness (D/W) versus EDV in patients with normal left ventricular function (○), patients with HOCM (●), COCM (×), aortic regurgitation (□), mitral regurgitation (■) and aortic stenosis (△)

right. The approximately linear correlation between D/W and EDV illustrated that ventricles with COCM could not be separated from dilated ventricles with aortic or mitral regurgitation. This means that COCM and chronic volume overload led to the same degree of dilatation and hypertrophy (as measured from D/W). Therefore, hypertrophy in these cases of COCM seemed to be as appropriate as in other dilated left ventricles. Hypertrophy, however, might be considered inadequate in COCM, inasmuch as an additional increase of preload is neccessary to maintain a normal stroke work.

On the contrary, in some ventricles with HOCM, D/W was smaller than in ventricles with aortic stenosis with similar pressure overload. Assuming that in these cases of HOCM the myocardial wall was thickened abnormally with regard to the pressure load, this condition might rather be called "inappropriate hypertrophy."

Summary

In HOCM systolic ventricular function and systolic myocardial function at rest were normal. On the average, diastolic ventricular compliance and, to a certain degree, myocardial compliance of the posterior wall were reduced.

In COCM a pronounced reduction of systolic, ventricular, and myocardial function was found; diastolic compliance was diminished only in a few cases.

The increased pressure load in HOCM was compensated by hypertrophy and increased preload. In COCM the poor myocardial function was also compensated by an increase of wall thickness and myocardial preload.

Hypertrophy in COCM seemed to be similar to that in ventricles with pressure and volume overload. Ventricles with HOCM, however, were more hypertrophied than other ventricles with nearly the same pressure loads. Therefore the term "inappropriate hypertrophy" seemed to be more suitable in HOCM.

References

1. Diamond, G., Forrester, J.S., Hargis, J., Parmley, W.W., Danzig, R., Swan, H.J.C.: Diastolic pressure-volume relationship in the canine left ventricle. Circulat. Res. *29*, 267 (1971)
2. Dodge, H.T., Sandler, H., Baxley, W.A., Hawley, R.R.: Usefulness and limitations of radiographic methods for determining left ventricular volume. Amer. J. Cardiol. *18*, 10 (1966)
3. Ferrans, V.J., Massumi, R.A., Shugoll, G.I., Ali, N., Roberts, W.C.: Ultrastructural studies of myocardial biopsies in 45 patients with obstructive or congestive cardiomyopathy. In: Cardiomyopathies. Bajusz, E., Rona, G. (eds.). Munich: Urban und Schwarzenberg 1974
4. Goodwin, J.F.: Congestive and hypertrophic cardiomyopathies. Lancet *1970/I*, 731
5. Goodwin, J.F., Oakley, C.M.: The cardiomyopathies. Brit. Heart J. *34*, 545 (1972)
6. Gotsman, M.S., Lewis, B.S., Mitha, A.S., Bakst, A.: Left ventricular performance in congestive cardiomyopathy. In: Cardiomyopathies. Bajusz, E., Rona, G. (eds.). Munich: Urban und Schwarzenberg 1974
7. Grant, C., Raphael, M.J., Steiner, R.E., Goodwin, J.F.: Left ventricular volume and hypertrophy in outflow obstruction. Cardiovasc. Res. *4*, 346 (1968)
8. Hamby, R.I., Catangay, P., Apiado, O., Khan, A.H.: Primary myocardial disease. Amer. J. Cardiol. *25*, 625 (1970)
9. Klein, M.D., Lane, F.J., Gorlin, R.: Effect of left ventricular size and shape upon the hemodynamics of subaortic stenosis. Amer. J. Cardiol. *15*, 773 (1965)
10. Kreulen, T.H., Gorlin, R., Herman, M.V.: Ventriculographic patterns and hemodynamics in primary myocardial disease. Circulation *47*, 299 (1973)
11. Mathes, P., Just, H.: Die diastolische Dehnbarkeit des linken Ventrikels bei Kardiomyopathie. Verh. dtsch. Ges. Kreisl.-Forsch. *39*, 137 (1973)
12. Oakley, C.M.: Clinical recognition of the cardiomyopathies. Circulat. Res. *34,35*, Suppl. II, 152 (1974)
13. Roberts, W.C., Ferrans, V.J.: Pathological aspects of certain cardiomyopathies. Circulat. Res. *34,35*, Suppl. II, 128 (1974)
14. Wong, A.Y.K., Rautaharju, P.M.: Stress distribution within the left ventricular wall approximated as a thick ellipsoidal shell. Amer. Heart J. *75*, 649 (1968)

16. Regional Left Ventricular Wall Motion in Congestive Cardiomyopathy

P. MATHES, W. DELIUS, H. SEBENING, A. WIRTZFELD, and H. BLÖMER

Introduction

The hemodynamic classification of CMs in hypertrophic, hypertrophic-obstructive, and congestive forms is generally accepted [7, 13, 18]. HOCM represents a homogeneous, probably genetically determined disease [5, 18]. In contrast, the COCM is almost certainly a highly heterogeneous condition. The end result of almost any cause of myocardial cell damage is likely to be a failure of systolic contraction. It has been suggested that the COCM be redefined as "heart muscle disorder of unknown cause or association" in order to emphasize the necessity of searching for an etiologic agent [17]. COCM is characterized by an increased ventricular volume in the presence of a reduced systolic performance, which is not explained on the basis of coronary or valvular heart disease. Thus, in this heterogeneous group, clinical course and prognosis vary considerably. The present investigation was undertaken to define criteria for clinical course and prognosis on first examination. To achieve this goal, left ventricular cineangiograms were analyzed in detail, with emphasis on alterations in regional wall motion.

Methods

We examined the left ventricular cineangiograms of 36 patients aged 28–56 y. suffering from COCM. Exertional dyspnea was the most common symptom, whereas angial symptoms were present only in a minority of patients. All patients had regular sinus rhythm. The left ventricular cineangiogram was performed via the femoral route. Selective coronary angiography was performed in all patients; the absence of coronary arterial disease was a prerequisite for admission to the study.

The normal pattern of radial motion was established in a group of 16 normal persons in whom a selective coronary angiogram had to be performed to exclude coronary artery disease, despite application of all available noninvasive methods. Cardiac output was determined by the direct Fick principle or by dye-dilution (Indocyanin Green). The ventricular volumes were determined by the area-length-method of Dodge *et al.* [4].

The left ventricular cineangiogram was performed in the 30° RAO position. Via a pigtail catheter 8F (Cordis-Ducor), 25–30 ml of 76% amidotrizoe-acid (Urografin) were injected into the left ventricle. The flow rate varied between 8 and 12 ml/s. The camera speed was 50 or 90 frames/s. Within the first five beats following injection of contrast material, two consecutive sinus beats were used for analysis. None were postextrasystolic. To define the radial motion of the ventricular wall, the center of the left ventricle was determined in the following manner. From the borders of the aortic valve, two lines were drawn to the maximally distant segment of the apical region. Then a line was drawn from the center of the aortic valve to the point where the two lines crossed. The latter line served as the long axis of the ventricle, the midpoint as the center of the ventricle. The axes and the center were determined for the enddiastolic and endsystolic frame and then superimposed. The center (Fig. 1) served as the 0 reference point for the polar coordinate system. The entire ventricular silhouette was divided into sections of 30° each (Fig. 1). The difference between endsystolic and

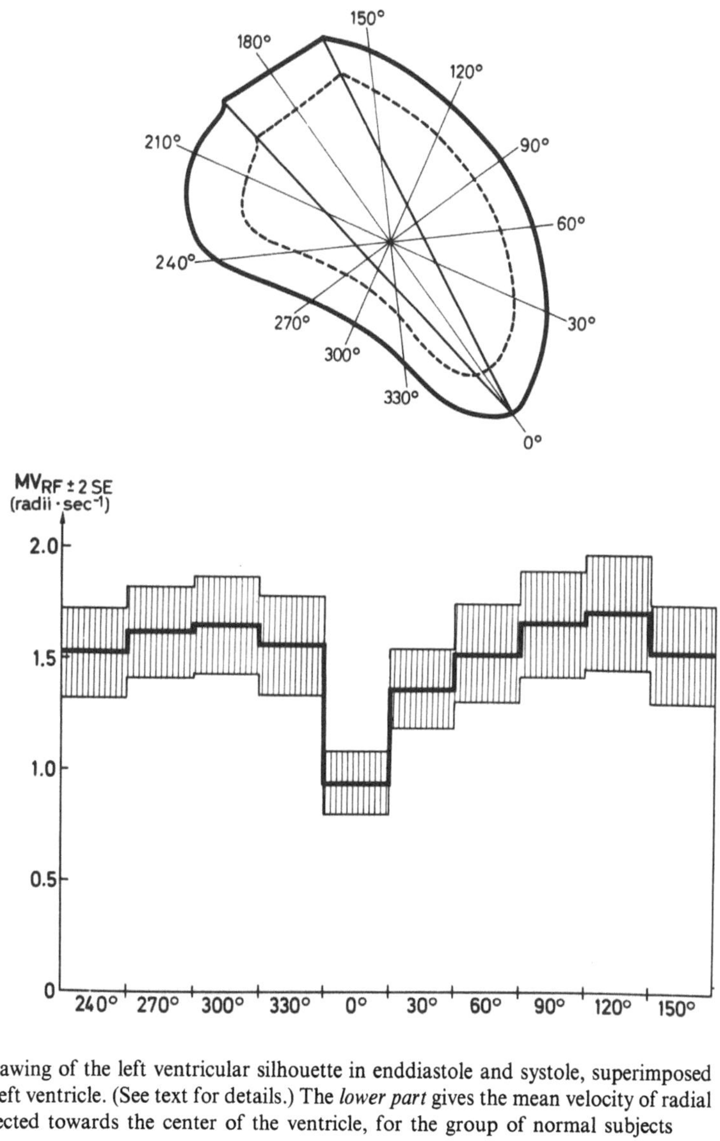

Fig. 1. Schematic drawing of the left ventricular silhouette in enddiastole and systole, superimposed at the center of the left ventricle. (See text for details.) The *lower part* gives the mean velocity of radial motion ±2SE, directed towards the center of the ventricle, for the group of normal subjects

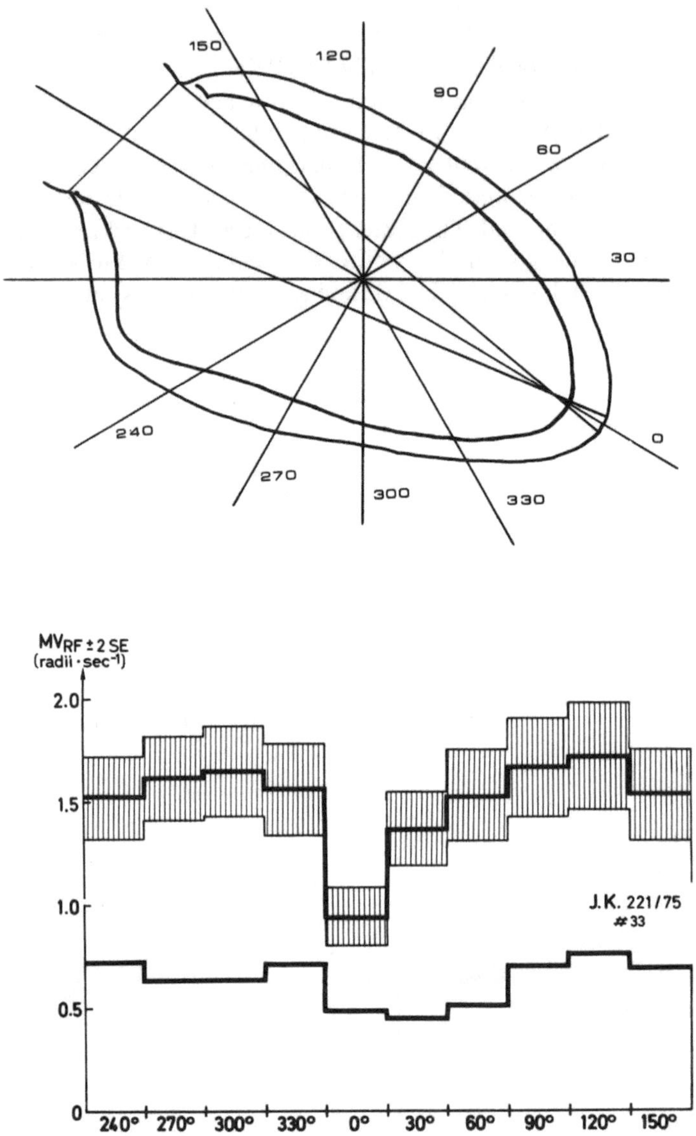

Fig. 2. Example of a COCM without regional akinesis. There is a uniform reduction in the extent and mean rate of radial fiber shortening in comparison to the normal pattern (*lower panel*)

enddiastolic radius was defined as percent shortening, and the ratio of percent shortening to ejection time was defined as the mean velocity of radial fiber shortening (mV_{rf}). The 10 segments (240°–150°) representing the muscular section of the ventricular silhouette were defined as 100%, each 30° section as 10% of the ventricle.

Results

The normal pattern of radial motion is shown in Figure 1. The mean rate of radial fiber shortening is relatively uniform in the region of the anterior (30°–150°) and inferior (240°–330°) wall of the ventricle, whereas the apical region (0°) shows a lower rate of radial fiber shortening. In patients with COCM, two different patterns of wall motion abnormality were observed. In 19 patients, a rather uniform, generalized decrease in radial wall motion was observed (see Fig. 2). The other 17 patients demonstrated akinetic segments of varying extent (Fig. 3) in

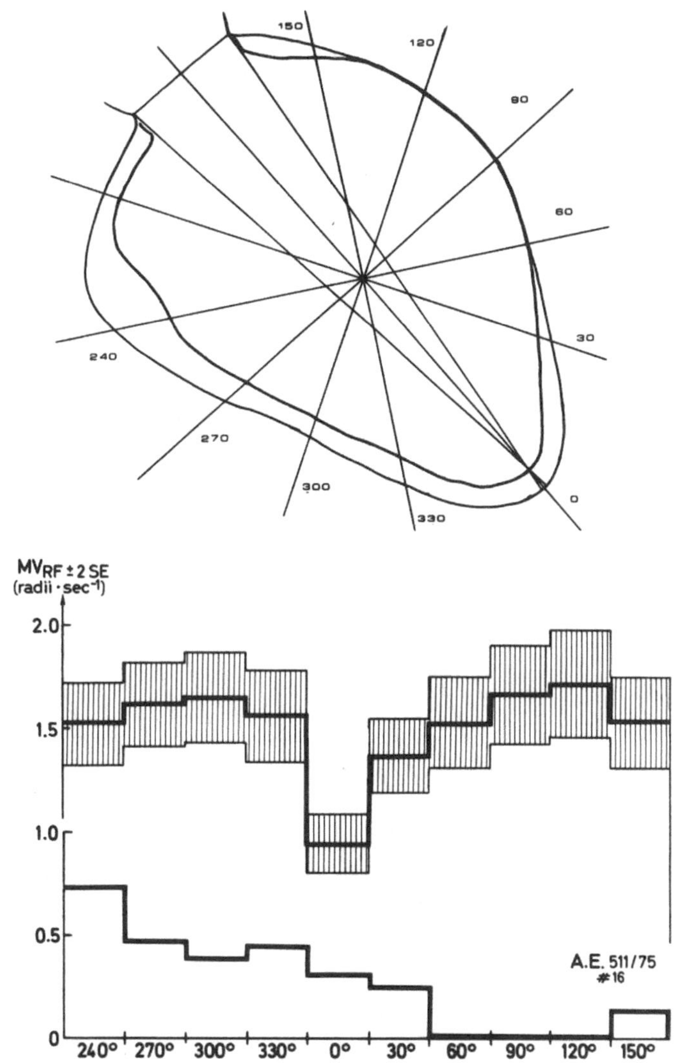

Fig. 3. Example of a COCM with an akinetic segment in the anterior wall. The severe reduction in motion in the other segments in comparison to the normal group is apparent as well

addition to the reduced extent of wall motion in the remaining segments. Figure 3 depicts an akinetic segment, comprising 30% of the ventricular circumference.

The influence of akinetic segments on ventricular hemodynamics at rest is shown in Figure 4. The cardiac index is already reduced in cases with generalized hypokinesis and shows a further reduction in the group with an akinetic segment of more than 30% of the ventricular circumference. The left ventricular filling pressure at rest shows a tendency to increase with the extent of akinetic segments.

Figure 5 shows the influence of the presence of akinetic segments on measures of ventricular function. EF is reduced in the group without akinetic segments, whereas a further reduction is observed in patients with additional akinetic segments. The mean rate of radial fiber shortening of all examined segments shows a marked reduction in COCM, with a further decline in cases with akinetic segments.

The mV_{rf} also decreases markedly in patients with COCM, again decreasing further in the presence of akinetic segments (Fig. 6). The left ventricular EDV is increased in patients with COCM; a further significant increase is observed in patients with akinetic segments in excess of 30% of the left ventricular circumference.

The mean follow-up period was 21 months, ranging from 6 to 70 months. Among the 15 patients without akinetic segments, 9 were in functional class II (NYHA) and remained unchanged during the period of observation. Six were in functional class III. Two showed improvement of cardiac symptoms, and

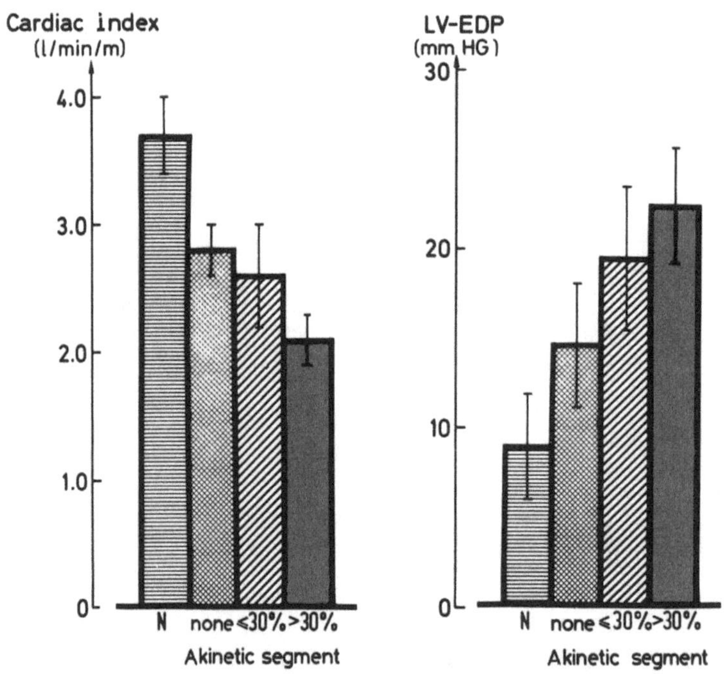

Fig. 4. Hemodynamics in COCM. With increasing size of the akinetic segment, there is a reduction in cardiac index and an increase in left ventricular filling pressure to be observed. *N*, normal group

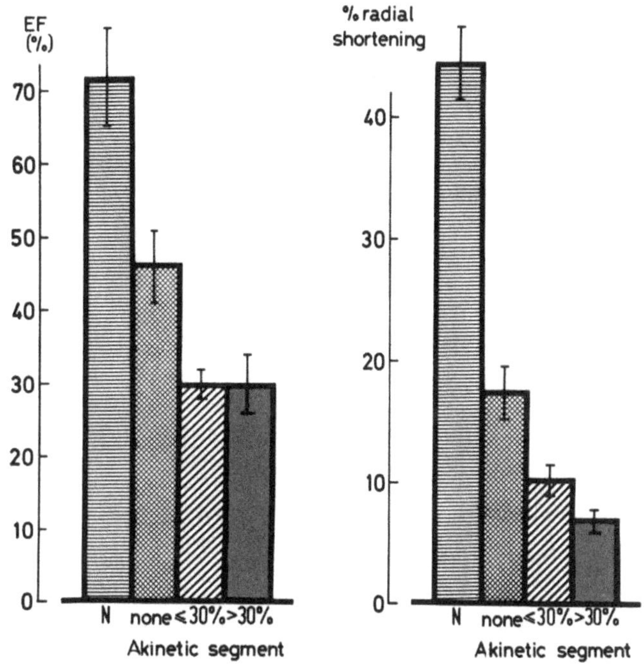

Fig. 5. Ventricular function in COCM. In cases with akinetic segments, a further reduction in *EF* and mV_{rf} is observed

the others remained stable. Among the nine patients with akinetic segments of less than 30% of the ventricular circumference, six were in functional class II at the time of examination. One of them deteriorated; the others remained stable. Among the 12 patients with akinetic segments in excess of 30% of the ventricular circumference, 11 were in functional class III at the time of the initial examination; 4 deteriorated to class IV; 5 of those patients died during the period of observation (mean observation period 13 months, ranging 12–15 months).

A complete LBBB in 7 of the 12 patients with akinetic segments of more than 30% of the ventricular circumference was seen in the ECG. In four cases a pattern suggestive of myocardial infarction (loss of R waves with a resulting QS pattern) was observed, the location corresponding with the akinetic segment in the ventriculogram. In the group without akinetic segments a complete LBBB was observed in two cases; ECG patterns suggestive of myocardial infarction were not observed.

Discussion

A quantitative analysis of regional left ventricular wall motion poses considerable problems since wall motion during contraction occurs in all three planes. Moreover, the cardiac chambers rotate during contraction, and there is considerable variation within each chamber. For these reasons, extracardiac reference points

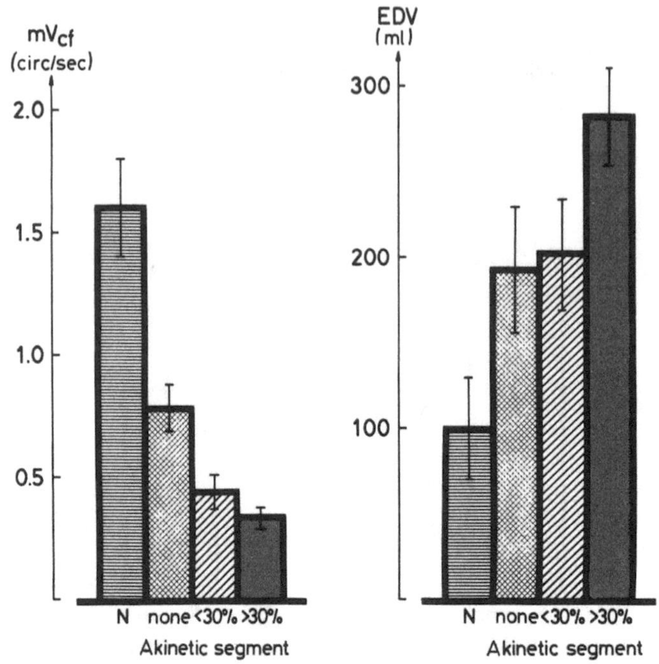

Fig. 6. Ventricular function in COCM. The group of CMs is characterized by a decrease in mV_{cf} and an increase in EDV. In the presence of akinetic segments, these changes are more pronounced than in cases without akinetic segments

do not permit a realistic assessment of regional ventricular wall motion. To define a fixed intracardiac reference point, Sniderman [22] proposed to leave a catheter in the coronary sinus in order to compensate for the rotation of the heart. However, since the catheter itself will participate in the cardiac motion it cannot serve as a reliable reference point. Leighton *et al.* [14] proposed to divide the ventricle into two areas of equal size; however, since the long axis will move toward the region of abnormal wall motion, the extent of abnormal wall motion will be underestimated.

This study uses a coordinate system based on reference points at the aortic valve and the left ventricular apex. These points were chosen because they are the most clearly defined intracardiac anatomic landmarks that persist throughout systolic contraction. The midpoint of the long axis was chosen as the common reference point, and it was assumed that wall motion occurs in a radial manner toward this center. This assumption is based on an analysis of fiber orientation throughout the wall of the left ventricle [20, 23].

In contrast to the marked differences in regional wall motion in coronary heart disease, COCM is regarded as a generalized disease of the myocardium, affecting all areas to the same extent [1, 7, 9, 10, 13, 17]. Roughly half of our patients showed demonstrable regional differences in contractile behavior, an observation previously made by Kreulen *et al.* [12] and Leighton *et al.* [14]. There is no clear explanation at present for the occurrence of these akinetic segments.

In pathologic-anatomic studies, Roberts and Ferrans [21] demonstrated extensive endocardial and myocardial scarring in COCM. Mural thrombi, in the process of organization and fibrosis could also cause a regional decrease in ventricular wall motion. Embolization of major coronary arteries was excluded by selective coronary angiography.

In approximately 15% of patients with COCM, a pattern suggestive of myocardial infarction (loss of R waves with a resulting QS complex) is observed [2,6,11,19,24]. These changes were seen in six of our patients; the location corresponded to the angiographically determined area of akinesis. The majority of patients did not show such a correlation, possibly as a consequence of the high incidence of complete LBBB in cases with large akinetic segments.

A correlation between cardiac index, EF, and left ventricular filling pressure could not be observed, possibly as a consequence of an alteration of diastolic compliance in COCM [3,15]. However, hemodynamic parameters and indices of ventricular function were decreased in patients with akinetic segments. Among the 24 patients without akinetic segments or with akinesis of less than 30% of the left ventricular circumference, 20 remained stable. Clinical deterioration was observed in only four patients. There were no deaths in this group. Among the 12 patients with akinetic segments of more than 30% of the left ventricular circumference, four showed clinical deterioration, and five died during the period of observation; only three patients remained stable. Apparently, the occurrence of extensive akinesis in COCM indicates an advanced stage of the disease, with an unfavorable prognosis.

Summary

Regional analysis of the left ventricular angiogram obtained at diagnostic cardiac catheterization was undertaken in 36 patients with COCM and in 16 healthy subjects. Applying the concept of radial wall motion, directed towards the center of the left ventricle, areas of akinesis comprising 20%–50% of the left ventricular circumference were found in more than half of the cases with COCM. The greater the area of akinesis, the greater the reduction in hemodynamic parameters and left ventricular function. The health of nearly all patients with akinetic segments in excess of 30% of the left ventricular circumference deteriorated in the subsequent period of observation (6–70 months, averaging 21 months). In contrast, in patients without akinetic segments, the clinical condition remained stable. A large akinetic area in COCM indicates a severe reduction in left ventricular function and is an unfavorable prognostic sign.

References

1. Baxley, W.H., Reeves, T.J.: Abnormal regional myocardial performance in coronary artery disease. Prog. cardiovasc. Dis. *13*, 405 (1971)
2. Delius, W., Sebening, H., Weghmann, N., Oversohl, K., Wirtzfeld, A., Mathes, P.: Klinik und Verlauf der kongestiven Kardiomyopathie ungeklärter Ätiologie. Dtsch. med. Wschr. *101*, 635 (1976)

3. Diamond, G., Forrester, J.S.: Effect of coronary artery disease and acute myocardial infarction on left ventricular compliance in man. Circulation *45*, 11 (1972)
4. Dodge, H.T., Baxley, W.H.: Left ventricular volume and mass and their significance in coronary artery disease. Amer. J. Cardiol. *23*, 528 (1969)
5. Emanuel, R., Wither, R., O'Brien, K.: Dominant and recessive modes of inheritance in idiopathic cardiomyopathy. Lancet *1971/II*, 1065
6. Gau, G., Goodwin, J.F., Oakley, C.M., Raphael, M.J., Steinter, R.E.: Q-waves and coronary angiography in cardiomyopathy. Brit. Heart J. *32*, 554 (1970)
7. Goodwin, J.F.: Congestive and hypertrophic cardiomyopathies. A decade of study. Lancet *1970/I*, 733
8. Hamilton, G.W., Murray, J.A., Kennedy, J.W.: Quantitative angiocardiography in ischemic heart disease. Circulation *45*, 1065 (1972)
9. Herman, M.V., Gorlin, R.: Implications of left ventricular asynergy. Amer. J. Cardiol. *23*, 538 (1967)
10. Herman, M.V., Heinle, R.A., Klein, M.D., Gorlin, R.: Localized disorders in myocardial contraction. Asynergy and its role in congestive failure. New Engl. J. Med. *277*, 222 (1967)
11. Hollister, R.M., Goodwin, J.F.: The electrocardiogram in cardiomyopathy. Brit. Heart J. *25*, 357 (1963)
12. Kreulen, T.H., Gorlin, R., Herman, M.V.: Ventriculographic patterns and hemodynamics in primary myocardial disease. Circulation *47*, 299 (1973)
13. Kübler, W., Kuhn, H., Loogen, F.: Die Kardiomyopathien. Z. Kardiol. *62*, 3 (1973)
14. Leighton, R.F., Wilt, S.M., Lewis, R.P.: Detection of hypokinesis by quantitative analysis of left ventricular cineangiograms. Circulation *50*, 121 (1974)
15. Mathes, P., Just, H.: Veränderte Elastizität der linken Herzkammer bei Kardiomyopathie. Z. Kardiol. *63*, 72 (1973)
16. Mathes, P., Delius, W., Sebening, H., Wirtzfeld, A., Blömer, H.: Das regionale Kontraktionsverhalten der linken Herzkammer bei kongestiver Kardiomyopathie. Dtsch. med. Wschr. *101*, 995 (1976)
17. Oakley, C.M.: Clinical definitions and classifications of cardiomyopathies. Postgrad. med. J. *48*, 703 (1972)
18. Oakley, C.M.: Clinical recognition of the cardiomyopathies. Circulat. Res. *34,35*, Suppl. II, 152 (1974)
19. Pruitt, R.D., Card, G.W., Leachman, R.: Simulation of electrocardiograms of apico-lateral myocardial infarction by myocardial destructive lesions of obscure etiology (myocardiopathy). Circulation *25*, 506 (1962)
20. Roberts, J.T.: Dynamics and circulation of heart muscle. In: Pathologic Physiology. Sodeman, Sodeman (eds.). Philadelphia-London: W.B. Saunders 1967, p. 314
21. Roberts, W.C., Ferrans, V.J.: Pathological aspects of certain cardiomyopathies. Circulat. Res. *34,35*, Suppl. II, 128 (1974)
22. Sniderman, A.D., Marpole, D., Fallen, E.: Regional contraction patterns in the normal and ischemic ventricle in man. Amer. J. Cardiol. *31*, 484 (1973)
23. Streeter, jr., D.D., Hanna, W.T.: Engineering mechanics for successive states in canine left ventricular myocardium. II. Fiber angle and sarcomere length. Circulat. Res. *33*, 656 (1973)
24. Tavel, M.E., Fisch, C.: Abnormal Q-waves simulating myocardial infarction in diffuse myocardial diseases. Amer. Heart J. *68*, 534 (1964)
25. Yu, P.N., Cohen, J., Schreiner, B.F., Murphy, G.W.: Hemodynamic alterations in primary myocardial disease. Prog. cardiovasc. Dis. *7*, 125 (1964)

17. Evaluation of the Ventricular Septum by Biventricular Cineangiography in Congestive and Hypertrophic Cardiomyopathies

W. DELIUS, A. WIRTZFELD, A. SCHINZ, P. MATHES, H. SEBENING, and H. BLÖMER

Recent echocardiographic findings have greatly increased the clinician's interest in the morphology and function of the interventricular septum. The ratio of the septal to the posterior left ventricular wall thickness has become an essential parameter for the diagnosis of asymmetric septal hypertrophy (ASH) [2, 3, 8, 10, 16, 17]. In addition, the thickness and the motion of the ventricular septum are of interest for evaluating septal regional function in patients with coronary heart disease [3], COCM [3, 6] and various forms of congenital heart disease [1, 3, 5, 18]. In addition to echocardiography, two other techniques for noninvasive evaluation of the ventricular septum have recently been developed: the gated radionuclide cardiac blood pool scan [1, 13, 14] and the myocardial perfusion imaging with thallium 201 [1, 13]. Although a large number of publications deal with noninvasive assessment of structure and function of the interventricular septum, only a few reports deal with septal delineation by biventricular angiography as a method of determining the size, shape, and function of the interventricular septum [4, 9, 16]. The purpose of our study, therefore, is to determine the feasibility of angiographic septal visualization for quantitative and qualitative analysis in patients with congestive and hypertrophic myocardiopathies and to compare the results with those obtained by echocardiography.

Methods

Biventricular angiographic studies were performed in 22 patients: 6 with COCM and 6 with HOCM, 3 with hypertensive heart disease, and 7 without evidence of cardiac disease. All patients suffering from COCM had greatly dilated left ventricular cavities with an EF below 30%. They had normal coronary arteries. The etiology of the disease was unknown. The diagnosis of HOCM was made on the basis of characteristic angiographic and echocardiographic findings (septal to posterolateral left ventricular free wall ratio of 1.3 or greater). All six patients with HOCM had an outflow tract gradient on provocation or at rest. Out of the three patients suffering from essential hypertension one had also a slight valvular aortic stenosis. The patients with normal hearts but atypical chest pain were studied to rule out coronary artery disease and were found to be free of heart disease. Prior to the angiograms, data including right and left ventricular pressures were recorded. Following left ventricular angiography in the RAO position patients were placed in an LAO position, and biventricular angiography for visualization of the ventricular septum was performed. Manual injections of contrast material into the right ventricle were used to determine the position most appropriate for septal visualization. Biventricular angiography was done by simultaneous injections into the left and right ventricular cavities; the left ventricular injection was made via a pigtail catheter 8 F (Cordis Ducor) using the Contrac-injector at a flow rate of 8–10 ml/s; the right ventricle was opacified by manual injection of 15–20 ml contrast material via a 7 F-Swan-Ganz catheter.

The method of analysis of the ventricular septum is depicted in Figure 1. The aortic valve and the apical and inferior aspects of both ventricular cavities were drawn on transparent paper in enddiastole (solid line) and in endsystole (dotted line). In addition, for analysis of the septal contraction process, the septal contours were delineated at intervals of 0.04 s using the "center of the left ventricle" as the reference point. The ventricular center was defined by the midpoint of a line connecting the center of the aortic valve with the left ventricular apex. This line was constructed according to the method previously described [12]: The border of the aortic valve was connected with the farthest point on the apical contour. Through the intersection of these two lines, another line was drawn starting from the center of the aortic valve; this was defined as the axis of the left ventricle.

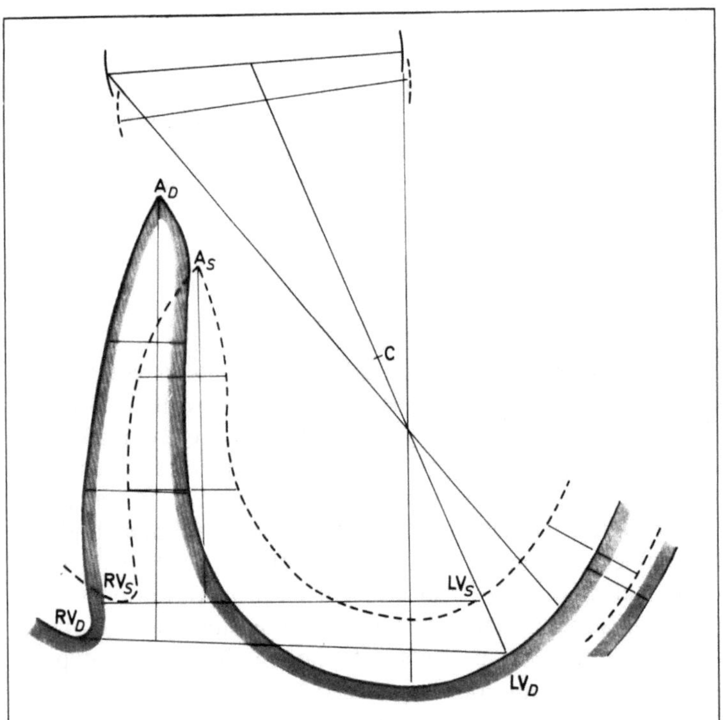

Fig. 1. Diagram showing the analysis of the interventricular septum by biventricular cineangiography. Enddiastolic (*solid line*) and endsystolic (*broken line*) contours of the ventricular septum and the apical right and left ventricular region in a normal individual. For detailed description, see text

This axis was constructed separately for the enddiastolic and the endsystolic frames (LV_D and LV_S). From the apical intersection of the ventricular axis a line was drawn to the apex of the right ventricle and a perpendicular line through the ventricular septum was constructed to determine the septal length and to divide the septum into three equal parts. These auxiliary lines were selected because it was relatively easy to find the appropriate reference points on the angiograms. The thickness of the free ventricular wall was measured at the junction of the middle to the lower third. For correction of X-ray magnification a graded scale was filmed at the end of the procedure which was placed according to the level of the ventricles. Using echocardiography, septal thickness was measured below the level of the distal margins of the mitral valve. Posterobasal left ventricular free wall thickness was measured with the transducer oriented so that part of the echocardiographic signal was reflected from the posterior mitral leaflet [10].

Results

Figure 2A represents an example of the enddiastolic frame of a normal ventricular septum visualized by biventricular angiography in a 45° LAO projection. Both ventricles are filled by contrast material; the mitral valve is still open. The left and right ventricular septal outlines are approximately parallel to each other in their middle sections, showing a slight convex bending towards the right ventricular cavity, and in their lower sections they diverge somewhat towards the apices. The free left ventricular wall is equal in thickness to the middle and upper parts of the septum.

The ventricular septum in patients with HOCM shows marked thickening. Figure 2B clearly shows the narrowing of the left ventricular outflow tract by the anterior systolic motion of the mitral leaflet. (The left ventricular anterior wall overlaps partially the lower section of the septum; on the original film the septal contour can be clearly recognized.) This example also shows the marked difference in the thickness of the septum as compared to the left ventricular free wall.

In COCM the septum appears disproportionately thin in relation to the size of the ventricular cavity. The left and right ventricular septal surfaces run parallel to each other (Fig. 2C).

The configurational changes of the ventricular septum occurring during systole are drawn in Figure 3 at intervals of 0.04 s. During systolic contraction the normal septum roughly maintains its shape; the right and left ventricular endocardial surfaces remain parallel (Fig. 3A). There is a shortening of the septal length with a corresponding increase of approximately 30% in its diameter. In addition, the septum moves towards the left ventricular cavity. In HOCM the septal motion is markedly reduced (Fig. 4A). In addition, as seen in Figure 3B, there is a systolic bulging of the septal surface into the left ventricular chamber. In patients with COCM (Fig. 3C) we found very few changes in configuration and motion of the ventricular septum during systole; the length and diameter of the septum showed only minimal alterations.

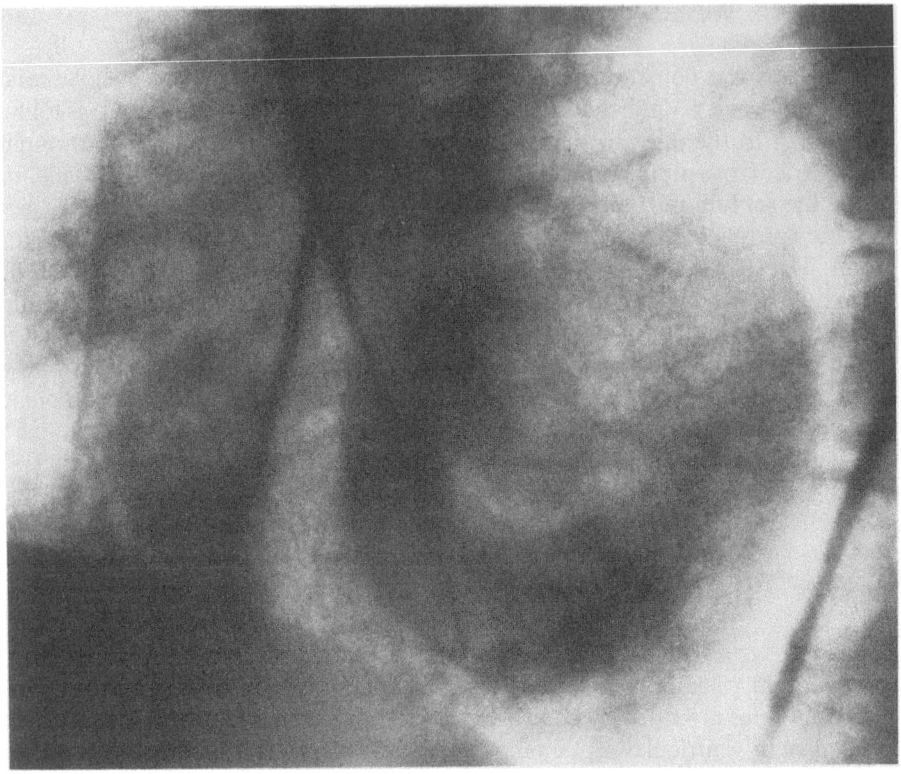
A

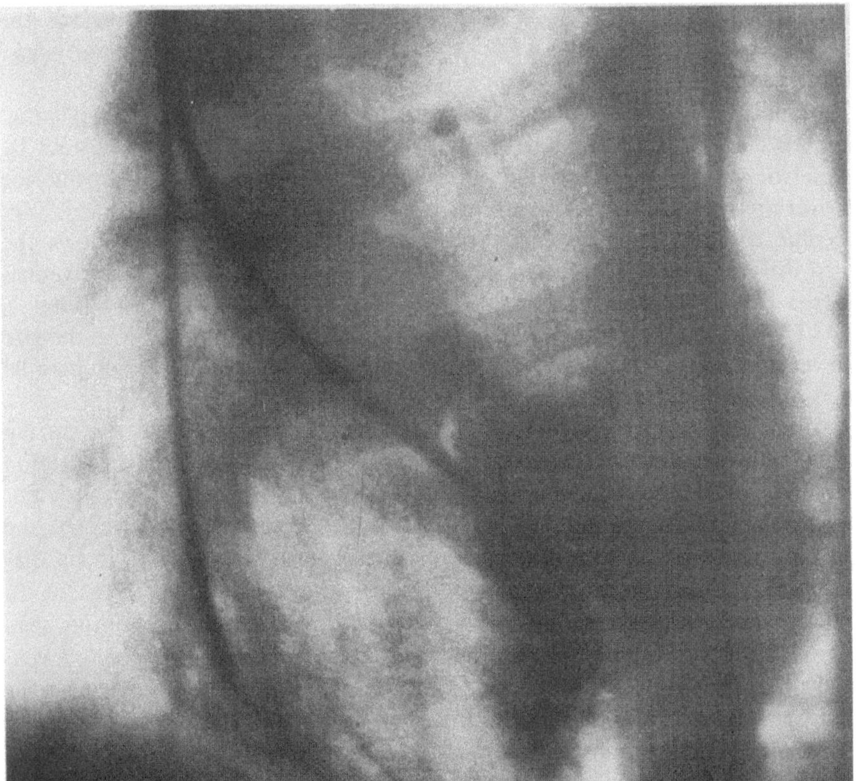
B

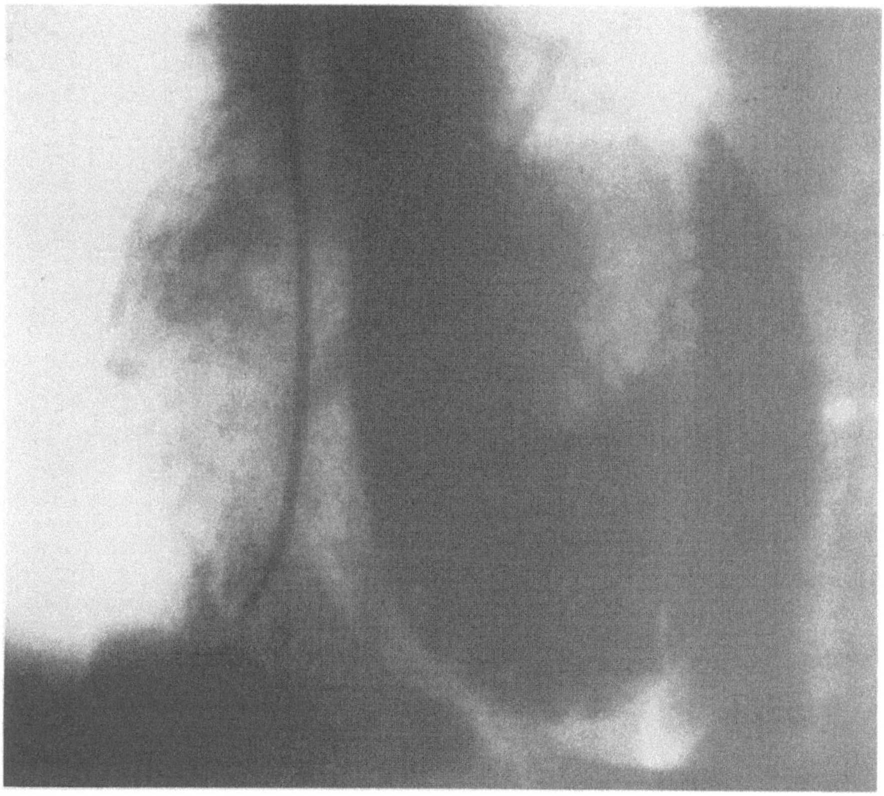

C

Fig. 2. Examples of biventricular angiograms. *A*. Normal interventricular septum in enddiastole. *B*. Septum of a patient with HOCM in endsystole showing narrowing of the left ventricular outflow tract due to systolic anterior movement of the anterior leaflet of the mitral valve. *C*. Enddiastolic frame of a patient with COCM showing a thin-walled elongated interventricular septum with parallel course of the right and left ventricular endocardial surfaces

As demonstrated in Figure 4, the configuration of the ventricular septum in a patient with HOCM (Fig. 4A) may look very similar to patients with generalized left ventricular hypertrophy secondary to essential hypertension or aortic stenosis (Fig. 4B). However, in patients with hypertrophy secondary to pressure overload, in contrast to HOCM, the thickness of the left ventricular free wall equals the mean septal thickness.

The enddiastolic septal diameter, as measured at the junction of the upper to the middle thirds (Fig. 1) amounted to 9.4 $\pm$0.5 mm in normal individuals, 8.6 $\pm$0.5 mm in patients with COCM, 21.1 $\pm$1.6 mm in patients with HOCM, and 14.9 mm in those 3 patients presenting with essential hypertension (Fig. 5). At the junction of the middle to the lower third of the septum the average diameters were 11.2 $\pm$0.6 mm for normals, 9.0 $\pm$0.5 mm for patients with COCM, 25.8 $\pm$1.1 mm in cases with HOCM, and 17.6 mm in essential hypertension. There is a statistically significant difference ($P < 0.001$) in septal thickness of patients suffering from HOCM as compared to normal controls. In patients with

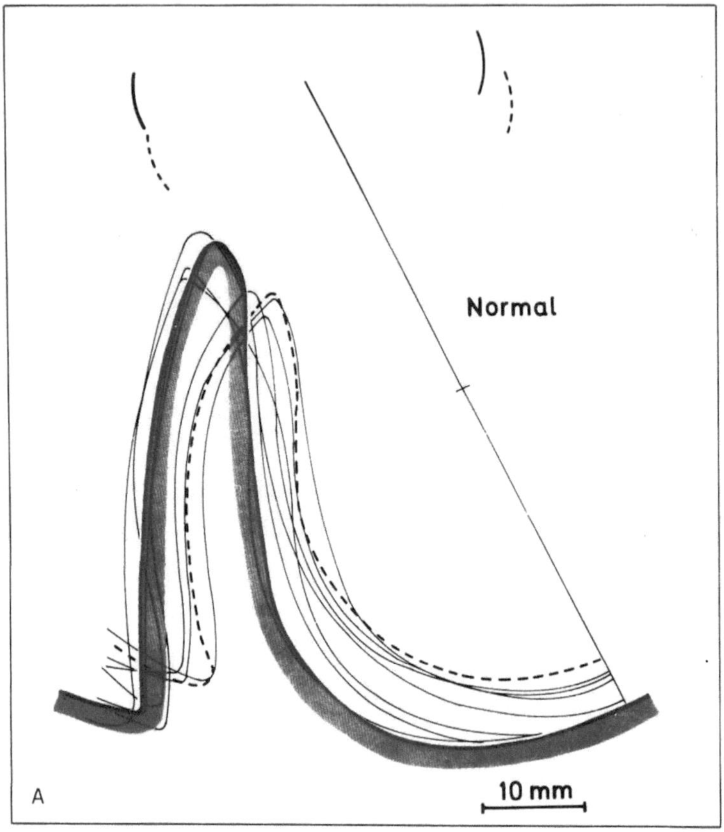

Fig. 3. Configurational changes of the interventricular septum occurring during systole: *A*. Normal septum. *B*. HOCM. *C*. COCM

COCM the upper septal diameter reached normal values, but the septal thickness at the lower level was significantly smaller ($P < 0.01$). The comparison of the septal diameters measured at the upper and lower levels confirmed the angiographic impression that in patients with COCM the endocardial surfaces remained parallel during systole, whereas in normal individuals there is a slight increase and in patients with HOCM a marked increase in the lower septal width.

Comparison of Angiographic and Echocardiographic Measurements of the Septal Width

Table 1 represents a summary of our data obtained on those patients in whom angiographic as well as echocardiographic studies were available. Because the number of cases examined with both techniques is relatively small, our data are also compared with those published by Henry *et al.* [10] (Table 2). In spite of the fact that in our patients with HOCM and in normals, echocardiographic

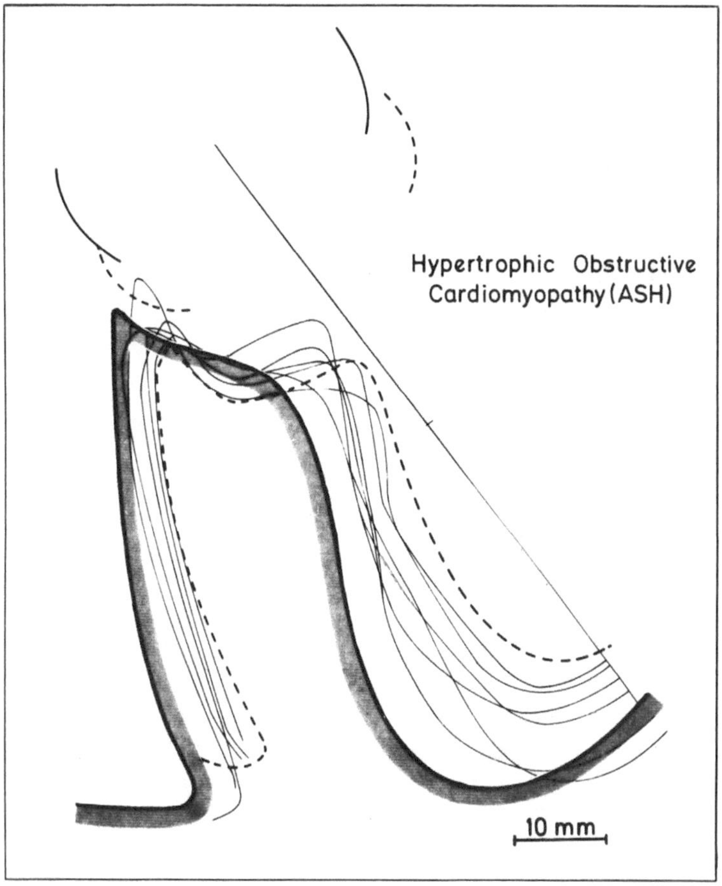

Fig. 3B

Table 1. Comparison of angiographic and echocardiographic data regarding the thickness of the interventricular septum and the left ventricular free wall in patients with HOCM and COCM and in normals.

Diagnosis	Patient	Septal thickness (mm)		Left ventricular free wall thickness (mm)		Septal: free wall thickness	
		Angio	Echo	Angio	Echo	Angio	Echo
HOCM	M.	20	20	12	11	1.6	1.8
	J.	21	19	14	10	1.5	1.9
	S.	21	22	12	11	1.7	2.0
	St.	23	19	14	10	1.6	1.9
COCM	G.	8	7	8	10	1.0	0.7
	R.	9	10	9	10	1.0	1.0
	P.	9	11	8	10	1.1	1.1
Normal (n = 7)		9.4 ±0.5	9.6 ±1.1	9.7 ±0.5	9.1 ±1.2	0.96	1.0

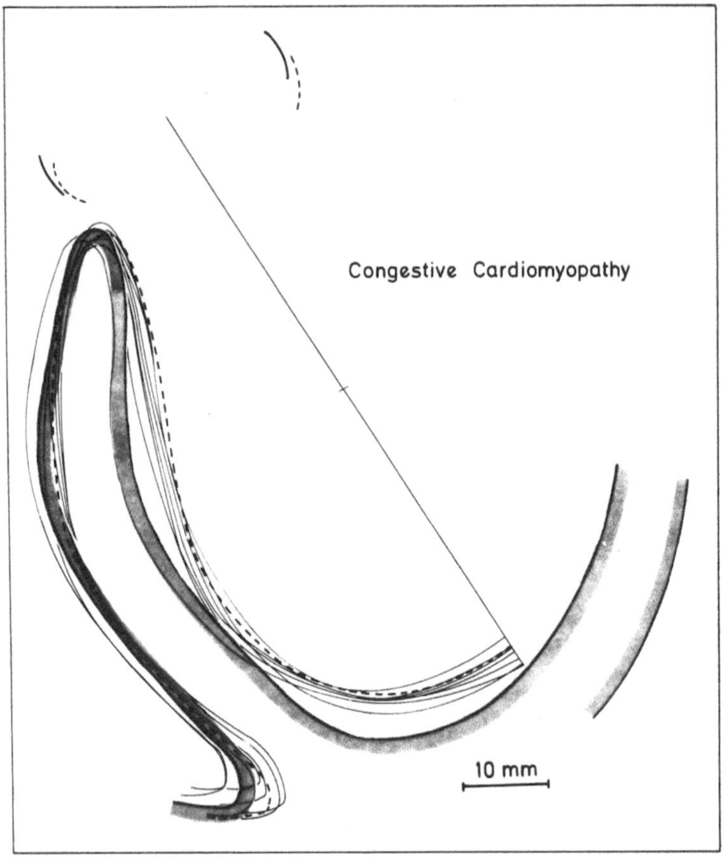

Fig. 3C

Table 2. Comparison of our data regarding septal and free ventricular wall thickness in HOCM with the echocardiographic data published by Henry *et al.* [*Circulation 50*, 447 (1974)].

	Normal		HOCM	
	Angio	Echo	Angio	Echo
Septal thickness (mm)	9.4 ±0.5	9.9 ±0.1	21.1 ±1.6	23.2 ±0.9
Left ventricular free wall thickness (mm)	9.7 ±0.5	9.5 ±0.1	13.3 ±0.6	12.0 ±0.3 13.3 ±0.4
Septal thickness / Free wall	0.96	1.0	1.6	1.9 1.8

measurement of the left ventricular free wall thickness was somewhat smaller than the angiographic measurement, there is a good overall agreement in the data obtained by both techniques (Table 1). Accordingly, the ratio between septal and left ventricular free wall thickness is slightly higher when determined echocardiographically. This ratio determined by angiogram and by echocardiography (our data in parentheses) amounts to 0.96 and 1.0 (1.0) in normals, 1.6

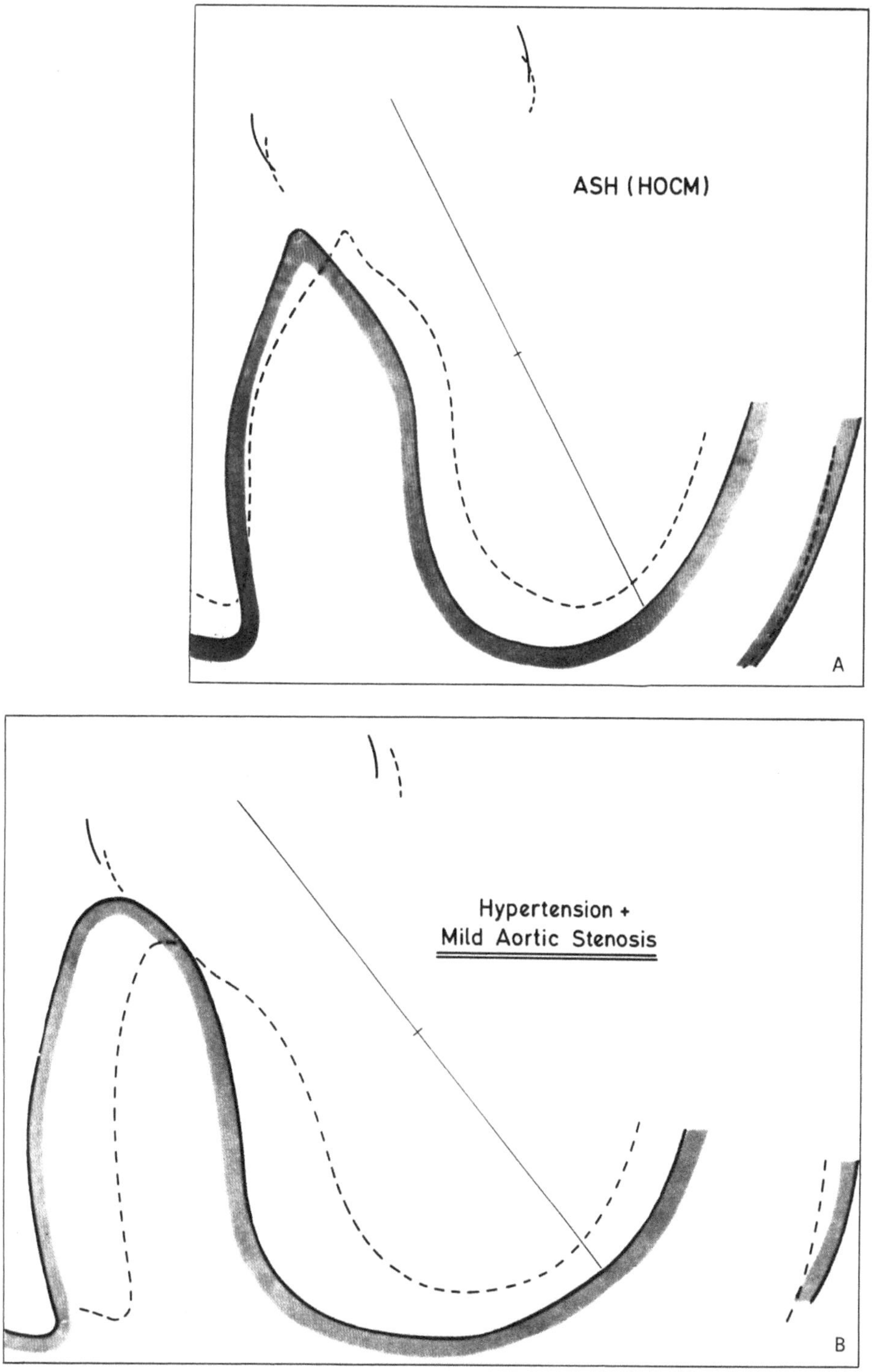

Fig. 4. Comparison of septal and left ventricular free wall thickness in (*A*) a patient with obstructive cardiomyopathy and (*B*) a patient with left ventricular hypertrophy secondary to essential hypertension and mild aortic stenosis. Notice the asymmetrical hypertrophy of the ventricular septum in *A* and the equal hypertrophy of the septum and the posterior left ventricular free wall in *B*

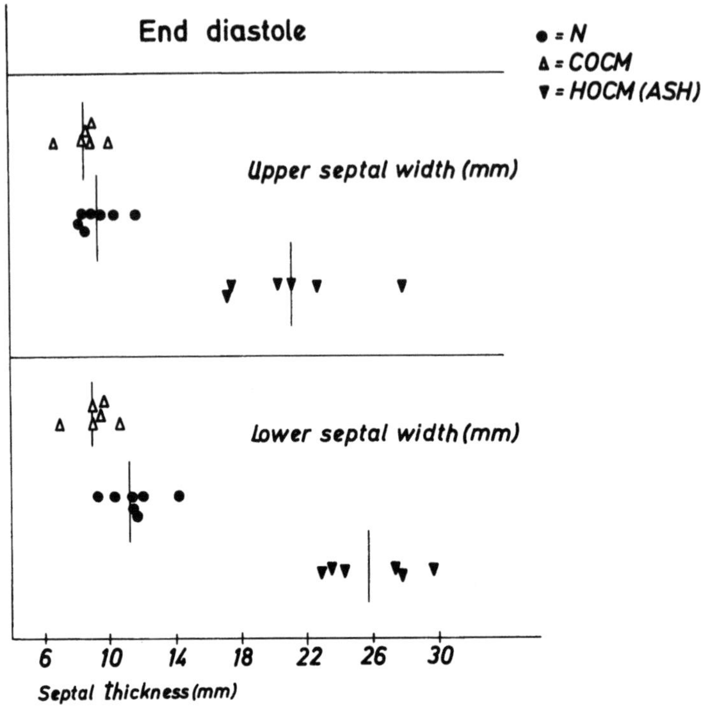

Fig. 5. Enddiastolic septal thickness in normals (N), patients with congestive cardiomyopathy (COCM), and those with hypertrophic obstructive cardiomyography (HOCM)

and 1.8 (1.9) in patients with HOCM, 1.0 and (0.9) in patients with COCM, and 0.9 in essential hypertension, respectively. These data also demonstrate that the ratio determined by either technique is significantly higher ($P < 0.001$) in patients with HOCM than in the other groups.

In normal individuals the systolic shortening of the interventricular septum in its longitudinal axis amounted to 21%, while in patients with COCM and HOCM there was only minimal shortening of 7%–8%.

Discussion

There are three methods available today to demonstrate abnormalities of the interventricular septum: echocardiography, biventricular angiography, and radioisotopic scanning techniques. The method most widely employed is echocardiography, by means of which the diagnostic significance for the evaluation of the ventricular septum in patients with various forms of CM has clearly been demonstrated. Even if for various reasons echocardiography should turn out to be superior in the analysis of ventricular septal function, for the time being it seems important that results obtained by invasive and noninvasive methods are compared. According to the criteria established by echocardiography the ratio of septal to posterobasal left ventricular free wall thickness is highly sensitive in distinguishing hearts with HOCM and hypertrophic cardiomyopathy without obstruction (HCM) from both normals and hearts hypertrophied secondary to left ventricular pressure overload [8, 10, 17]. A ratio equal to or greater than 1.3 is considered to indicate HOCM or HCM [10]. The validity of this concept has recently been limited by findings in healthy newborns [18] and in patients with right ventricular hypertrophy [5] who also may present with a septal to free wall ratio of 1.3. When comparing the angiographic visualization of the ventricular septum we must bear in mind that for technical reasons, echocardiographic measurement of the ventricular free wall is made at the posterobasal portion directly behind the posterior mitral leaflet, whereas in angiocardiograms usually the inferior part of the ventricular wall is measured. This difference may be important in patients with HCM since the posterobasal left ventricular free wall is normal in thickness and the free wall may become markedly thickened inferior to the posterior mitral leaflet. Therefore the septal to free wall ratio determined by echocardiography may be greater than 1.3, but may be smaller in the same patients when determined angiocardiographically [10, 15]. In patients with COCM echocardiographic analysis of the ventricular septum is less meaningful than in patients with HOCM or HCM. According to Corya *et al.* [3] mean diastolic thickness in patients with COCM does not differ significantly from normal. However, a decreased thickening is considered evidence of generalized myocardial involvement.

The technique of biventricular angiography for delineation of the interventricular septum has been rarely used, and few reports are available in the literature: Desilets *et al.* [4], Harmjanz *et al.* [9], and most recently Redwood *et al.* [15]. In accordance with Redwood *et al.* [15] our study shows that asymmetric septal hypertrophy is a distinctive feature of HOCM which may clearly be demonstrated by biventricular angiography. Also, angiographic visualization of the ventricular septum is superior to echocardiography for assessment of the configuration and the changes in total septal shape occurring during systole. In normal individuals, the septum appears as part of the left ventricular wall; right and left ventricular endocardial surfaces roughly parallel to each other curving toward the right ventricle. During systole, septal shortening occurs and septal thickness increases. The septum in patients with COCM, however, represents a thin-walled structure with an exactly parallel course of both surfaces and a conspicuous reduction in motility with lack of systolic increase in thickness. The ventricular septum in HOCM is characterized by a striking increase in thickness which amounts to 2–3 times the normal diameter. Redwood *et al.* [15] have drawn attention to the roughly triangular appearance of the interventricular septum as a highly characteristic configurational abnormality. We were able to confirm these findings on enddiastolic frames which showed the lower septal portion to be significantly thicker than the upper portion. But during systole there was a reversal of this ratio in some cases because of a relatively greater increment in the upper and middle septal diameter than in the lower portion of the ventricular septum. The significance of this observation must be investigated in a larger number of patients.

Angiographic analysis of the interventricular septum, therefore, is basically in agreement with echocardiographic findings in normal individuals and in patients with COCM or HOCM. The same is true for quantitative data referring to septal thickness. Concerning the diameter of the free posterior wall, however, some differences may be encountered, probably due to the method of measurement. The essential advantage of echocardiography is the procedure for screening and following-up. The advantage of biventricular angiography, however, is that the configuration and the systolic motion of the entire septum can be analyzed precisely. The diagnostic reliability in the assessment of the patient's cardiac condition by biventricular angiography is significantly superior to only left ventricular injection alone. The possibility of the right or left ventricle overlapping the septum or the right ventricular outflow tract superimposed on the upper septal portion must be considered when analyzing the interventricular septum; this may prove unavoidable in some cases. By using a low flow setting on the injector the septal contour can clearly be outlined in the majority of cases, even if there is some overlap of the ventricular cavities.

Preliminary results of the other methods of septal visualization, the gated radionuclide cardiac blood pool scanning and the myocardial perfusion imaging with thallium 201, show that with these techniques, as with biventricular angiography, the entire profile of the interventricular septum can be visualized [1,13, 14]. The sensitivity of these methods as compared to echocardiography and angiography remains to be determined.

Summary

Patients with hypertrophic and congestive forms of CM have a characteristic configurational abnormality of the interventricular septum which may be demonstrated by echocardiography as well as by biventricular cineangiography. Only the latter procedure, however, allows the visualization of the entire septum, showing the typical asymmetric hypertrophy in cases of HOCM. In COCM, the septum is thin-walled with parallel surfaces, showing only minimal thickening during systole. In HOCM the septal diameter is 2–3 times the normal thickness and the lower portion is significantly thicker than the upper portion, giving the septum a characteristic "triangular" appearance; in some cases the systolic increase in septal thickness is more pronounced in the upper than in the lower parts. Angiographic and echocardiographic analyses of the interventricular septum basically yield similar results which complement each other in the evaluation of cardiac abnormalities involving the septum.

References

1. Bulkley, B.H., Rouleau, J., Strauss, H.W., Pitt, B.: Idiopathic hypertrophic subaortic stenosis: Detection by thallium 201 myocardial perfusion imaging. New Engl. J. Med. *293*, 1113 (1975)
2. Cooperman, L.B., Rosenblum, R., Cohen, M.V.: Abnormal septal contraction in idiopathic hypertrophic subaortic stenosis. Circulation *50*, Suppl. III, 29 (1974)
3. Corya, B.C., Rasmussen, S., Feigenbaum, H., Knoebel, S.B., Black, M.J.: Systolic thickening

and thinning of the septum and posterior wall in patients with coronary artery disease, congestive cardiomyopathy, and atrial septal defect. Circulation *55*, 109 (1977)
4. Desilets, D.T., Kadell, B.M., Ruttenberg, H.D., Goldberg, S.J., McAlpin, R.N.: Angiographic demonstration of the ventricular septum. Radiology *91*, 329 (1968)
5. Goodman, D.J., Harrison, D.C., Popp, R.L.: Echocardiographic features of primary pulmonary hypertension. Amer. J. Cardiol. *33*, 438 (1974)
6. Goodwin, J.F.: Congestive and hypertrophic cardiomyopathy. Lancet I, 732 (1970)
7. Hamilton, G.W., Murray, J.A., Kennedy, J.W.: Quantitative angiocardiography in ischemic heart disease. Circulation *45*, 1065 (1972)
8. Hanrath, P., Schweizer, P., Bleifeld, W., Effert, S.: Echokardiographische diagnostische Kriterien der idiopathischen hypertrophen subaortalen Stenose. Dtsch. med. Wschr. *100*, 1759 (1975)
9. Harmjanz, D., Boettcher, D.: Die angiographische Darstellung des normalen und des hypertrophen Ventrikelseptums. Verh. dtsch. Ges. Kreisl.-Forsch. *38*, 326 (1972)

Noninvasive Methods and Other Diagnostic Procedures

18. Echocardiography in the Diagnosis of Cardiomyopathies

P. HANRATH and W. BLEIFELD

In recent years echocardiography has proved to be useful in the diagnosis of the various forms of CM.

1. The method allows accurate measurement of wall thickness and dimensions.
2. The high time resolution (> 1000 impulses/s) permits functional analysis.
3. The noninvasive character of the method makes it suitable for follow-up and serial studies.

A classification of CMs is possible on the basis of structural alterations and functional abnormalities. They are roughly divided into dilated and nondilated types.

Dilated or Congestive Cardiomyopathy

The characteristic finding in this type of cardiomyopathy is an enlarged left ventricular cavity and a wide outflow tract (Fig. 1). The interventricular septum and posterior wall of the left ventricle are of equal thickness and have a decreased amplitude motion, reflecting the decrease of left ventricular contraction. The impaired contractility is also shown by the low peak of systolic endocardial fiver shortening velocity (Fig. 2) [1].

The low motion amplitude of both mitral valve leaflets as well as the prolongation of the AC interval, indicative of chronic increased left ventricular enddiastolic pressure, are often seen in this condition (Fig. 3).

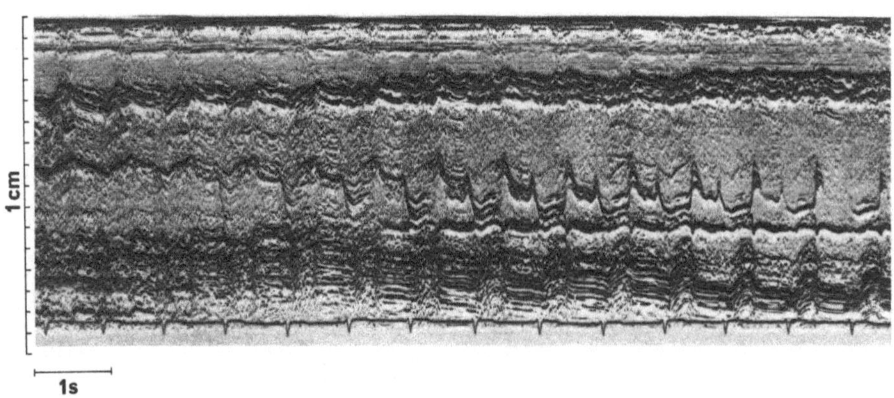

Fig. 1. Sector-scan-registration of a patient with dilative CM. Left ventricular dimension as well as left ventricular outflow tract are enlarged

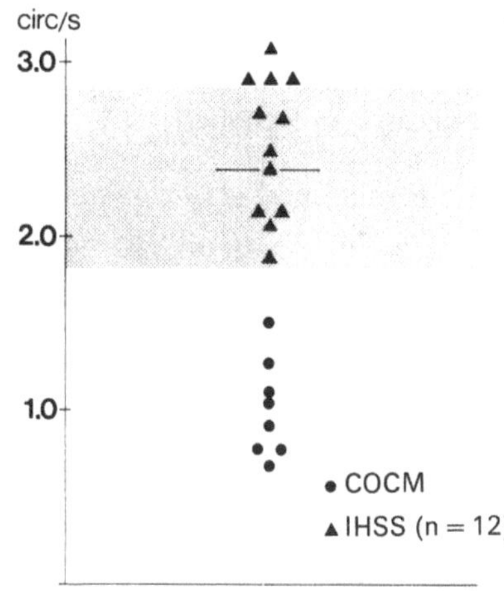

Fig. 2. Computer-aided analysis of maximal endocardial fiber shortening velocity in patients with IHSS (▲) and COCM (●). *Shaded area:* normal range

However, none of these signs absolutely indicates a diagnosis of dilated CM, since a dilated left ventricle with a decreased motion pattern of the septum and the posterior wall can also be observed in the end stage of valvular heart disease or in patients with diffuse coronary arterial disease. In patients with primary dilated CM the involvement is more diffuse, whereas it is more segmental in coronary artery disease. Echocardiographic findings in combination with the history and the clinical data allow differentiation in most cases of the various forms of heart disease.

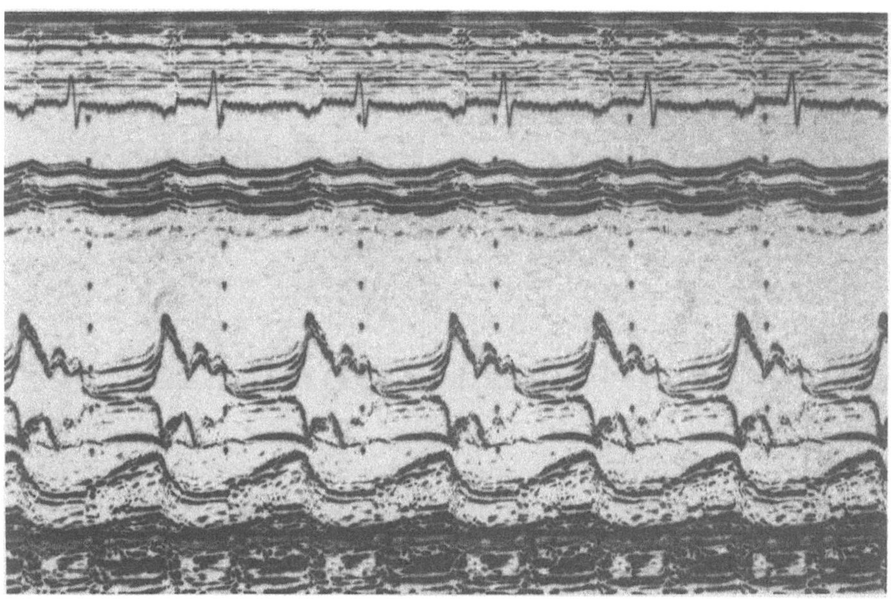

Fig. 3. Dilative CM: the systolic motion of the interventricular septum as well as the posterior wall are diminished due to decreased left ventricular contractility

Nondilated Cardiomyopathies

Concentric or Symmetrical Hypertrophy

This form of CM is rare and occurs in amyloidosis and other infiltrative diseases.

It is characterized by a normal or only slightly enlarged left ventricular cavity. The interventricular septum and posterior wall are thickened (Fig. 4). The echocardiographic changes associated with this type of CM can also be seen in patients with left ventricular pressure load (e.g. arterial hypertension, coarctation of the aorta, and valvular and subvalvular membranous aortic stenosis). In valvular and subvalvular membranous aortic stenosis the study of the aortic cusps and the left ventricular outflow tract can help differentiate these forms.

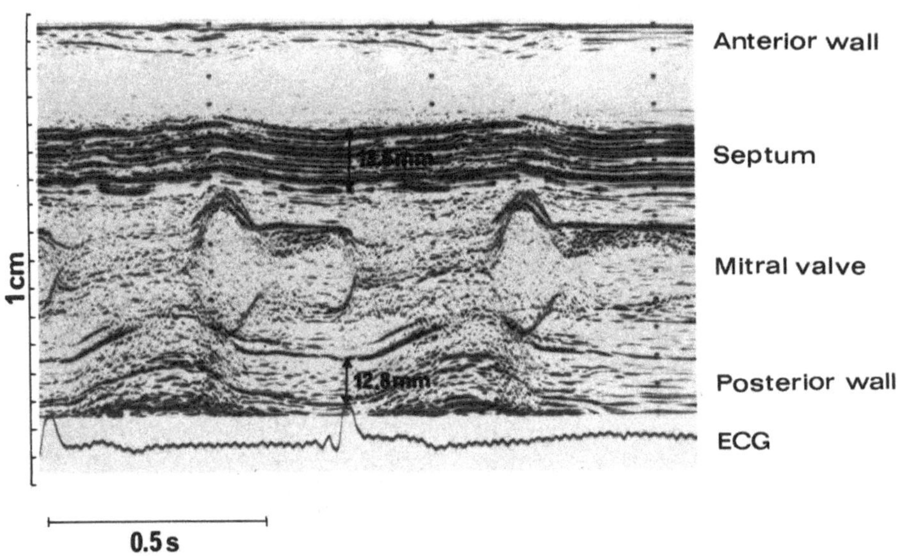

Fig. 4. Concentric hypertrophic CM: symmetrical hypertrophy of the interventricular septum (13.6 mm) as well as the left ventricular posterior wall (12.8 mm), the left ventricular enddiastolic dimension is slightly increased to 62 mm

Asymmetric Septal Hypertrophy Without and With Left Ventricular Outflow Abstruction (IHSS)

This disease is characterized by marked asymmetrical hypertrophy of the interventricular septum compared to the free posterior wall of the left ventricle. Echocardiography is accepted today as the easiest and most reliable method of detecting asymmetric septal hypertrophy (ASH). A ratio of septal to posterior wall thickness greater than 1.3 is diagnostic [5] (Fig. 5). However, the right ventricular endocardial surface of the interventricular septum may be difficult to delineate.

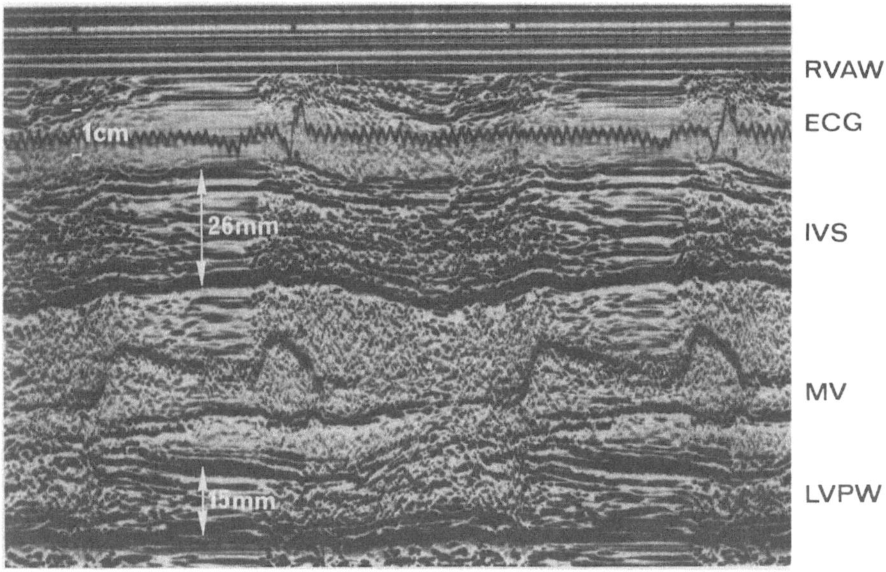

Fig. 5. Myopathic asymmetrical septum hypertrophy in a young patient with a septal to posterior wall ratio of 1.7. Note the low compliance motion pattern of the anterior mitral valve leaflet. *RVAW:* right ventricular anterior wall, *IVS:* interventricular septum, *MV:* mitral valve, *LVPW:* left ventricular posterior wall

The appearances of ASH are not necessarily diagnostic, because it can occur in patients with right ventricular pressure overload, or rarely in cases of aortic stenosis (Fig. 6), hypertension, or even in athletes.

Recent functional studies of the interventricular septum have shown that morphologic "asymmetry" of the septum may be accompanied by hypo- or akinesis. This can be explained by the destruction of the normal architecture of the muscle fibers. The posterior wall, less involved morphologically shows a hyperkinetic pattern which results in a normal systolic endocardial fiber shortening velocity (Fig. 2) [8].

In patients with ASH and left ventricular outflow obstruction (IHSS) the striking echocardiographic abnormality is the systolic anterior motion (SAM) of the anterior or both mitral valve leaflets. This, in combination with a primary narrow outflow tract, is considered to impede the ejection of blood from within the left ventricle (Fig. 7). The left ventricular outflow obstruction is functional, and SAM may therefore be observed intermittently or in various degrees (e.g., after provocation with amylnitrite or postextrasystolic augmentation of SAM. The systolic abnormal motion of the anterior leaflet is also the cause of concomitant mitral insufficiency. The exact mechanism of SAM is not clear, but a Venturi effect seems to be the most likely explanation.

SAM without ASH may be observed in other conditions such as mitral valve prolapse, pericardial effusion or in conditions in which the posterior left ventricular wall is hypercontractile.

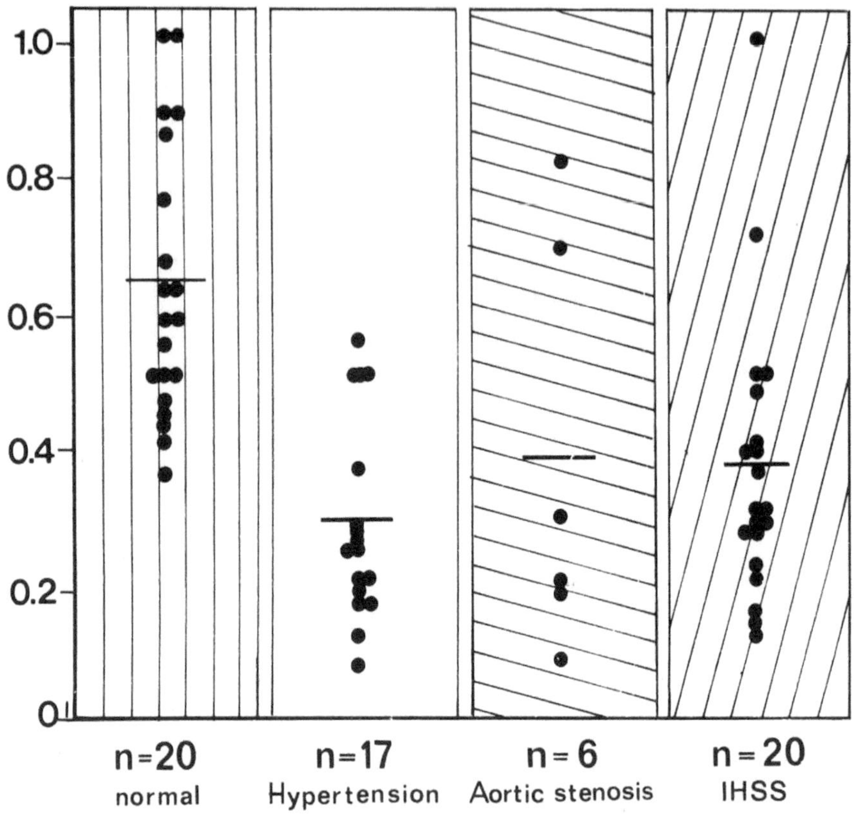

Fig. 6. Amplitude of the septum and the posterior wall motion during systole in patients with myopathic and nonmyopathic ASH. There is no significant difference in the motion pattern in these forms

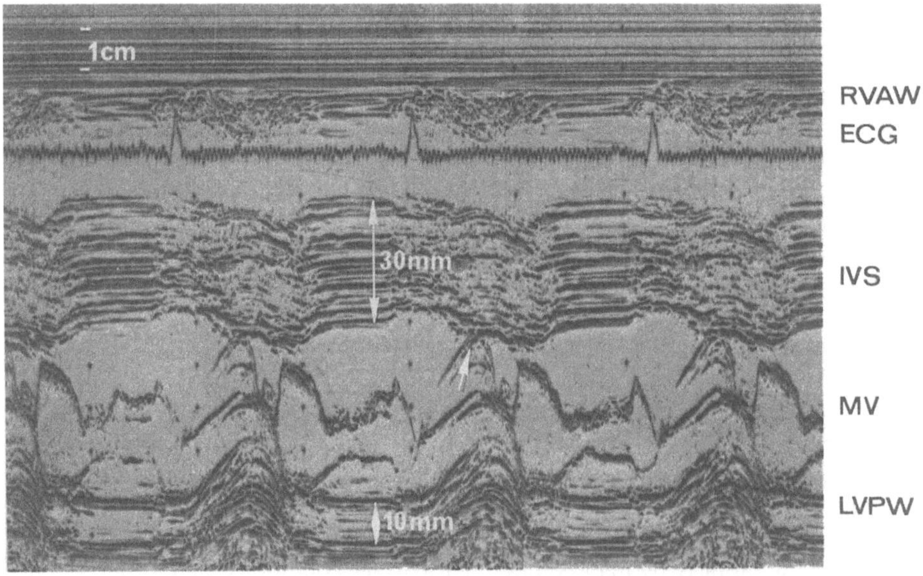

Fig. 7. Echocardiogram of a patient with ASH (ratio of septum to left ventricular posterior wall 3.0) and outflow obstruction, which is indicated by the systolic anterior movement of both mitral valve leaflets. *RVAW:* right ventricular anterior wall, *IVS:* interventricular septum, *MV:* mitral valve, *LVPW:* left ventricular posterior wall

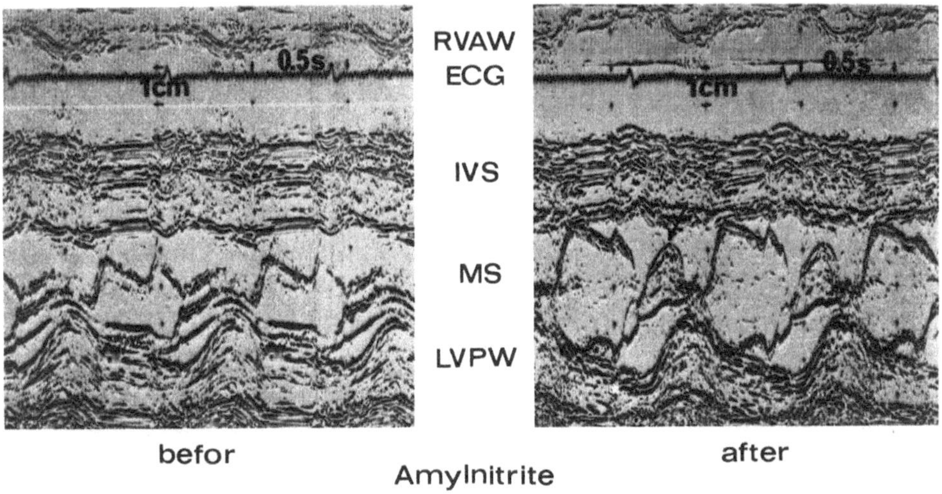

Fig. 8. Echocardiogram of a patient with malignant arterial hypertension. Note the asymmetrical septum hypertrophy with a reduced systolic motion pattern. After application of amylnitrite a sharp systolic anterior motion (SAM) of the anterior mitral leaflet can be documented as a sign of provocative subvalvular outflow obstruction. From the echocardiogram alone no decision can be made concerning the etiology of the ASH, whether myopathic or nonmyopathic

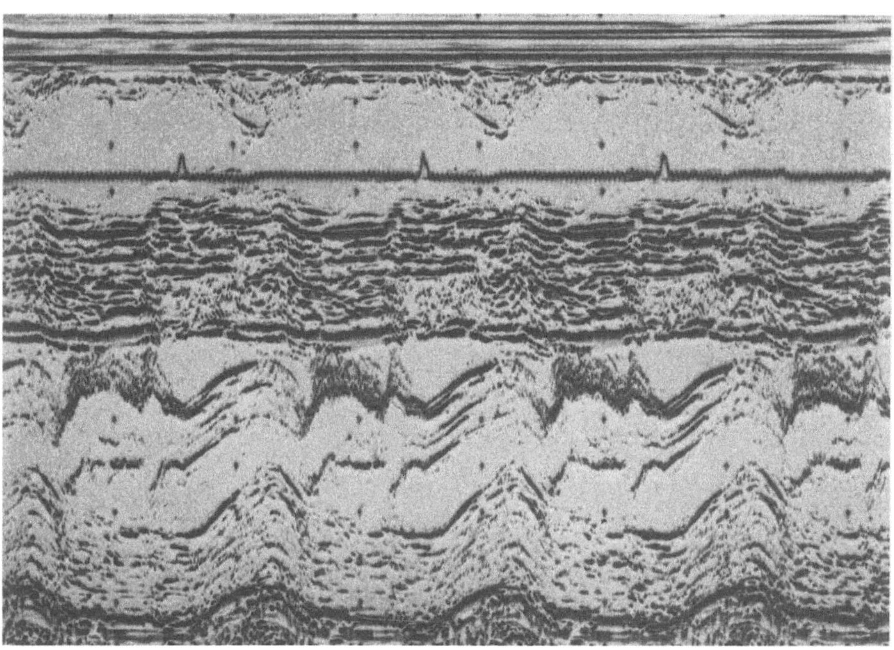

Fig. 9. Echocardiogram of a patient with combined aortic valve disease and dynamic subvalvular outflow obstruction. The high-frequency flutter of the anterior mitral valve leaflet is indicative of aortic regurgitation. Note the asymmetrical septal hypertrophy in relation to the hypertrophied left ventricular posterior wall

ASH, and rarely in combination with left ventricular outflow tract obstruction (Figs. 8 and 9) [3, 4, 6, 7], may also be observed in long-standing severe arterial hypertension and aortic stenosis. From the echocardiogram it is so far impossible to decide whether this is due to primary myopathic ASH associated with arterial hypertension or valvular aortic stenosis or whether it is secondary to non-myopathic asymmetrical septal hypertrophy, which in rare cases causes left ventricular outflow tract narrowing.

References

1. Corya, B.C., Feigenbaum, H., Rasmussen, S., Black, M.J.: Echocardiographic features of congestive cardiomyopathy compared with normal subjects and patients with coronary artery disease. Circulation *49*, 1153 (1974)
2. Hanrath, P., Figueireido, N., Bleifeld, W., Schweizer, P., Effert, S.: Ist die hypodyname Bewegung des interventrikulären Septums ein echokardiographisch spezifisches Kriterium einer myopathisch bedingten ASH? Zeitschrift f. Kardiologie Supp. *3*, 92 (1976)
3. Hanrath, P., Essen, R. v., Bleifeld, W., Effert, S.: Idiopathisch hypertrophe subaortale Stenose bei valvulärer Aortenklappenerkrankung. Diagnostik mittels Echokardiographie. Zeitschrift f. Kardiologie *65*, 964 (1976)
4. Hanrath, P., Bleifeld, W., Effert, S., Augustin, J., Gierlichs, A.: Morphologische und funktionelle Analysen des linken Ventrikels bei arterieller Hypertonie mittels Echokardiographie. Verhandlungen Dtsch. Ges. für Kreislaufforschung (1977). In press
5. Henry, W.L., Clark, C.E., Epstein, S.E.: Asymmetrical septal hypertrophy (ASH): The unifying link in the IHSS disease spectrum. Circulation *47*, 827 (1973)
6. Hironori, T., Yoshinori, H., Heniki, Y., Toshinori, A., Noboni, K.: Echocardiographic classification of hypertensive heart disease. Jap. Heart J. *16*, 377 (1975)
7. Nanda, N.C., Gramiak, R., Shah, P.M., Stewart, S., De Weese, J.A.: Echocardiography in the diagnosis of idiopathic hypertrophic subaortic stenosis coexisting with aortic valve disease. Circulation *50*, 712 (1974)
8. Rossen, R.M., Goodman, D.J., Ingham, R.E., Popp, R.L.: Ventricular septal thickening and excursion in idiopathic hypertrophic subaortic stenosis. Circulation (Suppl. III) *50*, 29 (1974)

19. Importance of Heart Volume Determination and Electrocardiography in Early Diagnosis of Cardiomyopathy

R. Hopf, M. Hopf, G. Kober, R. Lentz, H.E. Riemann, and M. Kaltenbach

Introduction

Symptoms of CM are often extremely variable and uncharacteristic. In patients with HOCM, 74% complained of dyspnea on exertion and 54% of typical angina pectoris. Among the patients with early COCM, 44% already had cardiac arrhythmias, 58% had precordial pain, and 44% complained of exertional dyspnea [2, 5, 6]. Advanced COCM was primarily characterized by congestive heart failure. It also appeared that physical examination alone was not very helpful diagnostically, particularly in cases of early CM.

Noninvasive screening methods, therefore, are needed to differentiate CM from other forms of organic heart disease as well as from purely functional cardiac disorders. The objective of the present investigation was to assess the diagnostic value of roentgenologic heart volume determination and of ECG, at rest and during exercise, in early and in advanced CM.

Material and Methods

Of 103 patients (aged 16–63 years; 15 females and 88 males), 91 suffered from COCM and 12 from HOCM. Diagnosis was established by cardiac catheterization, including ventricular and coronary angiography; in some cases myocardial biopsies were performed also.

In all patients conventional biplane (posteroanterior and lateral) chest roentgenograms were taken in upright position and were assessed by an experienced senior radiologist. In addition, roentgenologic heart volumes were determined from biplane teleroentgenograms with the patient in supine position, utilizing the method of Musshoff and Reindell [8]. Cardiac volume was quantified in milliliters and adjusted for 1.73 m^2 of body surface, the latter to correct for individual body size variablility. Mean values of normal heart volumes in supine position had been obtained by comparative assessment within a large population of noncardiac patients. Average heart volume was 620 + 170 ml/1.73 m^2 (mean + upper 2-sigma level) in males and 570 + 120 ml/1.73 m^2 in females. Accordingly, the heart volumes in our study were graded "normal," "slightly enlarged," "moderately enlarged," and "severely enlarged" (Table 1).

ECG at rest was carried out using 18 leads, i.e., 6 conventional limb and 6 chest leads as well as 6 additonal precordial leads attached two intercostal spaces above the usual Wilson leads. For exercise ECG, the 3 bipolar limb leads and the regular precordial leads V_4 through V_6 were employed. Electrodes were strapped to the patient's chest according to the method of Rosenkranz [9]. The patients exercised using the climbing step test [3].

During and following exercise, heart rate was continuously monitored and compared with normal reference data obtained from healthy males and females.

In the nondigitalized patients of our series, ECG ST-segment changes during and following exertion were evaluated according to standard criteria.

Table 1. Classification of heart size by supine biplane teleroentgenography.

Females		Males
570–690 ml/1.73 m²	Normal	620– 790 ml/1.73 m²
691–800 ml/1.73 m²	Slightly enlarged	791– 900 ml/1.73 m²
801–900 ml/1.73 m²	Moderately enlarged	901–1000 ml/1.73 m²
>900 ml/1.73 m²	Severely enlarged	> 1000 ml/1.73 m²

Results

Heart size of the 103 patients with CM was evaluated by conventional chest radiography in upright posture and by heart volume determination in supine position (Table 2). Routine chest films showed heart size to be normal in 33 patients, whereas the roentgenologic heart volume was normal only in 19 patients. Of the former 33 patients, 22 had definite heart volume enlargements when in supine position; the enlargement was severe in 6, moderate in 9, and slight in 7 patients. Conversely, the heart volume was found to be normal in 8 of 70 patients with increased heart size indicated by conventional techniques. In 30 of the 103 cases (29%), therefore, heart size was misjudged using conventional chest radiography.

The following two case histories further illustrate the definite superiority of heart volume determination in the diagnosis of CM. In both patients, conventional radiologic heart size was considered normal; detection of CM and indication for cardiac catheterization was based primarily on supine heart volume determination (Fig. 1 through 6).

Case 1. A 24-year-old, physically active female complained of intermittent extrasystolic heart beats. Conventional chest X-rays (Fig. 1) and ECG at rest (Fig. 2) were normal. Cardiac catheterization revealed an enlarged and

Table 2. Comparison of heart size determined by conventional chest radiography (upright position) and teleroentgenologic heart volume (supine position).

		Heart volume increase (supine)			
Patients (n = 103)	Heart size increase (standing)	None	Slight	Moderate	Severe
33	None	11	7	9	6
57	Left-sided	6	8	12	31
4	Right-sided	1	0	1	2
9	Bilateral	1	1	2	5

diffusely hypokinetic left ventricle with a reduced EF. Indication for cardiac catheterization was based on an enlarged supine heart volume of 985 ml/1.73 m^2 (Fig. 3).

Case 2. A 35-year-old male athlete whose ECG showed atrial fibrillation indicative of some underlying cardiac disorder. Again, routine upright chest X-rays (Fig. 4) werde judged normal, whereas the patient's heart volume of 1.063 ml/1.73 m^2 exceeded the 2-sigma level (Fig. 5). Cardiac catheterization revealed an increased left ventricular enddiastolic volume and an EF reduced to 43% (Fig. 6). Myocardial biopsy revealed severe myocardial hypertrophy, muscular degeneration, and interstitial fibrosis.

The ECG findings at rest and on exertion are summarized in Table 3. ECG at rest was normal in 21% of the cases. Pathologic ECG findings exceeded 100% since several patients exhibited more than one type of anomaly. In 79% of the patients pathologic axis deviation, hypertrophy, bundle branch block, and rhythm as well as conduction disturbances were observed. Of special importance is the finding of Q waves or QS complexes (Fig. 7) which tend to be misinterpreted quite frequently; often diagnostic differentiation between coronary heart disease and myocardial infarction then becomes particularly difficult. Such Q wave anomalies were found in 11% of patients with normal coronary angiograms.

On exertion 6% of the patients exhibited additional conduction or rhythm disturbances. In 23% of the cases increase in heart rate during exertion was inadequate. In 14% heart rate increased above normal, whereas in 9% of the cases

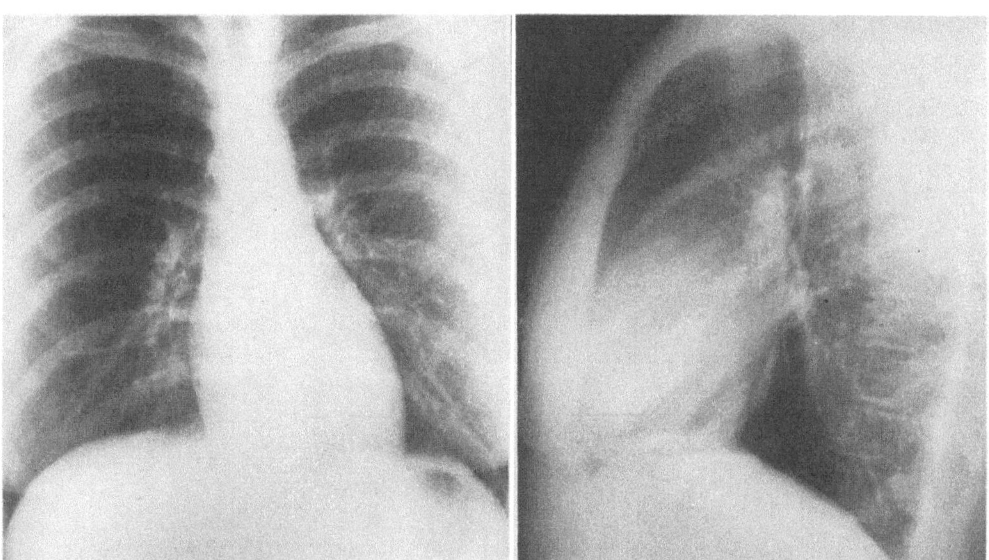

A
B

Fig. 1. Conventional chest X-rays taken in the posteroanterior (*A*) and left lateral (*B*) position. This 24-year-old female complaining of intermittent extrasystolic heart beats was judged to have a heart of normal size. Cardiac catheterization revealed an early COCM (compare with Fig. 2B)

Table 3. ECG anomalies found in 103 patients with COCM (91 patients) and HOCM (12 patients).

ECG at rest	(%)
Pathological axis deviation	23
Atrial hypertrophy	12
Right ventricular hypertrophy	6
Left ventricular hypertrophy	27
Right bundle branch block	11
Left bundle branch block	14
Signs of myocardial infarction	11
Sinus bradycardia (60 beats/min) or tachycardia (90 beats/min)	23
Extrasystoles	12
Atrial fibrillation	10
Supraventricular tachycardia	2
a-V block (different degrees)	
Exercise test	
Pathologic response of heart rate to exercise	24
Typical "ischemic reaction"	7
Questionable "ischemic reaction"	16
Rhythm and/or conduction disturbances	16

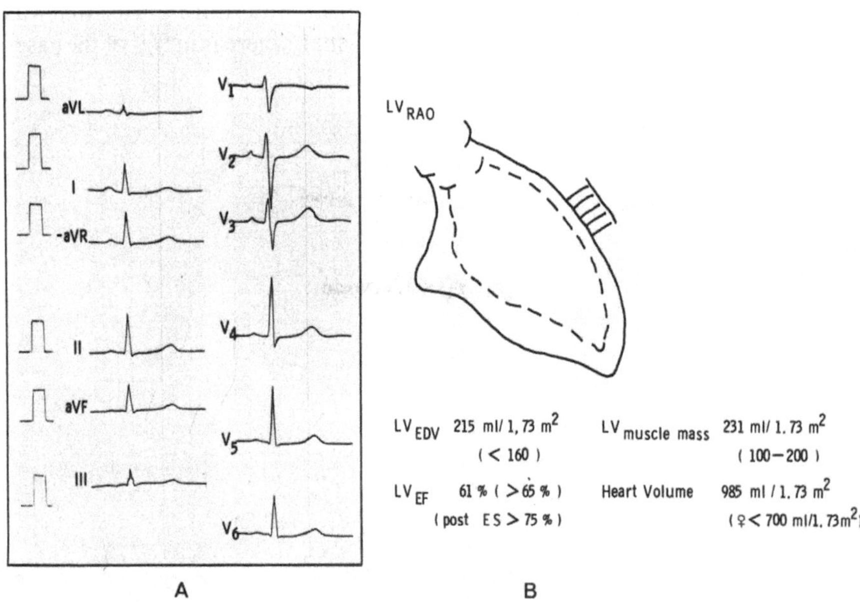

Fig. 2. (*A*) Normal ECG of the same patient as in Figure 1. (*B*) Left ventricular (LV) angiogram in the right anterior oblique (RAO) projection. Enddiastolic left ventricular dimensions are indicated by *solid lines*, endsystolic dimensions by *broken lines*. *Parallel lines* indicate left ventricular wall thickness. EDV, enddiastolic volume; EF, ejection fraction. Normal values are indicated in parentheses. Angiography revealed an enlarged and diffusely hypokinetic left ventricle with a reduced ejection fraction

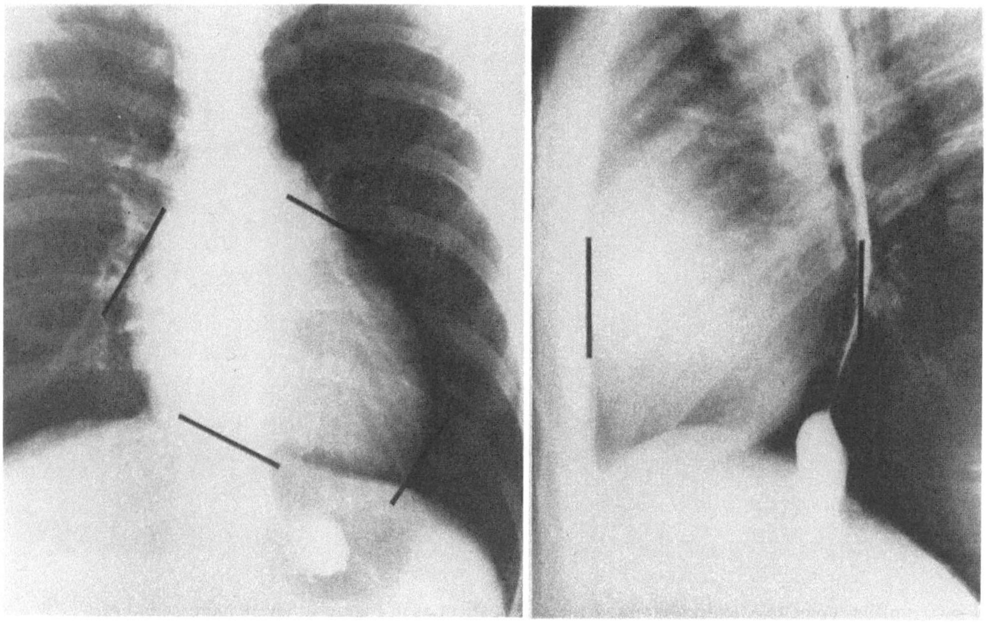

Fig. 3. Supine biplane teleroentgenogram. Same patient as in Figures 1 and 2. In contrast to normal conventional chest X-rays of Figure 1, heart volume determined from these films was increased to 985 ml/1.73 m^2 (normal upper limit in females: 690 ml/1.73 m^2)

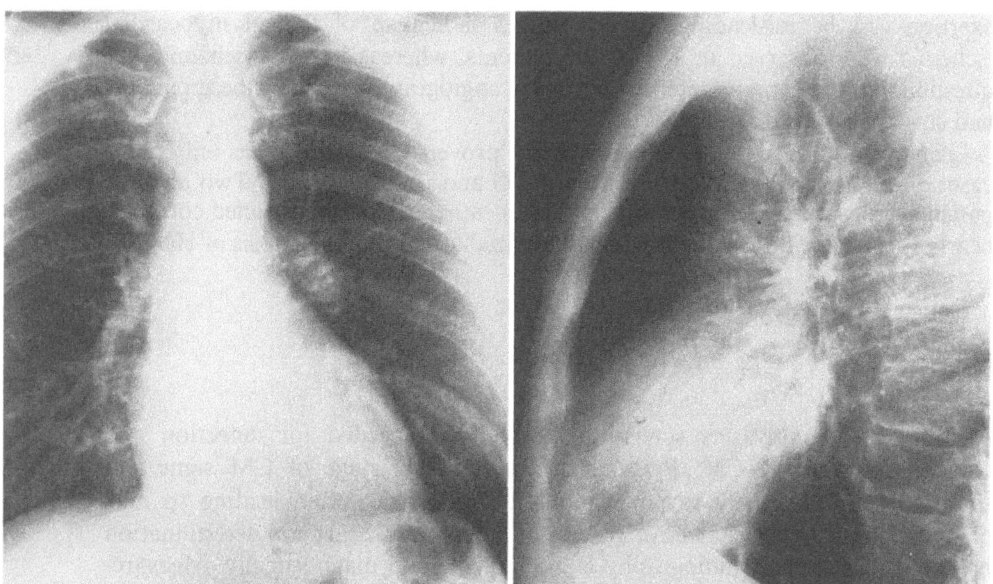

A
B

Fig. 4. Normal conventional biplane chest X-rays of a 35-year-old male with COCM. (*A*) Anterior and (*B*) left lateral positions

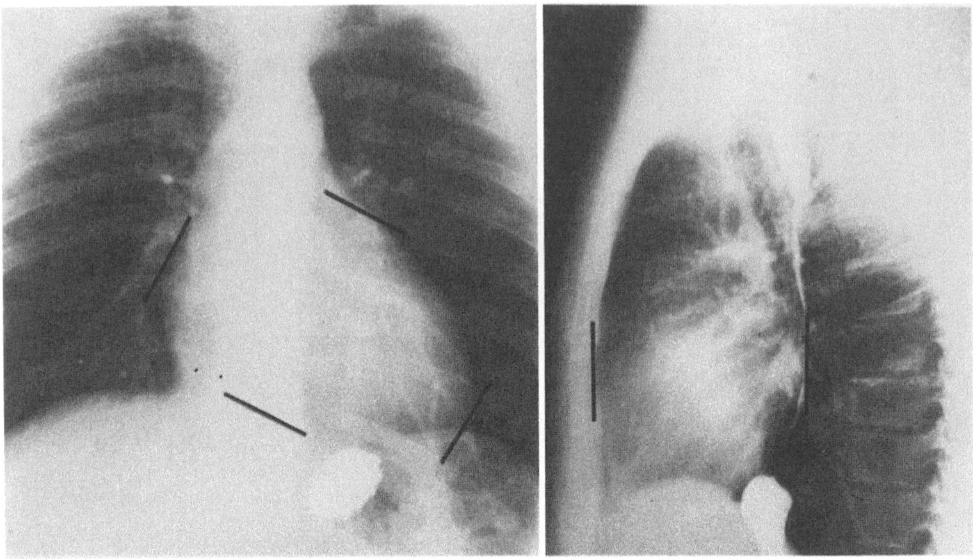

Fig. 5. Biplane supine teleroentgenogram of the same patient as in Figure 4. Severe increase in heart volume to 1.063 ml/1.73 m^2 (normal upper limit in males: 790 ml/1.73 m^2)

it was below normal. Two characteristic examples of pathologic increase in heart rate are presented in Fig. 8.

In the nondigitalized patient ST-segment depression during and following exertion can be misleading. ECG changes indicative of typical myocardial ischemia were observed in 7% of the patients, whereas in 16% ischemia was questionable. As demonstrated by coronary angiography, none of these patients had coronary heart disease.

Among all 103 cases of diagnostically proven CM there were only three cases of mild or early CM with normal ECG and roentgenogram. Two of these patients with severe angina pectoris had been catheterized for suspected coronary heart disease. The third patient was catheterized after initial diagnosis of HOCM.

Discussion

Reliable and noninvasive screening methods are needed for detection and clinical follow-up of CM. Particularly in the early stage of CM signs and symptoms are extremely variable and uncharacteristic, often leading to misdiagnoses. Due to the subjective criteria of assessment, heart size determination by conventional chest radiography is not very helpful diagnostically. Measurements such as the cardiothoracic ratio have not been generally accepted due to the enormous scatter of values under orthostatic influences. Conversely, roentgenologic heart volume determination with the patient in supine position allows exact quantification, provided criteria of assessment are strictly adhered

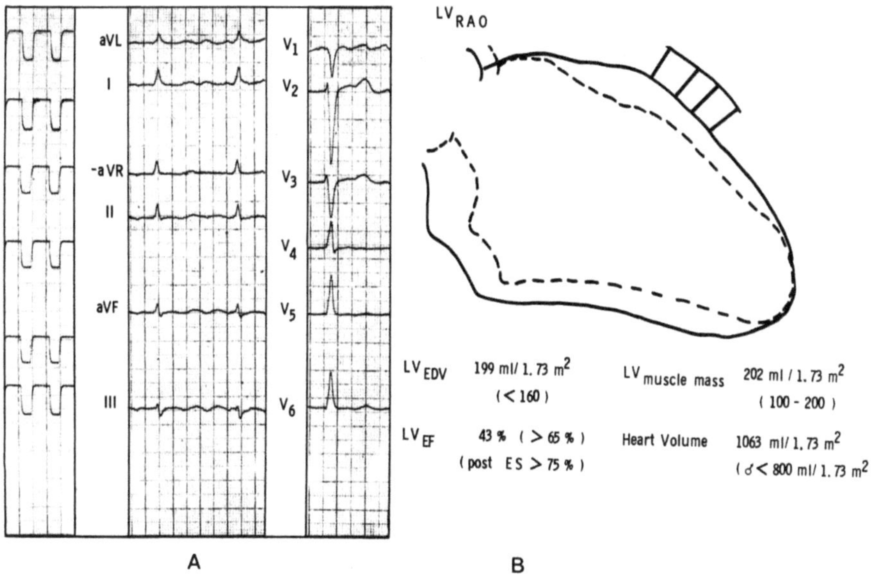

Fig. 6. ECG and left ventricular angiogram of the same patient as in Figure 4 and 5 in the right anterior oblique (RAO) projection. For further explanations see legend to Figure 2. The angiogram reveals regional hypokinesis and akinesis of the severely enlarged ventricle. The ejection fraction is severely reduced

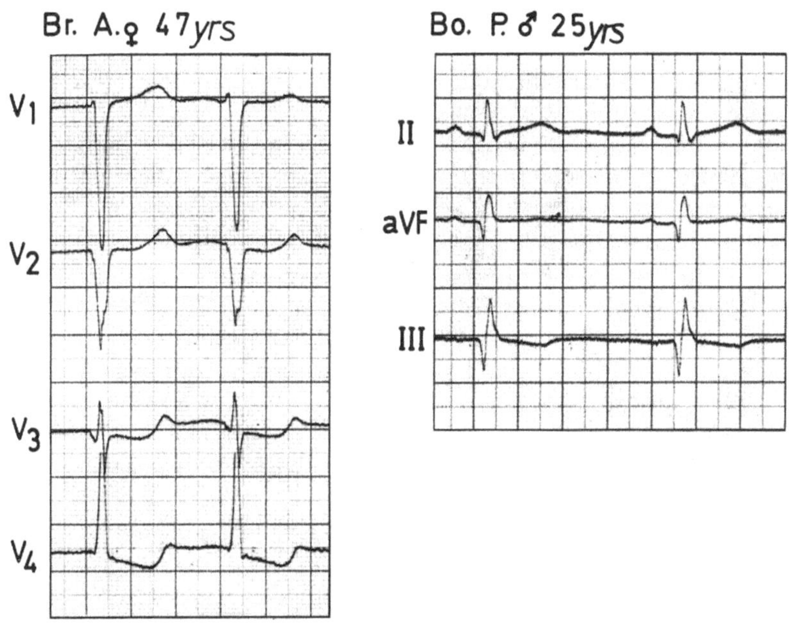

Fig. 7. ECGs of two patients with CM. While the ECG tracings were indicative of typical myocardial infarction, such event could be excluded by angiography

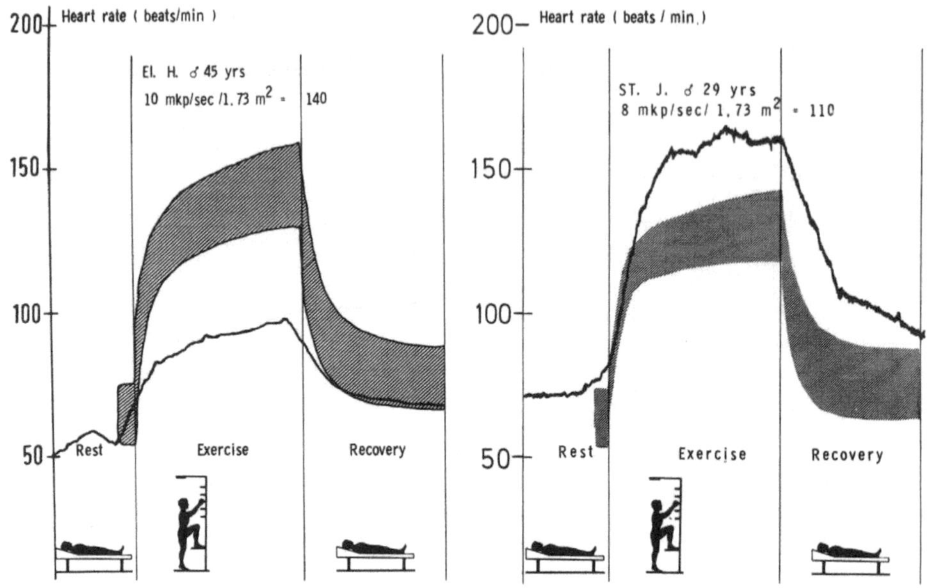

Fig. 8. Different forms of pathologic increases in heart rate due to exercise in two patients with CM. Both patients exercised on a climbing step. The cross-hatched area in each panel delineates the anticipated normal heart rate before, during, and following exercise. The patients' actual pulse curves are shown below (left panel) or above (right panel) this area

to. As could be demonstrated by paired analysis of the films by one or by several investigators [1,4,7], the variability of data remained well within the 5% limit. As opposed to conventional radiography, the risk of subjective error is negligible. Furthermore, orthostatic influences on heart size can be avoided by placing the patient in the supine position. The fact that heart size was misjudged in approximately one third of all patients indicates the superiority of supine heart volume determination. Parallel investigations in noncardiac patients further stress the validity of this technique. All of these patients had normal heart volumes. Conventional radiography, however, led to misinterpretation in 10% of the cases.

The ECG of the resting patient with CM is characterized by a high incidence of pathologic changes. Such changes, however, are unspecific and do not permit CM diagnosis. Arterial hypertension, valve diseases, and coronary heart disease should be excluded. Differential diagnosis tends to become particularly difficult in the presence of ECG changes "indicative" of myocardial infarction. Such infarction-like tracings have frequently been observed in patients with both COCM and HOCM. In the latter, the changes are induced by the underlying hypertrophy; in COCM, the changes coincide with the finding of large hypokinetic or akinetic areas of the left ventricle and thus probably constitute the equivalent of nonischemic scarring. Considering the overall incidence of coronary heart disease, coronary angiography is absolutely necessary for proper diagnosis of CM.

On exertion pathologic increases in heart rate are frequently observed in CM. Again, this finding is unspecific. Increase in heart rate above normal is mostly associated with reduction in left ventricular stroke volume, while in some cases of early CM such increase in heart rate is considered a sign of hyperkinetic dysregulation. Insufficient increase in heart rate, on the other hand, points to CM involvement of the conduction system.

An ST-segment depression is yet another change in the exercise ECG of patients with CM with and without anginal pain. These ST changes are associated with disturbances of the cellular myocardial metabolism following hypertrophy of the heart muscle and a reduction in peripheral coronary reserve. The relationship between large coronary artery diameter and muscle mass to be perfused is still normal. In the nondigitalized patient, coronary heart disease can be excluded through coronary angiography.

Roentgenologic heart volume determination as well as ECG at rest and on exertion have been found to provide objective and noninvasive screening methods for proper diagnosis of CM. For detection of early CM biplane teleroentgenography with the patient in supine position is the method of choice. Once the patient has become severely symptomatic, diagnosis can be adequately established by means of physical examination and conventional radiography.

According to current literature, long-term prognosis of CM is rather poor. This is mainly true for advanced CM. The course of early CM is hardly known due to the lack of adequate noninvasive screening methods. This gap is filled by roentgenologic heart volume determinations which provide a useful means for CM detection.

Summary

In 103 patients in whom the diagnosis of CM of various degrees was based on angiography and partly on myocardial biopsy, the specifity of the initially employed noninvasive screening tests was evaluated. When compared to conventional radiography, the technique of roentgenologic heart volume determination in supine position proved to be highly specific diagnostically. Heart size, as determined from conventional chest films, was misjudged in 29% of the patients.

ECG changes, both at rest and during exertion, were observed in 79% of the patients. The interpretation of these findings, however, was difficult, particularly in cases where coronary heart disease had to be excluded.

Only three patients had normal ECG and roentgenologic findings.

In the present investigation, the technique of roentgenologic heart volume determination has been demonstrated to provide a valuable means for detection of early forms of CM.

References

1. Axen, O., Lindgren, E., Malmström, G.: Metod for jnärtvolymbestämming. Nord. Med. *29*, 592 (1946)
2. Braunwald, E., Lambrew, C.T., Rockoff, S.D., Ross, J., Morrow, A.G.: IHSS. A description of the disease based upon an analysis of the 64 patients. Circulation *29*, 30, Suppl. IV, 8 (1964)
3. Kaltenbach, M.: Exercise Testing of Cardiac Patients. Bern-Stuttgart-Vienna: Hans Huber Publishers 1976

4. Lind, J.: Heart volume in normal infants et roentgenological study. Acta radiol. (Stockh.), Suppl. 82 (1950)
5. Loogen, F., Kuhn, H., Kübler, W.: Klinik der idiopathischen Kardiomyopathien. Therapiewoche *31*, 2420 (1972)
6. Meerschwam, J.S.: Hypertrophic obstructive cardiomyopathy – a clinical study. Excerpta Medica Foundation, Amsterdam, 1969
7. Meythaler, M., Fick, H., Haas, W., Schmidt, J.: Die klinische Größenbeurteilung des Herzens. Arch. Kreisl.-Forsch. *55*, 123 (1968)
8. Musshoff, K., Reindell, H.: Zur Röntgenuntersuchung des Herzens in horizontaler und vertikaler Körperstellung. Dtsch. med. Wschr. *81*, 1001 (1956) and *82*, 1075 (1957)
9. Rosenkranz, K.A., Drews, A.: Über eine modifizierte Ableitungsmethode zur Registrierung von Brustwandelektrokardiogrammen während dosierter körperlicher Belastung. Z. Kreisl.-Forsch. *61*, 673 (1972)

20. Left Bundle Branch Block in Patients With and Without Cardiomyopathy

L. SEIPEL, G. BREITHARDT, and H. KUHN

Electrocardiographic findings indicate that left bundle branch block (LBBB) is common in CM patients [2,3,5,12,17,18,21,26,30,49]. His-bundle studies revealed a dangerous impairment of intraventricular conduction in many patients with LBBB and COCM [3,26,38,51]. In some cases complete A-V block was observed [6,11,26,49]. The purpose of the study was to find out possible electrophysiologic and morphologic differences in patients with LBBB with and without COCM, which may have clinical significance. Therefore, His-bundle studies were done in different groups of patients with LBBB. In addition, right ventricular endomyocardial biopsy was performed in order to correlate the electrophysiologic and electron-microscopic findings.

Methods and Material

His-bundle electrography was performed in the conventional technique according to Scherlag *et al.* [42] using the femoral route [45]. His-bundle potentials were derived by a special 4-F bipolar catheter for single use (Cordis). Atrial stimulation was performed with a modified 5837 Medtronic stimulator or the Medtronic conduction system analyzer model 5325. The ECG and the intracardiac potentials were simultaneously recorded by a six-channel ECG recorder (Siemens Cardirex). The measurements of the conduction time in the His-bundle electrogram (HBE) were made according to Scherlag *et al.* [43]. Our normal value for the A-H interval is 89 $\pm$17.2 ms and for the H-V interval 43 $\pm$6.9 ms ($\bar{x}$ $\pm$s.d.) [46]. The V-RVA time was measured according to Castellanos *et al.* [10], our normal value being 5–25 ms. For determination of the different refractory periods we used the definition of Wit *et al.* [52], as previously detailed [47]. In many patients the study was repeated after application of atropine or different antiarrhythmic drugs (Ajmaline, Aprindine, Propafenone, Mexiletine).

Additionally, most of the patients underwent heart catheterization, including coronary arteriography, as well as measurement of the pulmonary arterial pressure during rest and exercise. Endomyocardial biopsy from the right ventricle using a Konno bioptome [25] was performed in 25 patients. For quantitation of the electron-microscopic findings a morphologic score was used [27]. Statistical analysis was done by the Wilcoxon test.

Of 72 patients with LBBB, 20 had COCM; 9 patients were suspected of having LCM as defined by normal clinical and angiographic findings, but the only pathological finding was elevated pulmonary arterial pressure during exercise (see Ch. 11). In an HOCM patient the LBBB pattern appeared after surgical excision from the hypertrophied ventricular septum. In 13 patients the LBBB was thought to be due to coronary heart disease, and in 7 cases, to rheumatic lesions. In 22 patients all other findings were normal. Therefore, the LBBB was declared to be of unknown etiology (Table 1). Sixty-six patients showed a normal sinus rhythm. Six patients showed atrial fibrillation. In 24 cases with sinus rhythm a first-degree A-V block was present. In 6 patients an intermittent higher-degree A-V block could be documented. In 57 patients a "constant" LBBB was registered at all observed frequencies; in 15 patients an intermittent block was present. The QRS width during LBBB pattern was 120–140 ms in 24 patients and greater than 140 ms in 48 patients. Seventeen cases showed left axis deviation (LAD), one case with right axis deviation (RAD), the others with normal QRS axis.

Furthermore, His-bundle studies were done in five cases with COCM and normal QRS complex.

Table 1. H-V intervals in 72 patients with left bundle branch block.

Etiology	H-V, normal		H-V, prolonged		Total			
	n	H-V ms	n	H-V ms	n	H-V ms		
COCM	1	56.0 –	19	81.3 ±29.1	20	80.5 ±28.8	$P < 0.01$	$P < 0.05$
LCM	4	49.0 ±4.2	5	69.2 ±14.2	9	60.2 ±14.9		
HOCM	0	–	1	60.0 –	1	60.0 –	$P < 0.10$	
KHD	2	50.0 ±8.5	11	79.8 ±13.2	13	75.2 ±16.6	$P < 0.05$	
Rheumatic HD	2	50.0 ±1.4	5	66.6 ±10.9	7	62.1 ±11.6		
Unknown	5	49.6 ±6.1	17	67.2 ± 7.4	22	63.2 ±10.3		

Results

During His bundle study and atrial pacing no patient showed abnormal sinus node function. In 12 patients the A-H interval was prolonged.

Fifty-seven patients had a constant LBBB pattern at all rates of stimulation. In 13 patients with intermittent LBBB the block occurred at increasing heart rates of shorter coupling intervals, whereas at low frequencies the ventricular complex was normal. In one patient the LBBB appeared only at long cycle lengths and disappeared with increasing frequency. One patient showed intermittent LBBB pattern without significant changes in heart rate.

The H-V intervals in patients with LBBB ranged from normal to extremely abnormal values. In 7 of 15 patients with intermittent LBBB the H-V interval was constant during normal and abnormal QRS pattern. In the remaining 8 cases the H-V interval showed a sudden prolongation when the bundle branch block appeared. There was no difference in H-V time in patients with LBBB and normal axis or LAD. The H-V interval was somewhat longer in patients with a QRS width greater than 140 ms (72.4 ±22.5) than in cases with ventricular complexes between 120 and 140 ms duration (66.8 ±14.8 ms). These differences were not significant. Patients with first-degree A-V block showed a longer H-V time

(81.5 ±28.4 ms) than patients with normal P-R interval (65.1 ±10.7 ms). However, even in patients with normal A-V conduction time in the ECG, abnormal H-V intervals were found, so the differences were not significant.

Table 1 shows the frequency of normal and abnormal H-V intervals in the groups of patients with LBBB of different etiology. With one exception only abnormal H-V intervals were found in patients with COCM, whereas in the other groups normal and abnormal values were measured. Even in patients with LBBB of unknown etiology abnormal H-V intervals were seen. Taking the entire group of patients with COCM, LCM, and LBBB of unknown etiology, the mean H-V interval in patients with COCM (80.5 ± 28.8 ms) was significantly longer than in the other two groups (60.2 ±14.9 ms and 63.2 ±10.3 ms, respectively). However, there was an overlapping of the single values, as shown in Figure 1. In this figure the group of patients with LBBB of unknown etiology is smaller than in Table 1 since only those patients who underwent a complete diagnostic procedure were taken into account. Therefore, the differences in the mean H-V interval between this small group and the patients with COCM is not significant.

In 25 patients with LBBB we were able to correlate the electron-microscopic findings from the myocardial biopsy specimen with the electrophysiologic data. Figure 2 shows that there is no correlation between the morphologic score and the H-V time. However, the only three patients with normal H-V intervals had a low

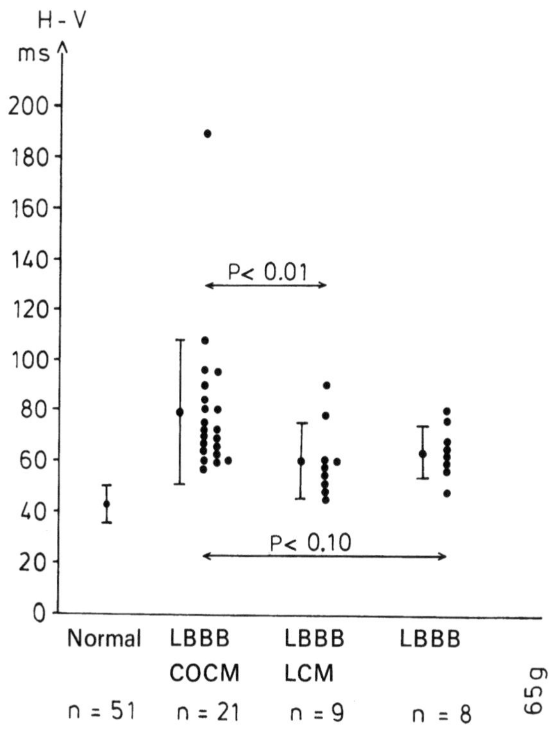

Fig. 1. H-V time in normal patients and in patients with LBBB and congestive cardiomyopathy (COCM), with LBBB and latent cardiomyopathy (LCM) and with LBBB without other abnormal findings

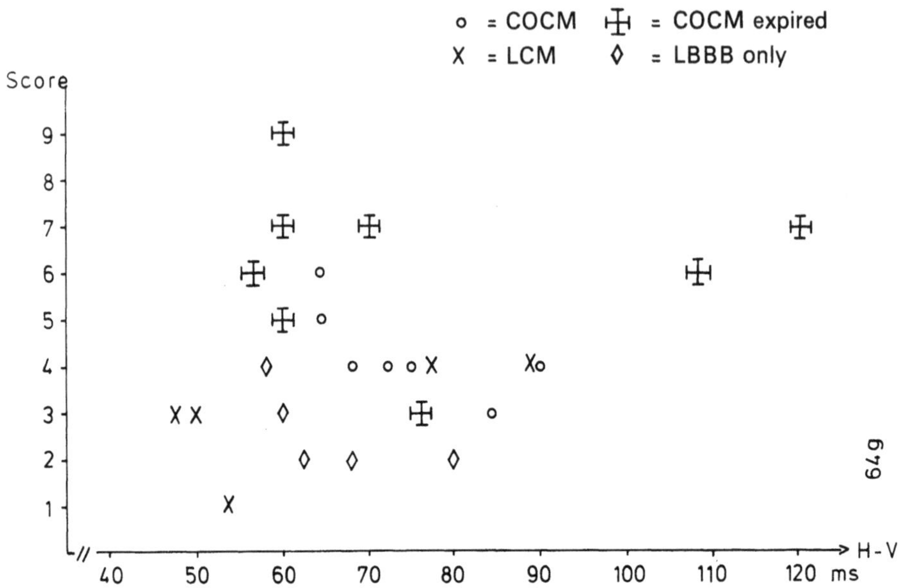

Fig. 2. Correlation between H-V intervals and electronmicroscopic findings (morphologic score) in 25 patients with LBBB

score (1–3 points), whereas every patient with a score of more than 3 points had a prolonged H-V time. In contrast to these findings some patients had a low morphologic score in spite of a prolonged H-V time.

From the five patients with COCM and a normal QRS complex, one had an H-V time of 40 ms, the others between 60 and 82 ms.

With one expection the V-RVA interval was prolonged up to 45 ms in all 25 patients with a prolonged H-V time in whom the V-RVA interval was measured (Fig. 3).

In 56 of the 66 patients with sinus rhythm, high-rate atrial pacing was performed. In most of the cases a block occurred above the level of His with increasing frequency. Only five patients showed a block distal to the H potential. In one patient a Wenckebach phenomenon within the His-Purkinje system was observed. In all other cases the block distal H occurred without measurable prolongation of the H-V time before block. The frequency at which the block distal H appeared was 100/min in two cases, 140/min in one case, 160/min in one case, and 180/min in two cases. In one patient a right bundle branch block pattern appeared in addition to the LBBB at a frequency of 140/min. However, the A-V block occurred within the A-V node at higher pacing rates.

In 25 patients programed atrial pacing was performed. At a basic cycle length of 750 ms five patients showed a distal His block, the effective refractory period of the His-Purkinje system (ERP H) ranging from 430 to 520 ms. In one patient a split His (H-H′) was observed at a coupling interval (A_1-A_2) of 320 ms and an H_1-H_2 interval of 440 ms. One patient showed in addition to the LBBB an RBBB pattern without A-V block if the H_1-H_2 interval was shorter than 450 ms

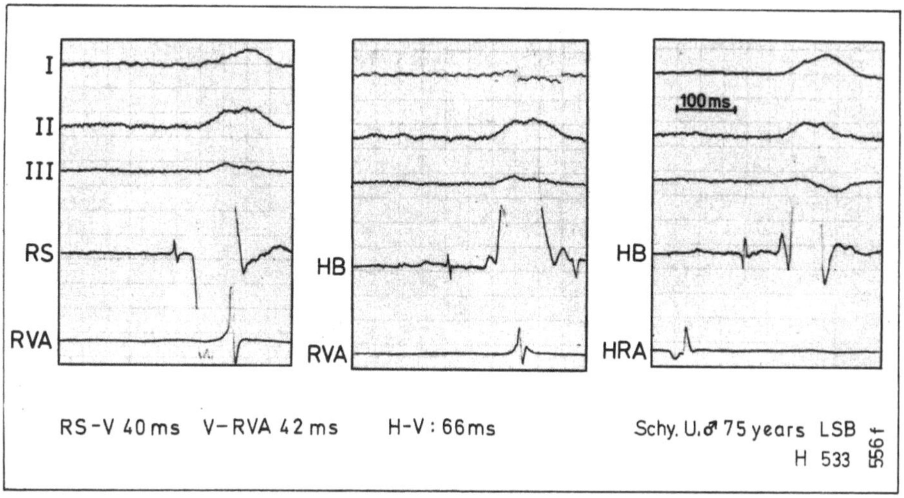

Fig. 3. Recordings of the ECG (lead D I–III), the right bundle branch (RS) and the His bundle (HB) potentials simultaneously with the activation of the right ventricular apex (RVA) and high right atrial potentials (HRA). In this patient with LBBB the H-V interval is prolonged as well as the V-RVA time

(Fig. 6, left side). The same phenomenon was observed during high-rate atrial pacing.

In one of the six patients with documented intermittent higher-degree A-V block the conduction at the level of the A-V node was extremely abnormal. The remaining five cases showed H-V intervals between 72 and 190 ms. In four of these five patients atrial stimulation was performed, leading in three cases to a block distal to the H potential at pacing rates between 100 and 140/min (Fig. 4). The fourth patient showed a bilateral bundle branch block pattern at a pacing rate of 140/min, as already described.

The different antiarrhythmic drugs tested showed a marked depressant effect on intraventricular conduction in many patients with LBBB, even after the administration of drugs which normally have only slight effects on the His-Purkinje system. Figure 5 shows a second-degree A-V block after injection of Disopyramide, whereas during control stimulation a one-to-one conduction was present. The block was located within the His-Purkinje system. Figure 6 demonstrates the same effect after application of Aprindine. Before drug injection the premature atrial impulses are conducted to the ventricle until the ERP of the A-V node is reached at a coupling interval of 310 ms. After administration of Aprindine the H-V interval is first prolonged with shorter coupling intervals. At an A_1-A_2 interval of 440 ms and an H_1-H_2 interval of 560 ms the ERPH is reached, leading to a block distal to the His potential.

No complication in any of the patients with LBBB was observed during His-bundle study. However, in three cases a higher-degree A-V block occurred during endomyocardial biopsy. Figure 7 shows the HBE immediately after biopsy. The block is located distal to the His potential. Due to the slow ventricular rate the

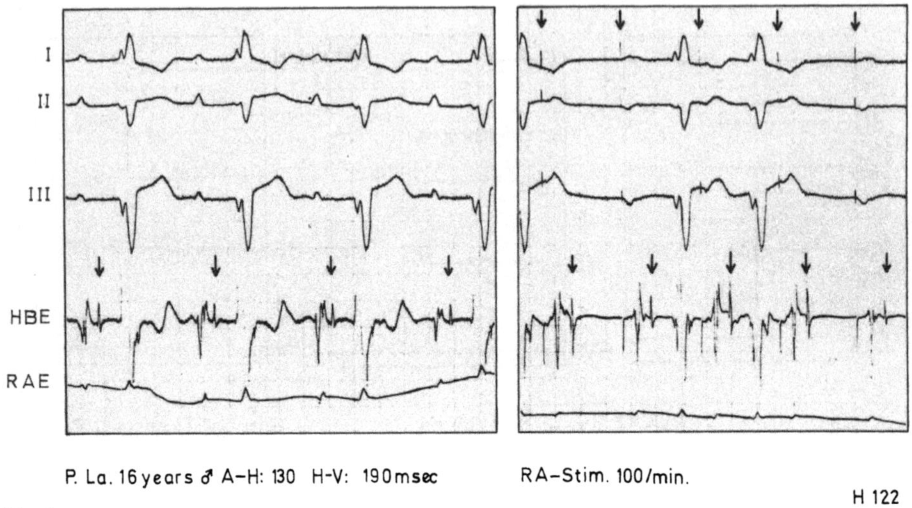
I
II
III
HBE
RAE
P. La. 16years ♂ A–H: 130 H–V: 190msec
RA–Stim. 100/min.
H 122

Fig. 4

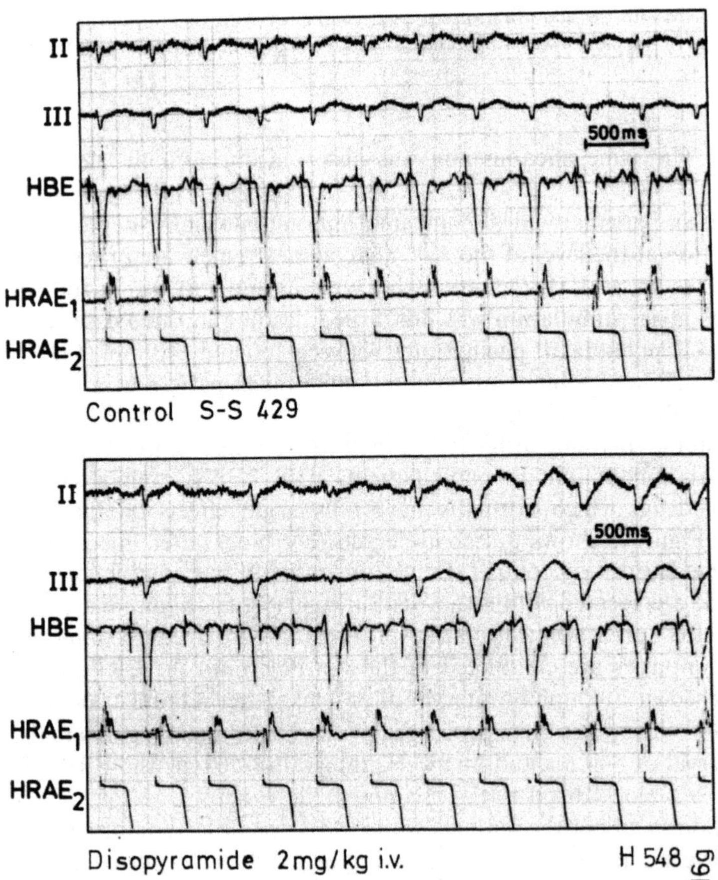
II
III
500ms
HBE
$HRAE_1$
$HRAE_2$
Control S-S 429
II
500ms
III
HBE
$HRAE_1$
$HRAE_2$
Disopyramide 2mg/kg i.v.
H 548
16g

Fig. 5

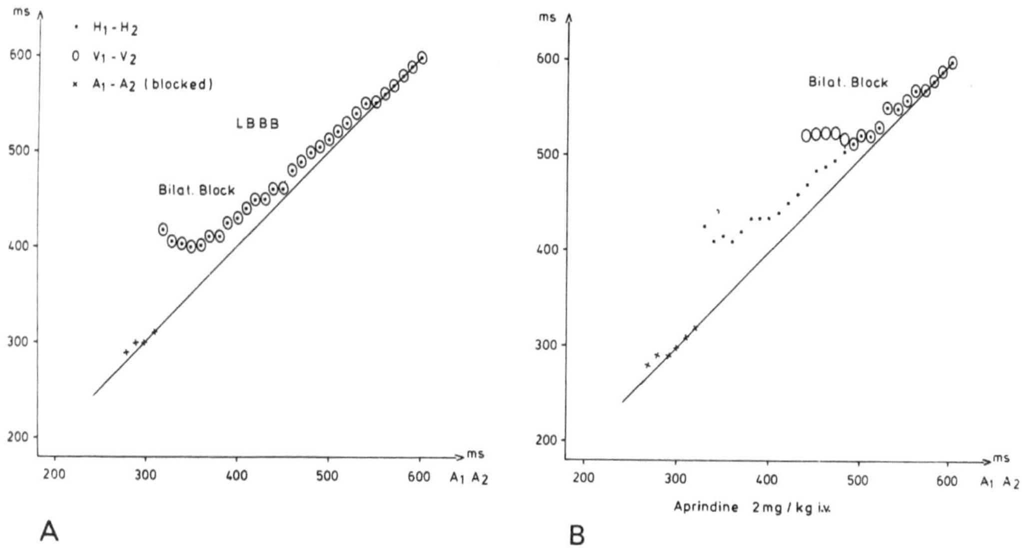

Fig. 6. Effect of Aprindine 2 mg/kg i.v. on A-V conduction in a patient with rate dependent LBBB. *A*. The result of programed atrial stimulation during control period. With shorter coupling intervals of the extrastimulus an LBBB pattern and in addition an RBBB pattern without A-V block is observed (bilateral block). Finally a block occurs after the A potential. After administration of Aprindine, the impulses are blocked distal to the H potentials at relatively long coupling intervals, indicating a prolongation of the ERP H by the drug (*B*)

QRS complexes were small, whereas in the normal ECG the patient had a "constant" LBBB during all frequencies registered. In all patients a one-to-one conduction reoccurred (Fig. 8).

Discussion

In our study LBBB pattern was often associated with cardiomyopathy, which is in agreement with some other studies [2, 3, 5, 12, 17, 18, 21, 26, 30, 49]. In some patients the LBBB seems to be the first manifestation of heart disease, COCM not developing until some years later [26]. The reason the left bundle branch is especially damaged in patients with COCM is unknown [3, 40]. Histologic studies of the conduction systems in patients with LBBB and COCM have shown

◁ Fig. 4. His bundle electrogram in a patient with LBBB and intermittent higher degree A-V block. During sinus rhythm there is a one-to-one conduction with a prolonged H-V time (left side). At atrial pacing rates of 100/min a block distal to the H potential is observed (right side)

Fig. 5. Effect of Disopyramide 2 mg/kg i.v. on intraventricular conduction in a patient with rate dependent LBBB. During control stimulation a one-to-one conduction with normal QRS complexes is documented. After administration of the drug, the impulses are intermittent blocked distal to the H potentials (left side) whereas during one-to-one conduction an LBBB pattern is present

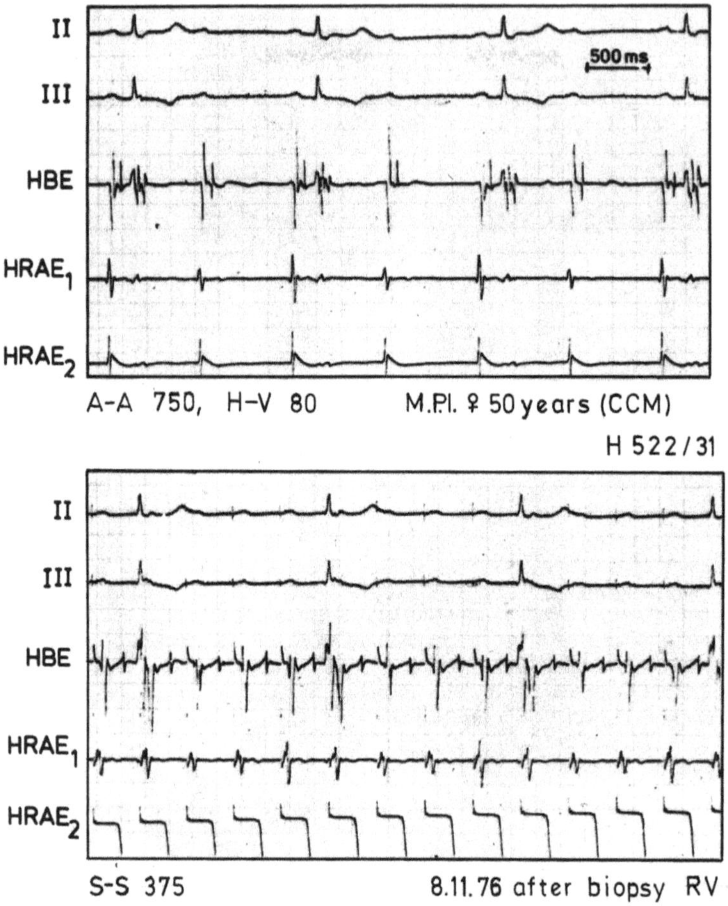

Fig. 7. Catheter-induced second degree A-V block during right ventricular myocardial biopsy. The block is located distal to the H potential in the HBE. Due to the slow ventricular rate the QRS complexes are small

changes varying from complete fibrosis of the left bundle branch up to morphologically normal findings [5].

Intraventricular conduction time studies in patients with LBBB show the same variation from normal to extremely prolonged values. According to previous findings [36] in our study a prolonged H-V interval was often seen in patients with first degree A-V block. However, as in other studies [28, 31, 34] a normal P-R interval did not exclude an abnormal H-V time. Neither the QRS axis [48] nor the width of the ventricular complex [38] was a good predictor for an abnormal H-V interval, which results were found by others [31, 51].

In the group of COCM patients nearly all showed a delayed H-V time, whereas in the other groups normal and abnormal values were found. The mean H-V interval in patients with COCM was significantly longer than the H-V time in patients with LCM or with LBBB of unknown etiology. Even in most patients

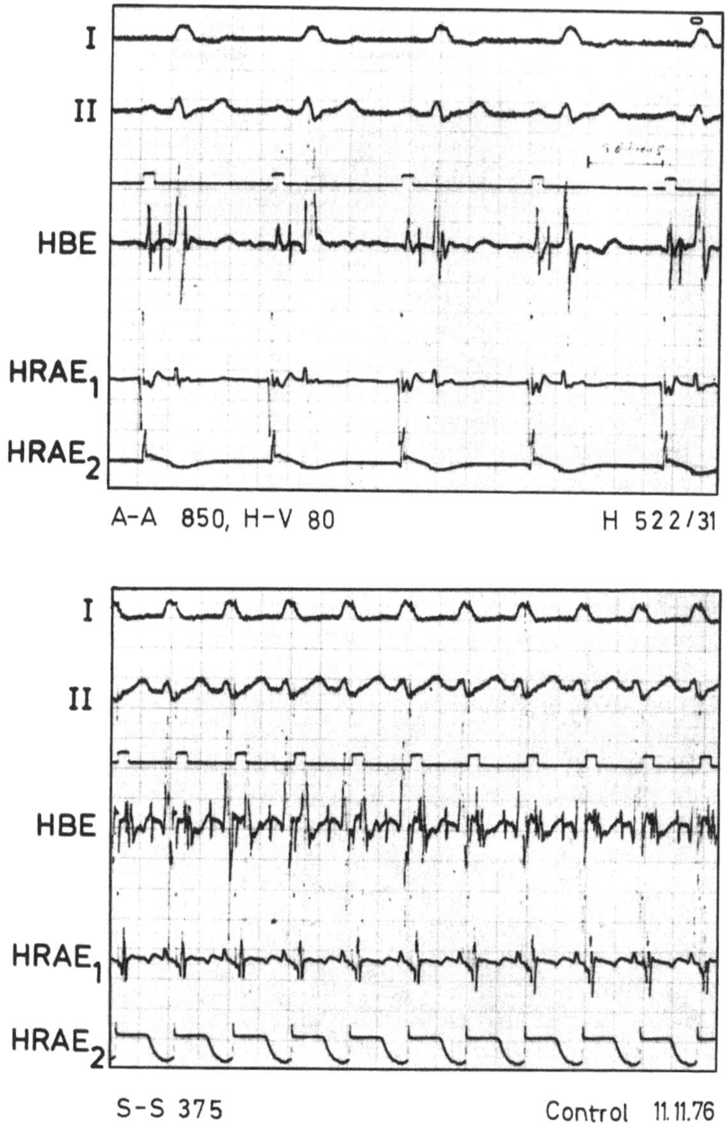

Fig. 8. Reoccurrence of one-to-one conduction in the same patient. A constant LBBB pattern is now registered during all frequencies

with COCM without LBBB the H-V time was markedly prolonged. The same was found by Waisser *et al.* [51], which indicates that in nearly all cases with COCM the conduction system is involved in the underlying myocardial process whether LBBB is or is not present. However, even in patients with LBBB without any other sign of heart disease prolonged H-V times were found. The abnormal morphologic findings in the right ventricular myocardium of these patients suggest that both the conduction system and the ordinary myocardium are involved in the same pathologic process. One can only speculate that perhaps these patients with a prolonged H-V interval will develop a COCM in the future. In contrast to other findings [38], there was no difference in the mean H-V interval of patients with CHD and COCM.

From the electrophysiologic point of view the interpretation of a prolonged H-V interval in LBBB is controversial. Some authors argue that a prolongation of the H-V time up to 20 ms can be explained by a "physiologic" delay in the activation of the interventricular septum after blockade of the left bundle branch [9,20]. However, experimental [1,15] and clinical data [32,37] indicate that in LBBB the activation of the septum from the right side occurs with a minimal delay of some milliseconds if at all. Therefore, a marked prolongation of the H-V interval in LBBB is considered to be due to an additional conduction delay within the His bundle or the right bundle branch [4,7,16,19,31,36,41,50,53], indicating a truncular of trifascicular disease. In nearly all our patients with LBBB and prolonged H-V interval a delay between the first recorded septal activation and the depolarization of the right ventricular apex (V-RVA) was found, which seems to underscore this interpretation. Such a prolonged V-RVA interval is described in patients with complete right bundle branch block [10,23]. Castellanos *et al.* [10] found normal V-RVA intervals in their patients with LBBB, but the authors did not give any comment on the H-V time in these patients. In addition, the constant normal H-V time in some patients with intermittent LBBB as observed in our study and by others [8,13] demonstrates that the occurrence of block within the left bundle branch does not necessarily prolong the H-V time.

Postmortem histologic examinations were performed only on a few patients with LBBB who underwent His-bundle studies. Rosen *et al.* [38] found in three patients with LBBB and a prolonged H-V time a severe damage of the His bundle and/or the right bundle branch in addition to the left bundle alterations. From our study only a correlation between the findings from the myocardial biopsy and the electrophysiologic data is possible. If the morphologic score of the electron-microscopic studies is compared with the H-V time, no correlation exists. However, all three patients with a normal H-V interval had only 1–3 points, whereas each patient with a score greater than 3 points showed a prolonged H-V interval. On the other hand, a long H-V time was not necessarily combined with a high morphologic score. In spite of that, the data may indicate an involvement of the interventricular conduction system in the myocardial process in many patients with a prolonged H-V time. Further studies are needed to support this thesis.

In addition to the conduction time the refractory nature of the intraventricular conduction system is a determinant factor in bundle branch block. Unfortunately, programed and high rate atrial pacing is of limited value in determinating the refractory nature of the His-Purkinje system. The first problem is that the occurrence of an LBBB pattern can be due to a delay or a block within the left bundle branch. Therefore, it is impossible to measure the ERP of the left bundle. For example, in a patient with complete LBBB an additional RBBB pattern without A-V block was observed during stimulation, which demonstrates the incomplete nature of some complete bundle branch blocks [54].

A second problem is that even in patients with LBBB the ERP of the His-Purkinje system exceeds the ERP of the A-V node only in a few cases. In five patients we were able to measure the ERP H by programed atrial stimulation, showing values between 430 and 520 ms. Even if no normal data concerning the ERP H exist we can assume, in agreement with Narula [31], that values of about 500 ms are critically prolonged. In three of the five cases a block distal H occurred even during rapid atrial pacing. This phenomenon is favored by the fact that in some patients with LBBB the refractory periods of the His-Purkinje system are paradoxically unchanged or prolonged with increasing heart rate. The same was reported by others [13, 33, 44]. A block distal to the H potential at frequencies up to 160/min occurred only in patients with a very long H-V interval. Normally a Mobitz type II block was observed. Only once were we able to demonstrate a Wenckebach phenomenon within the His-Purkinje system, which is rare even in patients with bundle branch block [35].

In previous studies no high degree A-V block occurred in patients with a prolonged H-V interval [3, 38, 51]. Waisser *et al.* [51] stated that the prognostic implications of H-V prolongation remain undefined in patients with COCM. This holds true even in our study. In spite of this statement we think that a group of especially endangered patients can be selected by His bundle recordings and atrial pacing. In all patients with documented higher degree A-V block extremely abnormal conduction times were found, in one patient within the A-V node, in the others within the His-Purkinje system. In addition, all patients tested showed abnormal behavior during atrial pacing. All these patients received a pacemaker. A prolonged H-V time in patients with bundle branch block indicates a bilateral conduction disease even if the refractory periods are normal. Because of the possible functional dissociation of conduction time and the refractory nature of the His-Purkinje system, a short ERP H does not exclude an intraventricular conduction defect [32]. The observation of Dhingra *et al.* [14] that many patients with a prolonged H-V interval die of their underlying heart disease is in agreement with our findings. However, this is not contradictory to the statement that prolonged H-V interval is a precursor of intraventricular block. In most of the patients with COCM pacemaker implantation does not improve the bad prognosis.

Another clinical problem is that patients with LBBB often need antiarrhythmic drugs for suppression of dangerous dysrhythmias. These drugs may lead to an additional impairement of the intraventricular conduction. Even drugs which normally have only slight effects on conduction time and the refractory nature of the His-Purkinje system may induce a block in patients with LBBB. Therefore, antidysrhythmic drugs should be tested under safe condition before ambulatory treatment in these patients.

It is noteworthy that no complication occurred during the studies in patients with LBBB. Stiff multipolar catheters may damage the His bundle or right bundle branch leading to A-V block [31]. This complication, documented in the literature [22, 24, 29], occurred in our laboratory only during the introduction of the stiff biotome into the right ventricle. Therefore, we use only small flexible electrodes for recording of His bundle potentials.

In summary, His bundle recording and myocardial biopsy make it feasibile to correlate electrophysiologic and morphologic findings in patients with LBBB of different etiology. The H-V interval in patients with LBBB and COCM was significantly longer than in cases with LCM or LBBB of unknown etiology. However, even in some patients with LBBB without any other sign of heart disease, prolonged H-V intervals were found. The abnormal morphologic findings in the right ventricular myocardium of the patients with a prolonged H-V interval suggest that both the conduction system and the ordinary myocardium are involved in the same pathologic process.

In addition, His bundle studies in patients with LBBB are of clinical value in that the results can influence the indication for pacemaker implantation and the treatment with antiarrhythmic drugs. Using a flexible thin bipolar catheter, the method seems to be without risk even in patients with LBBB.

References

1. Amer, N.S., Stukey, J.M., Hoffman, B.F., Cappelletti, R.R., Domingo, R.T.: Activation of the interventricular septal myocardium studied during cardiopulmonary bypass. Amer. Heart J. *59*, 224 (1960)
2. Banta, D.H., Estes, E.H.: Electrocardiographic and vectrocardiographic findings in patients with idiopathic myocardial hypertrophy. Amer. J. Cardiol. *14*, 218 (1964)
3. Bashour, T.T., Fahdul, H., Cheng, T.O.: Multifascicular block in cardiomyopathy. Cardiol. (Basle) *61*, 89 (1976)
4. Berkowitz, W.D., Lau, S.H., Patton, R.D., Rosen, K.M., Damato, A.N.: The use of His bundle recordings in the analysis of unilateral and bilateral bundle branch block. Amer. Heart J. *81*, 340 (1971)
5. Blondeau, M.: Complete left bundle branch block with marked left axis deviation of QRS. In: Recent Advances in Ventricular Condition. Cerqueira-Gomes, M. (ed.), p. 25. Basle: Karger 1975
6. Cannom, D.S., Hancock, E.W.: A syndrome of congenital cardiomyopathy with mitral regurgitation, complete heart block and atrial arrhythmias. Amer. J. Med. *56*, 261 (1974)
7. Cannom, D.S., Goldreyer, B.N., Damato, A.N.: Atrioventricular conduction system in left bundle branch block with normal QRS axis. Circulation *46*, 129 (1972)
8. Cannom, D.S., Goodman, D.J., Harrison, D.C.: Electrophysiological studies in patients with rate-related intermittent left bundle branch block. Brit. Heart J. *36*, 653 (1974)
9. Castellanos, A.: H-V intervals in LBBB (Letter). Circulation *47*, 1133 (1973)
10. Castellanos, A., Agha, A.S., Befeler, B., Castillo, C.A., Berkovitz, B.V.: A study of arrival of excitation at selected ventricular sites during human bundle branch block using close bipolar catheter electrodes. Chest *63*, 208 (1973)
11. Chmielewski, C.A., Riley, R.S., Mahendran, A., Most, A.S.: Complete heart block as a cause of syncope in asymetric septal hypertrophy. Amer. Heart J. *93*, 91 (1977)
12. Delius, W., Sebening, H., Weghmann, N., Oversohl, K., Wirtzfeld, A., Mathes, P.: Klinik und Verlauf der kongestiven Kardiomyopathie ungeklärter Ätiologie. Dtsch. med. Wschr. *101*, 635 (1976)
13. Denes, P., Wu, D., Dhingra, R.C., Amat-y-Leon, F., Wyndham, C., Rosen, K.M.: Electrophysiological observations in patients with rate-dependent bundle branch block. Circulation *51*, 244 (1975)
14. Dhingra, R.C., Denes, P., Wu, D., Wyndham, C.R., Amat-y-Leon, F., Town, W.D., Rosen, K.M.: Prospective observations in patients with chronic bundle branch block and marked H-V prolongation. Circulation *53*, 600 (1976)
15. Durrer, D., Van Dam, T., Freud, G.E., Janse, M.J., Meijler, F.L., Arzbacher, R.C.: Total excitation of the isolated human heart. Circulation *41*, 899 (1970)
16. Fleischmann, D., Mathey, D., Bleifeld, W., Irnich, W., Effert, S.: His-Bündel-Electrographie bei Patienten mit intraventrikulären Leitungsstörungen. Klin. Wschr. *51*, 1066 (1973)

17. Flowers, N.C., Heran, L.G.: Electrocardiographic and vectorcardiographic features of myocardial disease. In: Myocardial Disease. Fowler, N.O. (ed.), p. 181. New York: Grune & Stratton 1973
18. Forrester, J.S., Kemp, H.G., Gorlin, R.: Primary myocardial disease. Distinction from coronary heart disease. Circulation *39*, *40*, Suppl. III, 81 (1969)
19. Guérot, C., Coste, A., Valere, P.E., Motté, G., Tricot, R.: Enregistrement de l'activité du tronc du faisceau de His et de ses branches dans les troubles de conduction intraventriculaire. Arch. Mal. Cœur *66*, 269 (1973)
20. Haft, J.I., Weinstock, M., De Guia, R., Gupta, P.K., Fano, A.: Assessment of atrioventricular conduction in left and right bundle branch block using His bundle electrograms and atrial pacing. Amer. J. Cardiol. *27*, 272 (1971)
21. Hamby, R.I., Raia, F.: Electrocardiographic aspects of primary myocardial disease in 60 patients. Amer. Heart J. *76*, 316 (1968)
22. Jacobson, L.B., Scheinman, M.: Catheter-induced intra-Hisian and intrafascicular block during recording of His bundle electrogram. Circulation *49*, 579 (1974)
23. Kastor, J.A., Goldreyer, B.N., Moore, E.N., Shelburne, J.C., Manchester, J.H.: Intraventricular conduction in man studied with an endocardial electrode catheter mapping technique. Circulation *51*, 786 (1975)
24. Kimbris, D., Dreifus, L.S., Linhart, J.W.: Complete heart block occurring during cardiac catheterization in patients with preexisting bundle branch block. Chest *65*, 95 (1974)
25. Konno, S., Sakakibara, S.: Endomyocardial biopsy. Dis. Chest *50*, 345 (1963)
26. Kuhn, H., Breithardt, L.K., Breithardt, G., Seipel, L., Loogen, F.: Die Bedeutung des Elektrokardiogramms für die Diagnose und Verlaufsbeobachtung von Patienten mit kongestiver Kardiomyopathie. Z. Kardiol. *63*, 916 (1974)
27. Kuhn, H., Breithardt, G., Knieriem, H.J., Loogen, F., Both, A., Schmidt, W.A.K., Stroobandt, R., Gleichmann, U.: Die Bedeutung der endomyokardialen Katheterbiopsie für die Diagnostik und die Beurteilung der Prognose der kongestiven Kardiomyopathie. Dtsch. med. Wschr. *100*, 717 (1975)
28. Lang, K.: Klinik der AV-Überleitungsstörungen. Herz-Kreisl. *9*, 82 (1977)
29. Levites, R., Toor, M., Haft, J.I.: Progressive improvement of His-Purkinje conduction during recovery from catheter-induced heart block. Amer. Heart J. *91*, 79 (1976)
30. Massumi, R.A., Rios, J.C., Gooch, A.S., Nutter, D., Devita, V.T., Dailow, D.W.: Primary myocardial disease. Circulation *31*, 19 (1965)
31. Narula, O.S.: Intraventricular conduction defects. In: His Bundle Electrocardiography and Clinical Electrophysiology. Narula, O.S. (ed.), p. 177. Philadelphia: Davis Comp. 1975
32. Narula, O.S., Javier, R.P., Samet, P., Maramba, L.C.: Significance of His and left bundle recordings from the left heart in man. Circulation *42*, 385 (1970)
33. Neuss, H., Thormann, J., Schlepper, M.: Electrophysiologic findings in frequency-dependent left bundle-branch block. Brit. Heart J. *36*, 888 (1974)
34. Puech, P.: Corrélations entre les enregistrements de surface et l'électrogramme hisien. In: His-Bündel Elektrographie. Seipel, L., Both, A., Loogen, F. (ed.), p. 91. Stuttgart: Schattauer 1975
35. Ranganathan, N., Dhurandher, R., Phillips, J.P., Wigle, E.D.: His bundle electrogram in bundle-branch block. Circulation *45*, 282 (1972)
36. Rosen, K.M., Rahimtoola, S.H., Chuquimia, R., Loeb, H.S., Gunnar, R.M.: Electrophysiological significance of first degree atrioventricular block with intraventricular conduction disturbance. Circulation *43*, 491 (1971)
37. Rosen, K.M., Rahimtoola, S.H., Sinno, M.Z., Gunnar, R.M.: Bundle branch and ventricular activation in man. Circulation *43*, 193 (1971)
38. Rosen, K.M., Ehsani, A., Rahimtoola, S.H.: H-V intervals in left bundle-branch block. Circulation *46*, 717 (1972)
39. Rosen, K.M., Rahimtoola, S.H., Bharati, S., Lev, M.: Bundle branch block with intact atrioventricular conduction. Amer. J. Cardiol. *32*, 783 (1973)
40. Rosenbaum, M.B., Elizari, M.E., Lazzari, J.O., Kretz, A., DaRuos, H.O.: The clinical causes and mechanisms of intraventricular conduction disturbances. In: Advances in Electrocardiography. Schlant, R.C., Hurst, J.W. (eds.), p. 183. New York: Grune & Stratton 1972
41. Scheinman, M., Weiss, A., Kunkel, F.: His bundle recording in patients with bundle branch block and transient neurologic symptoms. Circulation *48*, 322 (1973)

42. Scherlag, B.J., Lau, S.H., Helfant, R.H., Berkowitz, W.D., Stein, E., Damato, A.N.: Catheter technique for recording His bundle activity in man. Circulation *39*, 13 (1969)
43. Scherlag, B.J., Samet, P., Helfant, R.H.: His bundle electrogram. Circulation *46*, 601 (1972)
44. Schlepper, M.: Contributions of intracardiac electrography to the understanding of normal and disturbed A-V conduction. In: Cardiac Pacing. Lüderitz, B. (ed.), p. 87. Berlin: Springer 1976
45. Seipel, L., Gleichmann, U., Loogen, F.: His-Bündel Elektrographie. Med. Technik *93*, 27 (1973)
46. Seipel, L., Both, A., Loogen, F.: Klinische Bedeutung der His-Bündel Elektrographie. Klin. Wschr. *53*, 499 (1975)
47. Seipel, L., Breithardt, G., Both, A.: Elektrophysiologische Effekte der Antiarrhythmika Disopyramid und Propafenon auf das menschliche Reizleitungssystem. Z. Kardiol. *64*, 731 (1975)
48. Spurrell, R.A.J., Krikler, D.M., Sowton, E.: Study of intraventricular conduction times in patients with left bundle-branch block and left axis deviation and in patients with left bundle-branch block and normal QRS axis using His bundle electrograms. Brit. Heart J. *34*, 1244 (1972)
49. Stapleton, J.F., Segal, J.P., Harvery, W.P.: The electrocardiogram of myocardiopathy. Progr. cardiovasc. Dis. *13*, 217 (1970)
50. Vera, Z., Mason, D.T., Fletcher, R.D., Awan, N.A., Massumi, R.A.: Prolonged His-Q interval in chronic bifascicular block. Relation to impending complete heart block. Circulation *53*, 46 (1976)
51. Waisser, E., Gaasch, W.H., Quinones, M.A., Alexander, J.K.: His bundle electrograms in patients with congestive cardiomyopathy. Europ. J. Cardiol. *2*, 343 (1975)
52. Wit, A.L., Wiss, M.B., Berkowitz, W.D., Rosen, K.M., Steiner, C., Damato, A.N.: Patterns of atrioventricular conduction in the human heart. Circulation Res. *27*, 345 (1970)
53. Wong, B.Y.S., Dunn, M.: Transient unifascicular, bifascicular and trifascicular block: Electrophysiologic correlations in a patient with rate-dependent left bundle branch block and transient right bundle branch block. Amer. J. Cardiol. *39*, 116 (1977)
54. Wu, D., Denes, P., Dhingra, R., Rosen, K.N.: Bundle branch block. Amer. J. Cardiol. *33*, 583 (1974)

21. Immunologic Investigation in Patients With Cardiomyopathies

H.-D. Bolte

Current procedures for the diagnosis of myocardial disease leave much to be desired. The terms congestive, hypertrophic (with or without obstruction) and restrictive are not sufficient for classifying all aspects of myocardial diseases. The definition of so-called primary CM does not include biochemical, morphologic or immunologic events, and therefore the borderline between primary and secondary CM is often vague. Thus for diagnosis and therapy all CMs should be further characterized clinically and by laboratory tests. Our present interest concerns primarily the relationship of cardiomyopathies to immunologic findings. In addition we have tried to correlate quantitative immunoglobulins, antibody determinations by immunofluorescence techniques using in some cases myocardial biopsy specimen, and the underlying myocardial disease of clinically examined patients [3].

Our primary focus was on the diagnostic relevance of myocardial antibodies demonstrated by immunofluorescence. In these techniques myocardium (human heart muscle, guinea pig, rat) serves as an antigen. Microscopic sections are covered with a patient's serum containing the antibody in question. The bound globulins of the serum are separated by rinsing the section with a phosphate-buffer medium. In order to visualize microscopically antigen-antibody binding, conjugates of antiglobulins with a fluorescent agent are used [1, 7] (see Fig. 1).

We used the indirect immunofluorescence test to examine sera and the direct test to examine myocardial biopsies. We used fluorescein-isothiocyanat-conjugated anti-human-globulins from rabbit (anti-IgG, anti-IgM) (Behring-Werke, Marburg). The sera of the patients were diluted 1 : 5. The conjugates were diluted 1 :10, 1 : 30, up to 1 : 40.

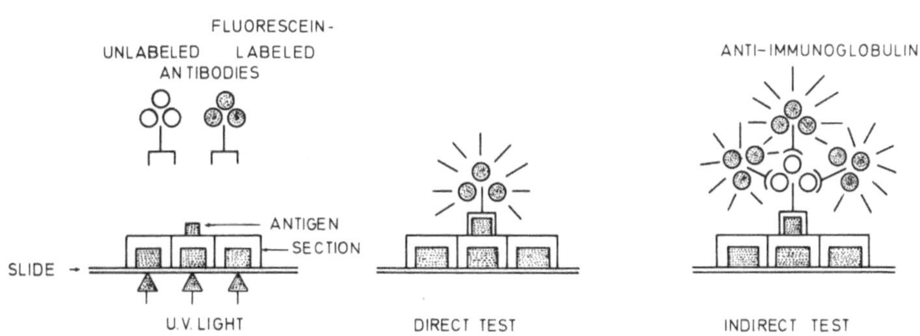

Fig. 1. The principal of direct and indirect immunofluorescence test

Results of the indirect immunofluorescence test in patients with various forms of CM are summarized in Figure 2. In agreement with other investigations [9, 14, 16], we found humoral myocardial antibodies (sarcolemmal localization) in postmyocardial infarction syndrome and in postcardiotomy syndrome. These results were important for the diagnosis of the disease and influenced the therapy.

In addition to positive results in patients with congestive CM of unknown etiology, the indirect immunofluorescence test was positive in 10 (41%) of 24 patients, i.e., 8 sarcolemmal type and 2 intermyofibrillar type. In the controls (30 clinically healthy persons), only one (3%) positive immunofluorescence test was observed. More quantitatively we demonstrated the same results by the antiglobulin consumption test which yielded an increased antiglobulin consumption directly proportional to concentration. The antiglobulin consumption test yielded titer decrease for congestive CM greater than those for controls by more than one step in 12 (50%). In the controls only 2 (10%) showed a titer decrease of only one step [10]. The positive antibody results coincided with more severe symptoms of congestive heart failure; those patients with negative antibody results did not have symptoms of congestive heart failure to the same extent. Furthermore the longer the duration of clinical symptoms, the higher the percentage of antibody coincidence: 36% in duration 0–5 years and 100% in duration 5–10 years.

Several groups have researched circulating heart reactive antibody. Robinson and co-workers noted an 11% incidence of heart reactive antibody [12]. Using an indirect immunofluorescence method Das and co-workers [8] found heart reactive antibodies in 6 of 35 patients (17%) with idiopathic cardiomegaly and in 1 of 43 control subjects. A similar coincidence of positive test result has been

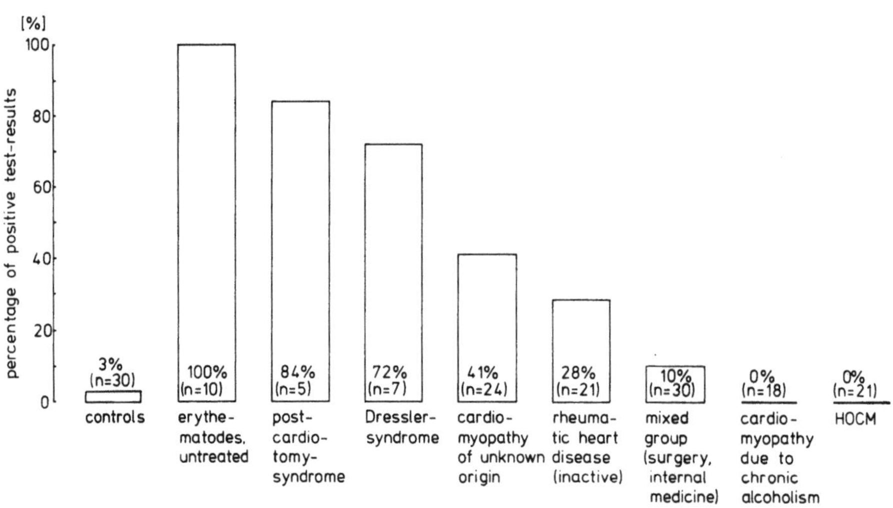

Fig. 2. Myocardial antibodies (indirect immunofluorescence test) in several myocardial diseases. The non existence of myocardial antibodies in alcoholic CM and in HOCM is remarkable in comparison to the other diseases

found in a study of 33 patients (12% of heart reactive antibodies) [6] and in a study of 68 patients, 60 of whom demonstrated antibodies against heart muscle sarcolemma [13].

These results indicate that immunologic evaluation is relevant to following the disease. However, it has not yet been decided whether the immune phenomena in CMs of unknown etiology have diagnostic significance only or if they can serve also as indicators of the underlying pathogenetic mechanism.

In this regard, we examined 22 patients with congestive CM due to chronic alcoholism. In all these patients we observed a negative myocardial antibody test, but in 95%, the IgA value was increased by 100% on the average. The existence of a congestive heart failure as the expression of congestive CM and the further symptoms of a negative immunofluorescence test and increased IgA value can serve as a guide to the diagnosis of CM due to chronic alcoholism. In the patients examined, there was no evidence for hepatic cirrhosis [2, 5].

Humoral myocardial antibodies could be detected in none of 21 patients with the characteristic symptoms of HOCM. All of the patients were examined clinically and by heart catheterization. We determined the typical intraventricular pressure gradient and, by angiography, the septical hypertrophy and outflow tract obstruction [4, 15].

For about a year and a half we have used in our department the Richardson bioptome for myocardial biopsy [11]. Our experience consists of biopsies of 30 patients, in which one to five biopsy samples were taken transvenously from the right ventricle. In two cases we took biopsies from the left ventricle, but we strongly prefer to take biopsies only from the right ventricle in order to prevent arterial embolism. To date we have had neither serious complications nor side effects except for two cases with some ventricular extrasystoles and intermittent bradycardia and one case with AV-block of degree III, reversible after 2 min.

Biopsy specimens were taken 1–2 days after angiography for histomorphologic and electron-microscopic analyses (E.G.J. Olsen, National Heart Hospital, London; E. Hübner, Pathologisches Institut, Universität München) and for immunologic evaluations.

Recently we performed the direct immunofluorescence test on biopsies from 15 patients with CM of various etiologies and hemodynamics. In all of them the biopsy was preceeded by pressure measurements by heart catheterization, left-ventricular angiography and coronary arteriography. There was no evidence of coronary heart disease, valvular heart disease or hypertension. All of the patients had indications of a disturbed myocardial function. In those of normal ejection fraction and normal enddiastolic volume, enddiastolic pressure was increased and/or pharmacologic function tests gave pathologic results (see Table 2).

Our results in myocardial biopsies of patients with CM are listed in Tables 1 and 2. The patients of Table 1 fulfilled in all hemodynamic and morphologic respects the criteria of congestive CM.

In 7 patients with congestive CM of unknown etiology we observed a high percentage (40%) of sarcolemmal antibodies. As documented in Table 1 these patients show a typically increased enddiastolic volume and a considerably lowered ejection fraction. For comparison we evaluated patients with secondary CM (Table 2). These patients had a remarkably lower hemodynamic degree than

Table 1. Congestive cardiomyopathy of inknown etiology. Immunologic results in myocardial biopsies.

Patient		Diagnosis	EF (%)	EDV (Ml)	Direct immunofluorescence[a] IgG	IgM
8.3.76	F.J.	COCM, unknown etiology	13	209	∅	∅
1.4.76	G.F.	COCM, unknown etiology	48	187	∅	∅
26.7.76	H.P.	COCM, unknown etiology	25	560	s+ I+	∅
30.8.76	D.M.	COCM, unknown etiology	44	297	s++	∅
31.8.76	S.A.	COCM, unknown etiology	25	288	s+	∅
20.10.76	B.R.	COCM, unknown etiology	10	339	∅	i+

[a] s, Sarcolemmal type; i, Intermyofibrillar type

Table 2. Secondary cardiomyopathies of various etiologies. Immunologic results in myocardial biopsies.

Patient		Diagnosis	EF (%)	EDV (Ml)	Direct immunofluorescence[a] IgG	IgM
21.1.76	S.G.	CM Polymyositis	71	130	∅	∅
20.1.76	G.U.	CM microangiopathy	78	163	∅	∅
7.5.76	W.A.	CM after virus infection	66	86	∅	∅
25.5.76	S.R.	Alcoholic CM	64	332	∅	∅
13.7.76	W.B.	Susp. myocarditis	74	128	∅	∅
8.9.76	J.E.	CM in cor pulmonale	60	192	s+	∅
10.9.76	F.E.	Viruscarditis	72	128	∅	s+
22.9.76	W.A.	CM in rheumatoid arthritis	76	130	∅	∅
23.9.76	F.A.	CM after coxsackie infection	75	132	s+	∅

[a] s, Sarcolemmal; i, Intermyofibrillar

those of Table 1 but showed pathologic results in pharmacologic function tests. In these patients we observed a remarkably lower percentage of bound immunoglobulins. A definite correlation of immunologic results to a virus disease could not be demonstrated despite the fact that in serologic analyses a virus infection could be documented. Both groups of patients demonstrated a low incidence of bound immunoglobulin M.

Fluorescent deposits were demonstrated in one of the patients (F.A., Table 2).

The relevance of these findings can not be definitely determined because of the low number of determinations. On the other hand it should be noted that a high percentage of demonstrated immunoglobulin G in congestive CM of unknown etiology is evidence of an immunologic process in which the myocardial disease seems to be involved.

Conclusion

Such immunologic methods as immunofluorescence tests and determinations of serum immunoglobulins (IgG, IgA, IgM) reveal important diagnostic criteria for differentiating several forms of congestive CM. In myocardial tissue of biopsy specimens, the relevance of immunoglobulin binding to immunologic determinants has not been analysed. However, it may be expected that an increased number of observations will reveal the criteria for the natural history of the disease and for therapy.

References

1. Bolte, H.-D.: Diagnostische Wertigkeit des indirekten Immunofluoreszenztestes zum Nachweis humoraler Antikörper gegen Myocard. Internist *16*, 180 (1975)
2. Bolte, H.-D.: Alkoholkardiomyopathie. Münch. Med. Wochenschr. *118*, 355 (1976)
3. Bolte, H.-D., Grothey, K.: Cardiomyopathies related to immunological processes. In: Myocardial Failure. Riecker, G., Weber, A., Goodwin, J. (eds.). New York-Heidelberg-Berlin: Springer-Verlag 1977 (in press)
4. Bolte, H.-D., Von Geldern, S.: unveröffentlicht (1977)
5. Bolte, H.-D., Milstrey, H.R., Tebbe, U., Rahlf, G.: Neuere Aspekte zur klinischen Diagnostik der Alkoholkardiomyopathie. Verh. Dtsch. Ges. Inn. Med. *80*, 1206 (1974)
6. Camp, T.F., Hess, E.V., Conway, G., Fowler, N.O.: Immunologic findings in idiopathic cardiomyopathy. Amer. Heart J. *77*, 610 (1969)
7. Coons, A.H., Creech, H.J., Jones, R.N.: Immunological Properties of an Antibody Containing a Fluorescent Group. Proc. Soc. Exp. Biol. Med. *47*, 200 (1941)
8. Das, S.K., Cassidy, J.T., Petty, R.E.: Antibodies against heart muscle and nuclear constituents in cardiomyopathy. Am. J. Cardiol. *25*, 91 (1970)
9. Engle, M.A., McCabe, J.C., Ebert, P.A., Zabriskie, J.: The Postpericardiotomy Syndrome and Antiheart Antibodies. Circulation *49*, 401 (1974)
10. Oevermann, W., Bolte, H.-D., Zwehl, W.: Indirekter Immunfluoreszenztest und indirekter Antiglobulinkonsumptionstest in der Diagnostik primärer Kardiomyopathien. Verh. Dtsch. Ges. Inn. Med. *79*, 1121 (1973)
11. Richardson, P.J.: King's endomyocardial bioptome. Lancet *1974/I*, 660
12. Robinson, J., Anderson, T., Grieble, H.: Serologic anomalies in idiopathic myocardial disease. Clin. Res. *14*, 335 (1966)
13. Sack, W., Sebening, H., Wachsmut, E.D.: Auto-Antikörper gegen Herzmuskelsarkolemm im Serum von Patienten mit primärer Cardiomyopathie. Klin. Wochenschr. *35*, 103 (1975)
14. Van der Geld, H.: Anti-Heart Antibodies in the Postpericardiotomy- and Postmyocardialinfarction-Syndromes. Lancet *1964/II*, 618
15. Von Geldern, S.: Immunologische Untersuchungen bei hypertrophischer obstruktiver Kardiomyopathie – Diss., Göttingen 1975
16. Zabriskie, J.B., Read, S.E., Ellis, R.J.: Cellular and humoral studies in diseases with heart reactive antibodies. In: Progress in Immunology. Amos, L. (ed.). New York: Acad. Pr. 1971

Congestive Cardiomyopathy

22. Prognostic Significance of Endomyocardial Biopsy in Patients With Congestive Cardiomyopathy

G. BREITHARDT, H. KUHN, and H.-J. KNIERIEM

Summary

A follow-up study was performed in 48 patients with clinically defined COCM in whom endomyocardial biopsy had been done. For the evaluation of the biopsy specimens, a semiquantitative morphologic score was used.

Overall mortality in these 48 patients was high (5-year cumulative survival rate after onset of symptoms: 66%, 10-year survival rate: 28%). By use of the morphologic score two groups of patients with a good prognosis (group I, ≤ 4 points, 2-year cumulative survival rate: 76%) and with a poor prognosis (group II, ≥ 5 points, 2-year cumulative survival rate: 36%) could be clearly seperated ($P < 0.01$). Hemodynamic data did not show the same prognostic significance when comparing these two groups. However, they were of somewhat better discriminative value when comparing those patients still alive to those deceased. The morphologic score was of special value in patients with a short duration of illness (less than 2 years), once again making a clear separation between surviving and dead patients possible.

Degenerative changes and alterations of mitochondria were the best indication of a poor prognosis. Thus, in patients with COCM, these changes probably signal late stages of myocardial hypertrophy related to exhaustion of cardiac reserves.

Previous studies on the prognosis of patients with CMs were restricted by the fact that no uniform definition existed which made a comparison of different studies difficult [7, 26, 41, 49, 56, 57]. Since the classification of CMs by Goodwin *et al.* [14, 15] clear clinical definitions exist which depend on hemodynamic and angiographic data. COCM is one of the main groups of CMs. It is characterized by an elevated EDV and ESV with impaired ventricular function. Diagnosis depends on the exclusion of valvular or coronary heart disease and of CMs of known causes [13, 14, 15, 25, 27, 32, 33].

The purpose of the present study was to correlate clinical and hemodynamic data as well as the results of endomyocardial biopsy to the clinical course of the patient. Preliminary data in a smaller group of patients have previously been reported [3, 29, 32, 34].

Patients and Methods

Forty-eight patients (40 male, 8 female) fulfilling the diagnostic criteria of COCM [14, 15, 24, 25, 27, 32, 33] were studied prospectively. In all patients endomyocardial biopsy was performed. Follow-up after biopsy had to be at least 6 months before a patient was included in this series. Besides biopsy from the right ventricle, right and left heart catheterizations, LV cineangiograms, coronary arteriography, chest radiography, ECG, phonocardiograms, apexcardiograms, external carotid pulse tracings, and laboratory test were obtained. From the LV cineangiograms, LVEDV and LVESV were estimated in 30° right anterior oblique projections considering the magnification and using the area-length method for calculation of ventricular volumes [8, 54]. From these data indices were derived, yielding the LVEDV index (LVEDVI) and the LVESV index (LVESVI) (unit: volume/m^2 surface area), and the ejection fraction (EF; %) was calculated. Teleroentgenograms in the p-a projection were used for estimation of cardiothoracic ratio. Endomyocardial biopsy was performed by the transfemoral approach using either the Konno's or the King's bioptome [22, 50, 53] as described elsewhere. There was no significant complication during this procedure which yielded one to three specimens for light and electron-microscopic examination (for technical details, see Ch. 8).

From the semithin and ultrathin sections a semiquantitative morphologic evaluation was done by one of us (H.-J. K.). The clinical data and the result of follow-up of the patient were unknown to him. The morphologic findings were estimated according to their frequency, their extent, and their severity using the following semiquantitative morphologic score that had already been used in earlier works [5, 33, 36, 38] (Table 1). Degenerative changes were considered to be myelin figures, frequent lipofuscin granules, increased number of lipid droplets, lysosomal changes, and lysis of myofilaments. Alterations of mitochondria consisted of extreme variation in size, abnormally large or small mitochondria, mitochondriosis, and abnormally configurated mitochondrias. Myofibrillar changes were considered to be present in case of abnormal arrangement of myofibers and myofibrils running in adverse directions, abnormal thickening of Z bands or irregular Z bands. Interstitial fibrosis was judged from

Table 1. Morphologic score for semiquantitative evaluation of myocardial biopsies.

		Points
1. Degenerative changes		
	rare–slight	1
	frequent–severe	2
2. Alterations of mitochondria		
	rare	1
	frequent	2
3. Myofibrillar changes		
	rare	1
	frequent	2
4. Interstitial fibrosis		
	moderate	1
	severe	2
5. Hypertrophy	slight	1
	moderate	2
	severe	3

the semithin sections. Myocardial hypertrophy was classified according to the size of myofibers; slight: 15–20 mμ, moderate: 21–25 mμ, severe: 26 mμ.

All patients were examined at regular intervals of 6 to 12 months in the outpatient clinic. No patient was lost to folow-up. January 10, 1977 was taken as the date for determining the outcome of each case. House physicians or local hospitals were contacted to report the condition of the patient during the weeks leading up to this date.

The following definitions were used: 1. duration of illness is the interval from the onset of symptoms to the date of myocardial biopsy; 2. follow-up period is the interval from the date of myocardial biopsy to January 10, 1977; 3. survival period is the interval from the date of biopsy to the death of the patient, or when still alive to January 10, 1977.

Cumulative survival curves were calculated using actuarial methods [5, 39]. Statistical analysis was performed by use of the Wilcoxon test for unpaired data.

Results

Mean age of all patients was 40.8 ±9.1 years, mean duration of illness prior to biopsy was 3.5 ±3.2 years (maximum 13 years, minimum 0.5 years), and mean survival period and follow-up period were 1.3 ±0.9 years and 2.1 ±1.1 years, respectively.

Figure 1 shows the cumulative survival rate of the 48 patients with COCM from the onset of illness to January 10, 1977 or the date of death. Five-year survival rate was 65.7%, ten-year survival rate only 28.1%.

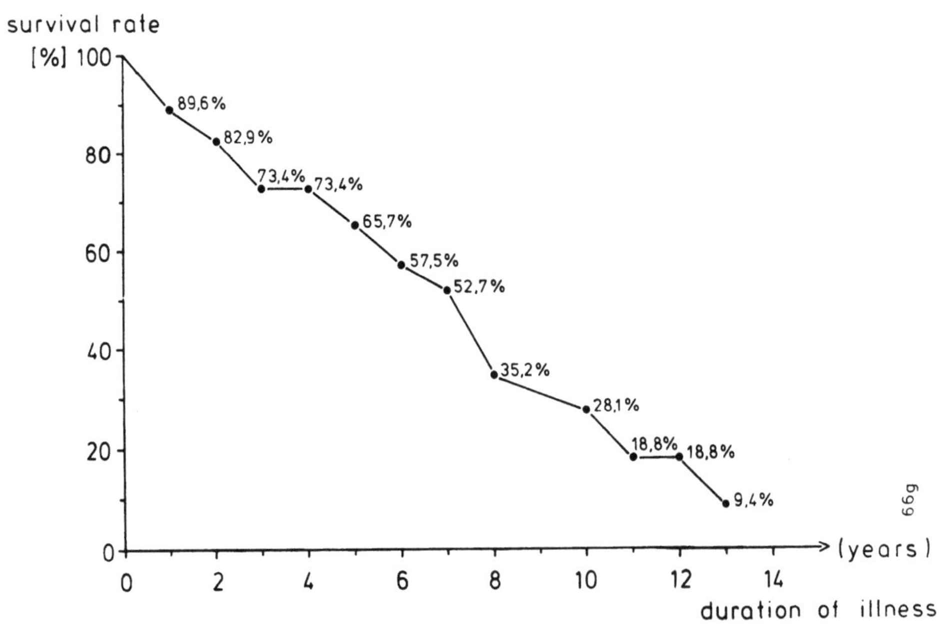

Fig. 1. Cumulative survival rate in 48 patients with COCM from the onset of illness to the end of the observation period

The frequency and extent of myocardial ultrastructural lesions varied considerably (Fig. 2). Interstitial fibrosis and myocardial hypertrophy were most frequently seen. Degenerative changes were found in 33 patients, alterations of mitochondria in 22 patients, and myofibrillar changes in 29 of them. Patients were then divided according to their morphologic score. Group I (n = 22) consisted of those patients with ≤4 points, group II (n = 26) of those with ≥5 points. In both groups, hypertrophy, interstitial fibrosis, and myofibrillar changes were seen with nearly identical frequency (Fig. 3). However, alterations of mitochondria were observed in only 9.1% of patients in group I and in 77% of patients in group II. Degenerative changes occurred in 41% of patients in group I and in 100% in group II. Mortality rate was highest in group II (17 out of 26 patients, 65%), and lowest in group I (6 out of 22 patients, 27%). Clinical and hemodynamic data were not significantly different between these two groups (Table 2), though cardiothoracic ratio and EDVI tended to be somewhat greater and EF tended to be lower in group II. Cumulative survival was lower at all intervals of follow-up in group II (Fig. 4). Survival rate after 4 years was 63% in group I and 18% in group II.

The prognostic significance of other parameters was tested by grouping the patients according to their final outcome independent of the morphologic score (Fig. 5). Mean age, duration of illness, survival period, and follow-up period were not significantly different when comparing those patients who died in the meantime, to those still alive. The morphologic score, cardiothoracic ratio, and EF were significantly different, the morphologic score having the lowest *P* value

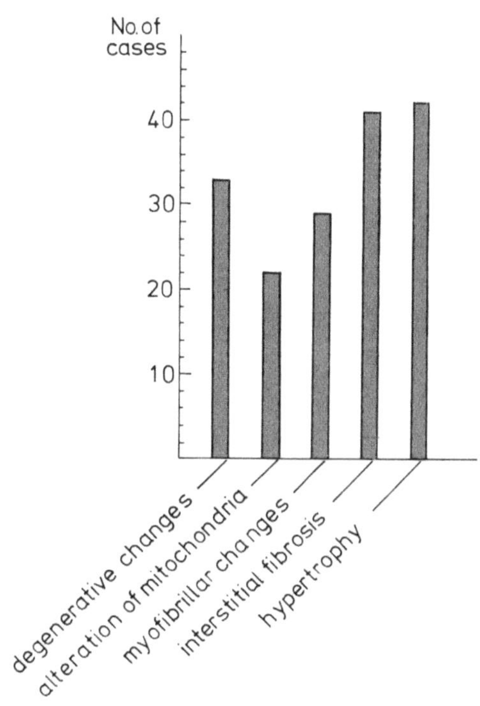

Fig. 2. Frequency of different morphologic alterations in 48 patients with COCM

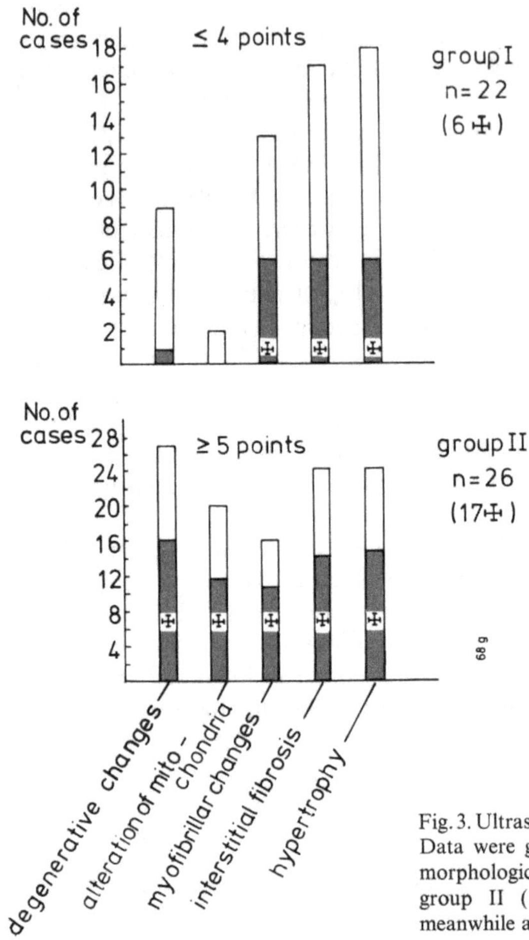

Fig. 3. Ultrastructural changes in 48 patients with COCM. Data were grouped according to the semiquantitative morphologic score into a group I (≤ 4 points) and a group II (≥ 5 points). Patients deceased in the meanwhile are indicated by *dark columns*

($P < 0.001$) and therefore the greatest significance in predicting the prognosis. EDVI was not significantly different, probably due to the great scatter of individual data, though the mean value was greater in those who died than in those still alive.

It might be supposed that the frequency and severity of morphologic changes depend on the duration of illness. Therefore, the morphologic score was compared to the duration of illness and the outcome of the case (Fig. 6). There was no significant correlation between morphologic changes and the duration of illness with an apparently great variation of data. Except for one patient, one or two points of the morphologic score were attributed only to patients with a duration of illness less than 5 years. However, when focusing on those patients with a duration of illness less than 2 years (n = 24), the survival could be predicted with great accuracy by the morphologic score (Fig. 7). Only one patient with ≤4 points died, whereas the survival rate at 1 year of follow-up was as low as 33% in those with ≥5 points. Some clinical data of this latter group of patients

Table 2. Morphologic score, clinical data and mortality in 48 patients with COCM.

	Morphologic score	Mean score	Age (mean)	Duration of illness	Mortality
Group I n = 22	≤4	2.8 ±1.0	39.0y. ± 9.8	4.1y. ±3.8	27% (n = 6)
Group II n = 26	≥5	6.3 ±1.2	42.3y. ± 8.8	3.0y. ±3.0	65% (n = 17)

	Morphologic score	H-T ratio	EF	EDVI
Group I n = 22	≤4	0.574 ±0.063	38.8% ±12.7	141 ± 35.4 ml/m²
Group II n = 26	≥5	0.595 ±0.05	36.3% ±17	198 ± 74.7 ml/m²

with a duration of illness ≤2 years are shown in Table 3. Mean duration of illness was somewhat lower in those patients with ≥5 points. The follow-up period was identical in both groups of patients, whereas the mean survival period was only 0.8 ±0.6 years in those with ≥5 points, and 1.8 ±1.0 years in those with ≤4 points. The differences in cardiothoracic ratio, EDVI, and EF did not reach statistical significance though there were similar trends as shown in Table 2.

Table 3. Clinical data and mortality in 24 patients with COCM and a duration of illness prior to biopsy less than 2 years.

Morphologic score	≤4 points	≥5 points
No. of patients	12	12
Age	37.8 ±10.7	42.9 ± 9.6yr
Duration of illness	1.3 ± 0.7	0.9 ± 0.7yr
Cardiothoracic ratio	0.565 ± 0.05	0.602 ± 0.06
EF	41.4 ± 6.1	35.3 ±18.3%
EDVI	136.2 ±31.6	194.1 ±80.6 ml/m²
Follow-up period	2.1 ± 0.9	2.0 ± 1.5yr
Survival period	1.8 ± 1.0	0.8 ± 0.6yr
Two-years cumulative mortality rate	7.3%	100%

Discussion

Recently, endomyocardial biopsy has been introduced for morphologic studies in patients with COCM. It has proved to be a relatively safe procedure (see Ch. 4). In patients with COCM, light and electron-microscopic studies did not reveal any specific findings in biopsy specimens thus obtained [11, 12, 20, 21, 32, 35, 44–46, 51, 52, 55, 59]. Hypertrophy, interstitial fibrosis, myofibrillar changes such as

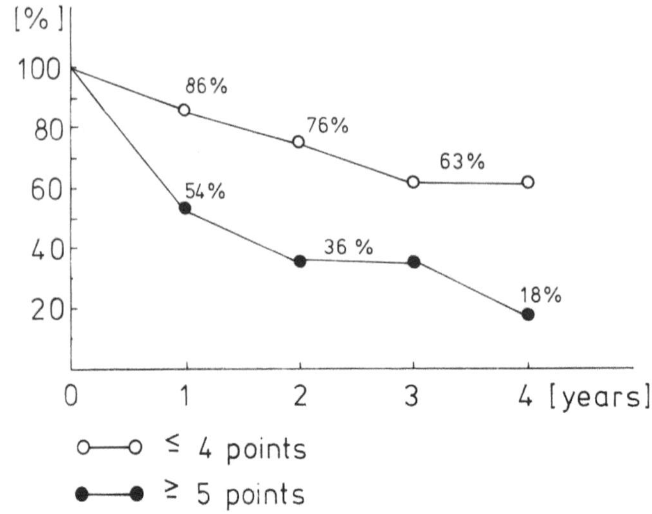

Fig. 4. Cumulative survival rate in 48 patients with COCM from the date of biopsy according to the morphologic score

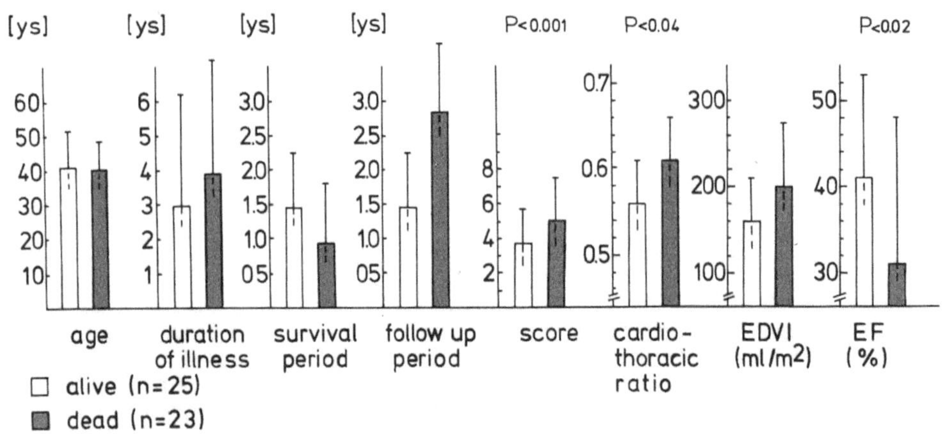

Fig. 5. Clinical and hemodynamic data and morphologic score in 48 patients with COCM. Patients alive (n = 25) indicated by *light columns*; patients dead (n = 23) indicated by *dark columns*. Mean ± standard deviation

disarray, Z-band anomalies, alterations of mitochondria, and degenerative changes were frequent findings.

COCM has a poor prognosis with a high mortality in the years following the clinical manifestation [1, 6, 14, 15, 18, 34]. The exact definition of the onset of the disease is difficult, as even patients with a depressed EF and enlarged heart on X-ray may be asymptomatic for long periods [6, 10, 32]. With these reservations in mind, our data confirmed the poor prognosis of patients with COCM from the onset of illness (Fig. 1). The speed with which the disease progresses may vary

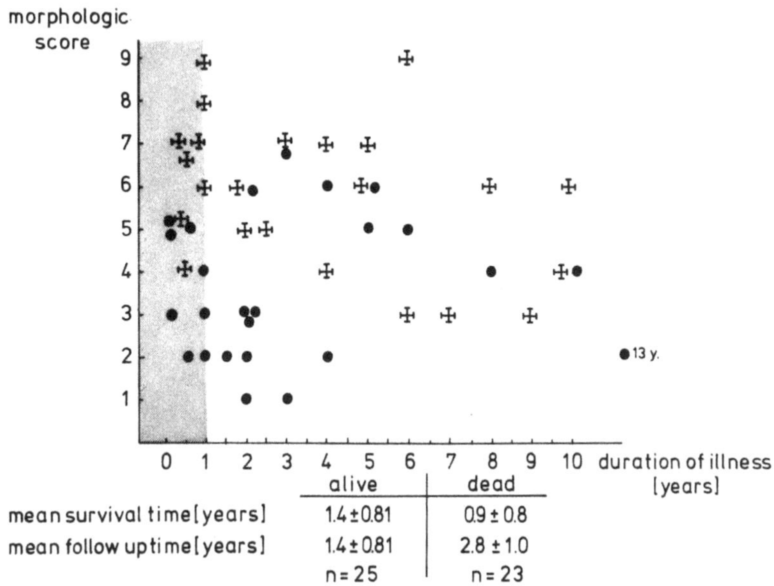

Fig. 6. A plot of the morphologic score vs. the duration of illness prior to biopsy in 48 patients with COCM. Patients alive indicated by *dark points;* patients dead indicated by *crosses*

considerably among a group of patients [1,6,14,15,17]. Hemodynamic and angiographic data have been used to predict the prognosis [1,6,9,10,29,32,43]. However, no single parameter has proved to be a reliable predictor of the course in the individual patient. In order to get more information on the prognosis in COCM, our study was undertaken to evaluate the prognostic significance of endomyocardial biopsy and to compare the results to clinical data. Except for one recent study [59], no similar study has been performed in a group of patients with COCM in whom the diagnosis has been made on the basis of presently accepted criteria. Biopsy specimens were studied by means of electron microscopy using a semiquantitative morphologic score that has been reported in a preliminary study [3,29]. In order to the minimize the subjective elements involved in use of a semiquantitative morphologic score, morphologic evaluation was done without the morphologist's knowing the patient or his final outcome.

In our study we were able to show that alterations of the myocardium were closely linked to the fate of the individual patient. Patients were divided into one group with ≤ 4 points (group I) and a second group with ≥ 5 points (group II). This delineation of the two groups had been done arbitrarily in our preliminary study [3,29]. The cumulative survival rates were significantly different between both groups, the survival rate after 4 years being 63% in group I and 18% in group II. Hypertrophy, interstitial fibrosis, and myofibrillar changes were frequent findings in both groups, and thus not of great importance for the outcome of the case. However, degenerative changes and mitochondrial abnormalities were found nearly exclusively in group II thus heralding a poor prognosis. Our data on the prognostic significance of morphologic changes were recently con-

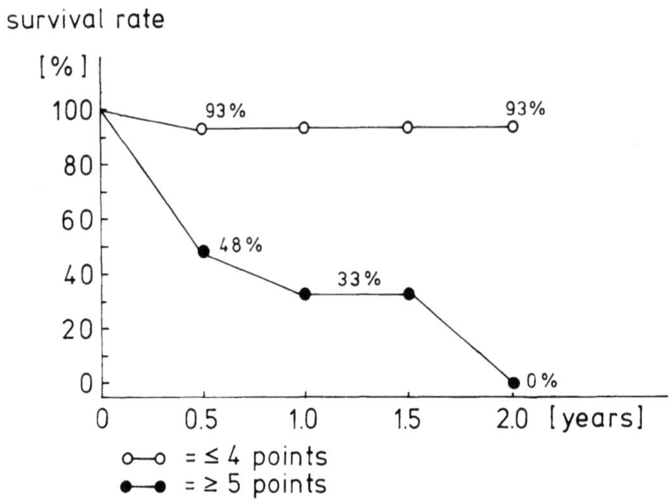

Fig. 7. Cumulative survival rate in 24 patients with COCM and a short duration of illness prior to biopsy (≤2 years). Patients were grouped according to the morphologic score

firmed by Bouhour *et al.* [59] who applied the morphologic score proposed earlier [3, 29]. In their group I (i.e. patients with ≤4 points) 3 out of 18 patients died, whereas in group II (≥5 points) there were 8 deaths in 20 patients.

In the two subsets of patients in our study who were grouped according to the morphologic score, other parameters were not significantly different, though cardiothoracic ratio and EDVI tended to be greater, and EF to be smaller in group II. However, grouping the patients in a different way (dead or alive) gives some prognostic significance to hemodynamic parameters (Fig. 5). These patients are still significantly different with respect to their morphologic score, but cardiothoracic ratio and EF were also significantly different. This was not the case with regard to EDVI though the mean value in patients still alive was lower than in deceased patients. EDVs over $2\frac{1}{4}$ times the maximum normal or EF less than 10% have been found to be of ominous significance [6, 10, 17, 23, 43]. In our study there was a great overlap of data which makes prognosis of the individual patient difficult. Generally speaking, a low EF, an elevated EDPI and EDVI are the surest hemodynamic and angiographic predictors of a poor prognosis.

The lower significance of hemodynamic data for seperating patients with different prognosis may be related to the variability of these parameters. They depend on the state of the patient, the degree of recompensation and the medication such as diuretics. Furthermore, it should be considered that in some patients the clinical course may show periods of remission [32, 34, 57]. Morphologic alterations are not subject to short-term changes except for swelling and vacuolation of mitochondria during hypoxia or after toxic actions, changes that were not seen in our study.

A patient with a short duration of illness presents a special problem. In these cases it seems most important to predict whether the patient will recover or whether his disease will progress. In a case with a short duration of illness a seronegative myocarditis cannot be excluded with certainty. Our data in patients with a duration of illness ≤ 2 years have provided new insight into the prognosis of these patients. By use of our semiquantitative morphologic score we were able to make a clear separation between those with a good prognosis (≤ 4 points; 2-year cumulative survival rate 92%) and those with a very poor prognosis (≥ 5 points; 1-year cumulative survival rate 33%, 2-year survival rate 0%). The duration of illness before biopsy was practically identical in both groups (Table 3). Hemodynamics of these two groups were different though they did not make a similarly distinct separation between both groups possible.

The greater prognostic ability of the morphologic score compared to hemodynamic data does not mean that the latter are of no significance. As a whole, there was a clear tendency of patients with a higher score to have poorer hemodynamics. However, as already discussed, hemodynamics may be more variable and subject to therapeutic intervention. It has been shown that other clinical findings are also related to the prognosis of the patient. A progressive increase in QRS duration with transition to LBBB and a leftward shift of the mean frontal plane vector to the left occurs with progression of the disease [6, 28, 30].

The question is whether the differences in the extent and kind of ultrastructural changes as observed in patients with poor or good prognosis represent different nosologic entities, or whether they merely represent different speeds of progression of the same disease which proceeds slowly in one patient, very rapidly in another. It might furthermore be suggested that these differences in prognosis are due to a different duration of illness. Hence, one would expect a patient with a long duration of illness to have more advanced alterations and a poorer prognosis. This was not the case as is shown by the fact that the mean duration of illness was not significantly different between group I and group II patients (Table 2).

From ultrastructural studies on experimental myocardial hypertrophy, it is well known that hypertrophy proceeds through different stages [38, 40]. In early stages acute adaptation to a severe stress is manifested by mitochondrial swelling, increase of the rough endoplasmatic reticulum and formation of new filaments [2, 47]. With further progression and adaptation, these changes may reverse. Later stages leading to myocardial failure are characterized by a decrease of the mitochondrial/myofibrillar ratio, irregularities of myofibrillar structure and the occurrence of degenerative changes [2, 37, 38, 40, 42, 47, 48, 58].

Similar observations on the relationship between the duration of myocardial overloading and the kind and extent of ultrastructural changes have also been reported in man. In patients with congenital heart disease associated with right ventricular outflow tract obstruction, changes directly related to hypertrophy, abnormalities of cellular or myofibrillar orientation, interstitial fibrosis, and degenerative changes were observed [19]. Degenerative changes correlated with increased age and elevated RVEDP. Patients without any obstruction to right ventricular outflow showed hypertrophy, but not cellular or myofibrillar disorientation or degeneration. This suggests that the occurrence of the latter changes is related to the degree and duration of myocardial overload. In a similar way, our findings suggest that hypertrophy, interstitial fibrosis, and myofibrillar disorientation represent early changes in the course of COCM, whereas the occurrence of mitochondrial abnormalities and degenerative changes herald a more advanced stage of the disease. Therefore, these changes are considered to be of greatest prognostic significance if the criteria of COCM are present. The latter is important as patients with normal angiographic findings and LBBB may also demonstrate some degenerative changes (see Ch. 26).

The cause of death in patients with COCM is attributed to heart failure in the majority of cases. In some cases, thromboembolic complications or arrhythmias are the event ultimately leading to death [1, 6, 14, 15, 17, 32]. Most of our cases died of progressive heart failure, but autopsies were performed in only a few cases since most patients died outside our hospital. In some cases embolic complications were suspected though these patients had also shown previous periods of heart failure. Anticoagulant therapy was advised in most patients, but it was discontinued in some cases by the house physician. Proof that therapeutic interventions are able to improve the long-term prognosis in these patients is merited. Long-term beneficial effect of neither digitalis nor of anticoagulation has been shown [16]. Prolonged bed rest has been advocated for some patients [4], but this also deserves the final proof before it is used as a common therapeutic tool, especially since special problems, such as thromboembolic complications, arise [4].

Concluding, endomyocardial biopsy from the right ventricle has proved to be of great significance for the prognostic evaluation of patients with COCM. Myocardial alterations do not represent specific findings, but they are closely related to the stage of myocardial hypertrophy and insufficiency. The different findings and courses of patients with COCM may indicate either different etiologies or different types of progression of the disease.

References

1. Blömer, H., Delius, W.: Prognostische Beurteilung von Patienten mit primärer Kardiomyopathie. Internist *16*, 548 (1975)
2. Bózner, A., Meessen, H.: Die Feinstruktur des Herzmuskels der Ratte nach einmaligem und nach wiederholtem Schwimmtraining. Virchows Arch. Abt. B *3*, 248 (1969)
3. Breithardt, G., Knieriem, H.-J., Kuhn, H., Loogen, F., Gleichmann, U.: Comparison of clinical data and ultrastructural findings in myocardial biopsy of patients with cardiomyopathies. In: Kölbel, F.: Adaptability of Cardiac Muscle, Symposium of the European Section of the International Study Group for Research in Cardiac Metabolism. Prague 1974 (in press)
4. Burch, G.E., Walsh, J.J., Black, W.C.: Value of prolonged bed rest in management of cardiomegaly. J. amer. med. Ass. *183*, 81 (1963)
5. Cutter, S.J., Ederer, T.: Maximum utilization of the life-table method in analyzing survival. J. Chronic. Dis. *8*, 699 (1958)
6. Delius, W., Sebening, H., Weghmann, N., Oversohl, K., Wirtzfeld, A., Mathes, P.: Klinik und Verlauf der kongestiven Kardiomyopathie ungeklärter Ätiologie. Dtsch. med. Wschr. *101*, 633 (1976)
7. Demakis, J.G., Rahimtoola, S.H., Sutton, G.C., Jamil, M., Proskey, A., Rosen, K.M., Gunnar, R.M.: The clinical course of cardiomyopathy associated with alcoholism. Amer. J. Cardiol. *29*, 259 (1972)
8. Dodge, H.T., Sandler, H., Baxley, W.A., Hawley, R.R.: Usefulness and limitation of radiographic methods for determining left ventricular volume. Amer. J. Cardiol. *18*, 10 (1966)

9. Dye, C.L., Genovese, P.D., Daly, W.J., Behnke, R.H.: Primary myocardial disease. Part II: Hemodynamic alterations. Ann. int. Med. *58*, 442 (1963)
10. Feild, B.J., Baxley, W.A., Russel, R.O., Hood, W.P., Holt, J.H., Dowling, J.T., Racklex, C.E.: Left ventricular function and hypertrophy in cardiomyopathy with depressed ejection fraction. Circulation *47*, 1022 (1973)
11. Ferrans, V.J., Morrow, A.G., Roberts, W.C.: Myocardial ultrastructure in idiopathic hypertrophic subaortic stenosis. Circulation *45*, 769 (1972)
12. Ferrans, V.J., Massumi, R.A., Shugoll, E.J., Ali, N., Roberts, W.C.: Ultrastructural studies of myocardial biopsies in 45 patients with obstructive or congestive cardiomyopathy. In: Cardiomyopathies. Bajusz, E., Rona, G. (eds.). Munich: Urban & Schwarzenberg 1974, p. 231
13. Fowler, N.O., Gueron, M.: Primary myocardial disease. Circul. *32*, 830 (1965)
14. Goodwin, J.F.: Congestive and hypertrophic cardiomyopathies. A decade of study. Lancet *1970/I*, 731
15. Goodwin, J.F., Oakley, C.M.: The cardiomyopathies. Brit. Heart J. *34*, 545 (1972)
16. Goodwin, J.F.: Treatment of the cardiomyopathies. Amer. J. Cardiol. *32*, 341 (1973)
17. Goodwin, J.F.: Prospects and predictions for the cardiomyopathies. Circulation *50*, 210 (1974)
18. Hamby, R.I., Catangay, P., Apiado, O., Khan, A.H.: Primary myocardial disease. Clinical, hemodynamic and angiocardiographic correlates in fifty patients. Amer. J. Cardiol. *25*, 625 (1970)
19. Jones, M., Ferrans, V.J., Morrow, A.G., Roberts, W.C.: Ultrastructure of crista supraventricularis muscle in patients with congenital heart diseases associated with right ventricular outflow tract obstruction. Circulation *51*, 39 (1975)
20. Knieriem, H.-J., Kuhn, H., Breithardt, G.: Zur Diagnostic der primären Kardiomyopathien mit Hilfe der Myokardbiopsie. Z. Kardiol., Suppl. *2*, 26 (1975)
21. Knieriem, H.-J., Kuhn, H., Breithardt, G.: Morphologische Befunde bei Myokard-Biopsien. Verh. dtsch. Ges. Path. *59*, 470 (1975)
22. Konno, S., Sakakibara, S.: Endomyocardial biopsy. Dis. Chest *50*, 345 (1963)
23. Kreulen, T.H., Gorlin, R., Herman, M.V.: Ventriculographic patterns and hemodynamics in primary myocardial disease. Circulation *47*, 299 (1973)
24. Kübler, W., Kuhn, H., Loogen, F.: Zur klinischen Einteilung der Kardiomyopathien. Dtsch. med. Wschr. *97*, 1834 (1972)
25. Kübler, W., Kuhn, H., Loogen, F.: Die Kardiomyopathien. Ihre Einteilung nach ätiologischen und klinischen Gesichtspunkten. Z. Kardiol. *62*, 3 (1973)
26. Kübler, W., Gleichmann, U., Loogen, F., Lück, J.: Natural history of idiopathic nonobstructive cardiomyopathy. In: Recent Advances in Studies on Cardiac Structure and Metabolism, Vol. 2, Cardiomyopathies. Bajusz, E., Rona, G. (eds.). Munich-Berlin-Vienna: Urban & Schwarzenberg 1974
27. Kuhn, H., Kübler, W., Loogen, F., Gleichmann, U.: Die congestive Cardiomyopathie. Med. Welt *24*, 996 (1973)
28. Kuhn, H., Breithardt, L.-K., Breithardt, G., Seipel, L., Loogen, F.: Die Bedeutung des Elektrokardiogramms für Diagnose und Verlaufsbeurteilung von Patienten mit congestiver Cardiomyopathie. Z. Kardiol. *63*, 916 (1974)
29. Kuhn, H., Knieriem, H.-J., Loogen, F., Both, A., Schmidt, W.A.K., Stroobandt, R., Gleichmann, U.: Die Bedeutung der endomyokardialen Katheterbiopsie für die Diagnostik und die Beurteilung der Prognose der kongestiven Kardiomyopathie. Dtsch. med. Wschr. *100*, 717 (1975)
30. Kuhn, H., Breithardt, G., Knieriem, H.-J., Seipel, L., Loogen, F., Both, A., Stroobandt, R.: Die Bedeutung des Elektrokardiogramms und der endomyokardialen Katheterbiopsie für Diagnose und Verlaufsbeobachtung der congestiven Cardiomyopathie. Verh. dtsch. Ges. inn. Med. *81*, 211 (1975)
31. Kuhn, H., Breithardt, G., Knieriem, H.-J., Seipel, L., Loogen, F.: Linksschenkelblock bei kongestiver Kardiomyopathie. Z. Kardiol., Suppl. *2*, 30 (1975)
32. Kuhn, H.: Die congestive Cardiomyopathie. Klinische und experimentelle Untersuchungen. Habilitationsschrift, Düsseldorf 1975
33. Loogen, F., Kuhn, H.: Kardiomyopathien ungeklärter Ätiologie (sog. primäre Kardiomyopathien). Internist *16*, 540 (1975)
34. Loogen, F., Kuhn, H.: Classification and natural history of primary cardiomyopathies. In: Myocardial failure. Eds. G. Riecker, A. Weber, J. Goodwin. Berlin-New York-Heidelberg: Springer 1977, p. 232

35. Maron, B.J., Ferrans, V.J., Henry, W.L., Clark, C.E., Redwood, D.R., Roberts, W.C., Morrow, A.G., Epstein, S.E.: Differences in distribution of myocardial abnormalities in patients with obstructive and nonobstructive asymmetric hypertrophy (ASH): light and electron microscopic findings. Circulation *50*, 436 (1974)
36. Maron, B.J., Ferrans, V.J., Roberts, W.C.: Myocardial ultrastructure in patients with chronic aortic valve disease. Amer. J. Cardiol. *35*, 725 (1975)
37. Meerson, F.Z., Zaletayeva, T.A., Lagutschev, S.S., Pshennikova, M.G.: Structure and mass of mitochondria in the process of compensatory hyperfunction and hypertrophy of the heart. Exp. Cell. Res. *36*, 578 (1964)
38. Meerson, F.Z.: The myocardium in hyperfunction, hypertrophy and heart failure. Circulation Res. Suppl. *25*, suppl. 2, 25 (1969)
39. Merrel, M., Schulman, L.E.: Determination of prognosis in chronic disease, illustrated by systemic lupus erythematodes. J. chron. Dis. *1*, 12 (1955)
40. Meessen, H.: Structural bases of myocardial hypertrophy. Brit. Heart J. suppl. ad *33*, 94 (1971)
41. Muehsam, G.E., Pschibul, F., Scerbo, J.E.: The natural history of idiopathic cardiomegaly. Amer. Heart J. *67*, 13 (1964)
42. Novi, A.M.: Beitrag zur Feinstruktur des Herzmuskels bei experimenteller Herzhypertrophie. Beitr. path. Anat. *137*, 19 (1968)
43. Oakley, C.: Ventricular hypertrophy in cardiomyopathy. Brit. Heart J. suppl. ad *33*, 179 (1971)
44. Olsen, E.G.J.: Diagnostic value of the endomyocardial bioptome. Lancet *1974/I*, 658
45. Olsen, E.G.J.: Results of endomyocardial biopsy. Histological, histochemical and ultrastructural analysis. Postgrad. med. J. *51*, 295 (1975)
46. Olsen, E.G.J.: Pathologie der „primären" Kardiomyopathien. Münch. med. Wschr. *118*, 735 (1976)
47. Onishi, S., Büchner, F., Zittel, R., Thermann, M.: Das elektronenmikroskopische Bild der Herzmuskelzelle des Hundes bei experimenteller Herzhypertrophie in der Anpassungsphase. Beitr. path. Anat. *139*, 94 (1969)
48. Poche, R., De Mello Mattos, C.M., Rembarz, H.W., Stoepel, K.: Über das Verhältnis Mitochondrien : Myofibrillen in den Herzmuskeln der Ratte bei Druckhypertrophie des Herzens. Virchows Arch. path. Anat. *344*, 100 (1968)
49. Rahimtoola, S.H., Demakis, J.G., Tobin, Jr., J.R., Gunnar, R.M.: The natural course of alcoholic cardiomyopathy. Ann. intern. Med. *80*, 293 (1974)
50. Richardson, P.J.: King's endomyocardial bioptome. Lancet *1974/I*, 660
51. Roberts, W.C., Ferrans, V.J., Buja, L.M., Ali, N.: Pathology of the dilated ventricular type of idiopathic cardiomyopathy: a gross, light microscopic and electronmicroscopic study. Circulation *48*, Suppl. IV, 207 (1973)
52. Roberts, W.C., Ferrans, V.J.: Pathological aspects of certain cardiomyopathies. Circulation Res. *34*, Suppl. II, 128 (1974)
53. Sakakibara, S., Konno, S.: Endomyocardial biopsy. Jap. Heart J. *3*, 537 (1962)
54. Sandler, H., Dodge, H.T.: The use of single plane angiocardiograms for the calculation of left ventricular volume in man. Amer. Heart J. *75*, 325 (1968)
55. Sekiguchi, M.: Electron microscopical observations of the myocardium in patients with idiopathic cardiomyopathy using endomyocardial biopsy. J. Mol. Cell Cardiol. *6*, 111 (1974)
56. Shugoll, G.I., Moore, J.P., Lenkin, M.L.: Follow-up observations and prognosis in primary myocardial disease. Arch. intern. Med. *129*, 67 (1972)
57. Stapleton, J.F., Segal, J.P., Harvey, W.P.: The electrocardiogram of myocardiopathy. Progr. Cardiovasc. Dis. *13*, 217 (1970)
58. Wollenberger, A., Schulze, W.: Über das Volumenverhältnis von Mitochondrien zu Myofibrillen im chronisch überlasteten, hypertrophischen Herzen. Naturwissenschaften *49*, 161 (1962)
59. Bouhour, J.B., Petitier, H., De Lajartre, A.Y., Almaza, M., Nicolas, G., Hoerau, J.: La biopsie myocardique dans les myocardiopathies congestives en apparence primitives. Arch. Mal. Cœur *69*, 485 (1976)

23. Correlations Between Clinical and Morphologic Findings and Natural History in Congestive Cardiomyopathy

B. KUNKEL, H. LAPP, G. KOBER, and M. KALTENBACH

Light- and electron-microscopic examinations of myocardial biopsies do not reveal pathognomic changes in COCM [1,2,4,5]. However, the morphologic changes differ markedly in severity and quantity. Therefore, this study was designed to demonstrate the course of disease and possible correlations between clinical stage and morphologic findings.

Material and Methods

Both myocardial hypertrophy and collagenous fiber content were calculated in biopsy specimen as described previously (Ch. 7). The results obtained were correlated with the stage of disease as classified by the NYHA (Fig. 2).

In order to compare electron-microscopic findings with clinical data a score-system was devised that allowed a semiquantitative analysis of electron-microscopic changes (Fig. 1). The score included nuclear, myofibrillar, and various mitochondrial alterations, as well as changes in structure and quantity of the sarcoplasmic reticulum, Golgi system and rough-surfaced endoplasmic reticulum, lipid-droplets, lysosomes, and interstitial changes. According to the estimated extent of changes due to hypertrophy, cellular degeneration, or interstitial fibrosis, all facts were included and scored with 1–4 points. Thus, the various electron-microscopic findings in myocardial biopsies could be summarized easily and could be compared to clinical data.

The results of these semiquantitative ultrastructural evaluations were correlated with the clinical stage of disease and the ejection fractions (Figs. 3 and 4). Patients were followed up over a 1–3 years period to establish the natural history of the disease. These results were compared with the morphologic data.

Results

The morphologically measured fibrous tissue content of the biopsy specimen was correlated to the stages of disease, as classified by the NYHA (Fig. 1). All clinical stages of disease involved an interstitial fibrosis of the myocardium. The mean amount of fibrous tissue increased with the severity of clinical symptoms. In stage I it amounts to 5.8%, in stage II to 7.7%, in stage III to 14.9%, and to 30% in patients of stage IV. A pronounced increase in fibrous tissue was found between clinical stages II and III and also between stages III and IV.

Comparison between clinical stage and mean cardiac muscle cell diameter showed an enlargement of cardiac fiber size with increasing severity of disease

ELECTRON MICROSCOPICAL SCORE IN CONGESTIVE CARDIOMYOPATHY

	points 1 - 4		points 1 - 4
Nuclear changes		Golgi apparatus	
Myofibrils:		Glycogen content	
lysis		Lysosomes	
loss		Lipofuscin granules	
disarray		Lipid droplets	
new formation		Interstitial fibrosis	
Mitochondria		Interstitial cells	
increase		Lymphocytes	
loss		Histiocytes	
dwarfed forms		Fibrocytes	
degeneration		Others	
Myelin figures		Cellular edema	
T - System		Interstitial edema	
hypertrophy			
dilatation			
Sarcoplasmatic reticulum			
hypertrophy			
dilatation			

Fig. 1

(Fig. 2). The mean cardiac muscle cell diameter was 14.7 μ in stage I, 18.3 μ in stage II, 20.1 μ in stage III, and 22.0 μ in patients with clinical stage IV.

A detailed analysis of the four different groups revealed that out of 17 cases studied in group I, 5 had a mild fibrosis and 8 had a mild hypertrophy. One patient showed an advanced hypertrophy; 8 patients had no or minor pathologic findings. Out of 17 biopsies of group II, 14 showed an increase of cardiac muscle cell diameter which, in four cases, was considered marked. An interstitial fibrosis was seen in nine cases and was classified as severe in two of them. Three cases from this group did not exhibit cardiac hypertrophy or interstitial fibrosis.

Biopsies of 28 patients of stage III showed cardiac hypertrophy, except in one case. Seven patients had no interstitial fibrosis.

All patients (n = 4) of clinical stage IV had a severe cardiac hypertrophy. An interstitial fibrosis was absent only in one patient.

Comparison of clinical stages and electron-microscopic score revealed an increase of points with increasing severity of illness (Fig. 3). The mean number of points was 10.6 in stage I, 15.1 in stage II, 23.5 in stage III, and 29.6 in stage IV.

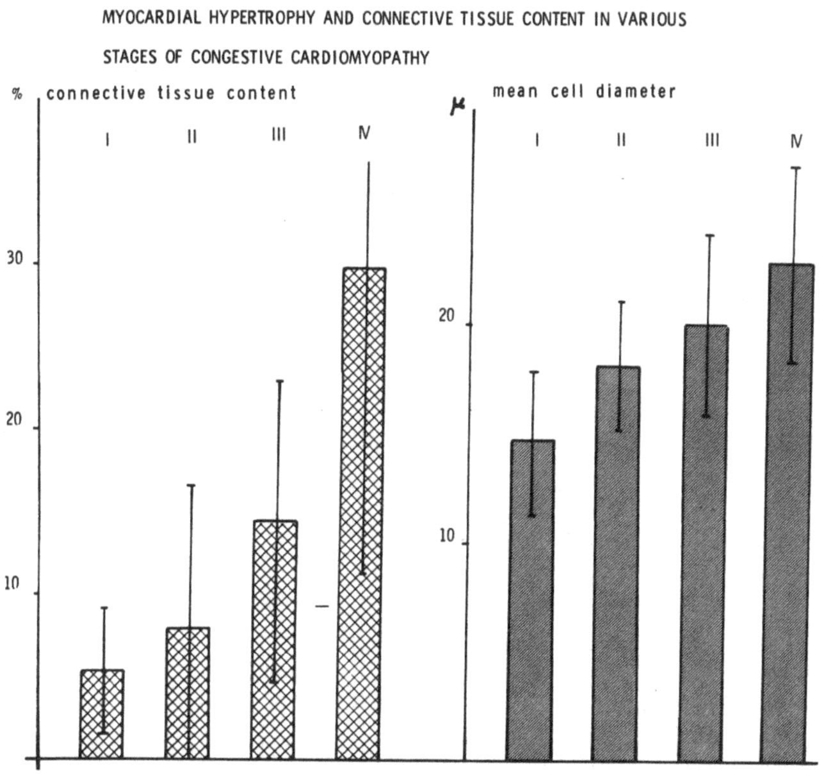

Fig. 2 Number of patients: I = 17; II = 17; III = 28; IV = 4

The score points counted in each group varied only minimally. Hence, morphologic and clinical findings correlated well.

Left ventricular ejection fraction in relation to the electron-microscopic score showed an increase in points with decreasing ventricular pump function (Fig. 4). Patients with normal or slightly decreased ejection fractions usually had minor pathologic changes. With decreasing left ventricular pump function massive ultrastructural changes due to hypertrophy or cellular degeneration occurred. In a few cases with early CM ultrastructural alterations of unusual degree were observed with a scoring much higher than could be anticipated according to mild clinical symptoms and data of heart catheterization. Generally, clinical impressions, hemodynamic, and light and semiquantitative electron-microscopic findings agree well. Some cases, however, present with severe myocardial alterations even in early stages of congestive cardiomyopathy. Figures 5 and 6 demonstrate characteristic clinical and morphologic findings in two patients with early and advanced congestive CM.

The natural history of the disease during a short 1–3 years/period of observation is shown in Figure 7. Of the patients with advanced congestive cardiomyopathy, 73% were unchanged after this time, whereas 27% of the patients had died. The patients in the last group exhibited extreme histologic and ultrastructural myocardial changes.

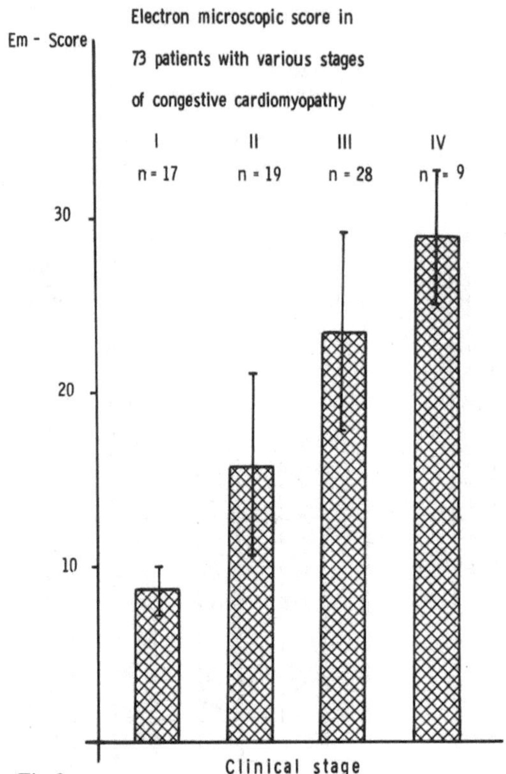
Em - Score
Electron microscopic score in
73 patients with various stages
of congestive cardiomyopathy
I
II
III
IV
n = 17
n = 19
n = 28
n = 9
30
20
10
Clinical stage

Fig. 3

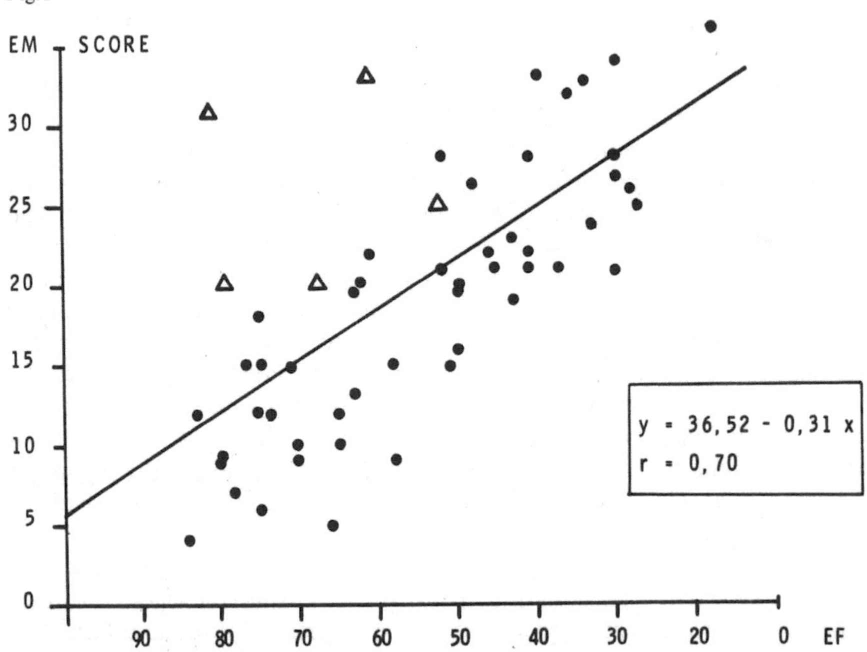
EM - SCORE
30
25
20
15
10
5
0
90
80
70
60
50
40
30
20
0
EF
y = 36,52 - 0,31 x
r = 0,70

Fig. 4

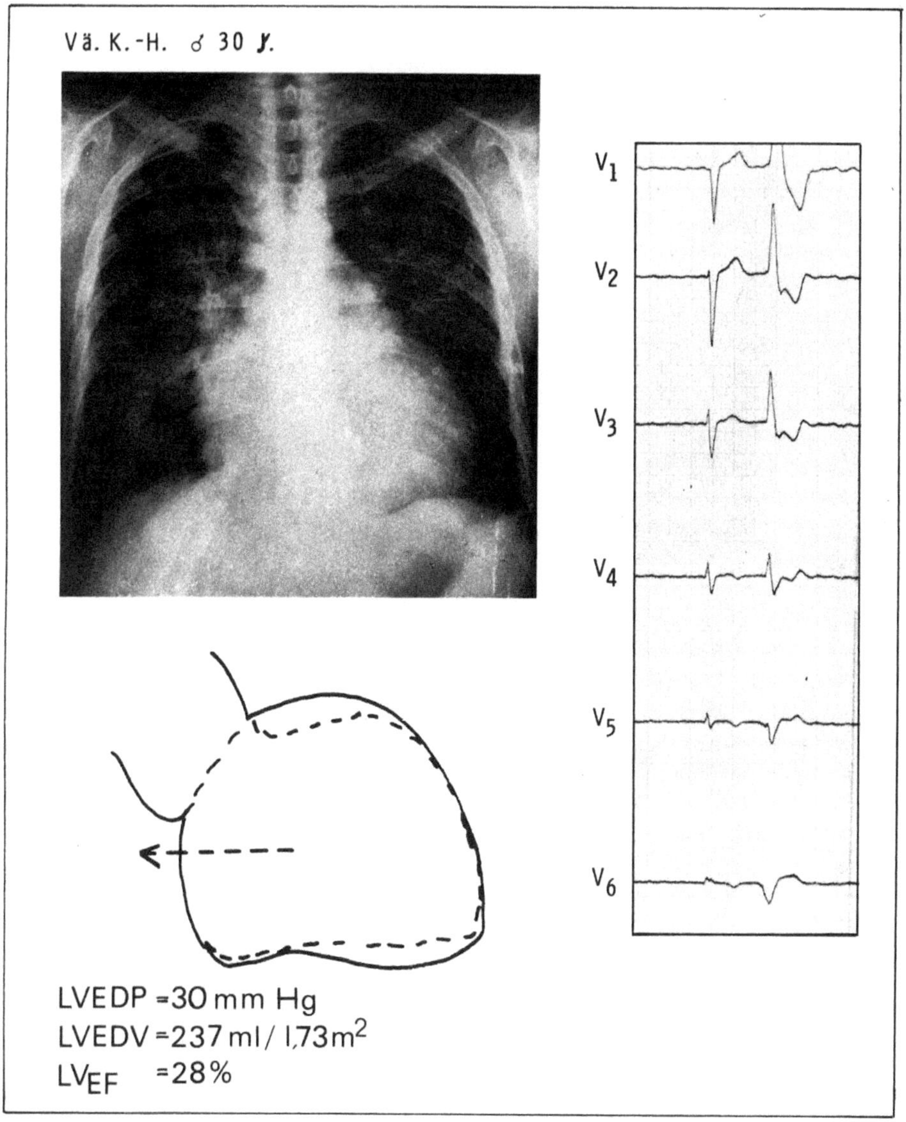

a

Fig. 5. Patient: Vä, male, 30y. (*a*) Clinical findings: Congestive heart failure for two years. X-Ray: severe cardiac enlargement. Pulmonary congestion. ECG: atrial fibrillation. Ventricular premature beats. Heart catheterization: Left ventricular enddiastolic pressure increased. Left ventricular end-diastolic volume markedly increased. Left ventricular ejection fraction markedly reduced. Course of disease: died 30 months after onset of symptoms. Myocardial biopsy: (*b*) Light microscopy: Severe cardiac hypertrophy and interstitial fibrosis (mean cardiac fiber size: 25 μ). (*c*) Electron microscopy: Late stage hypertrophy of cardiac muscle cells with loss of myofibrils and mitochondria. Mitochondrial degeneration

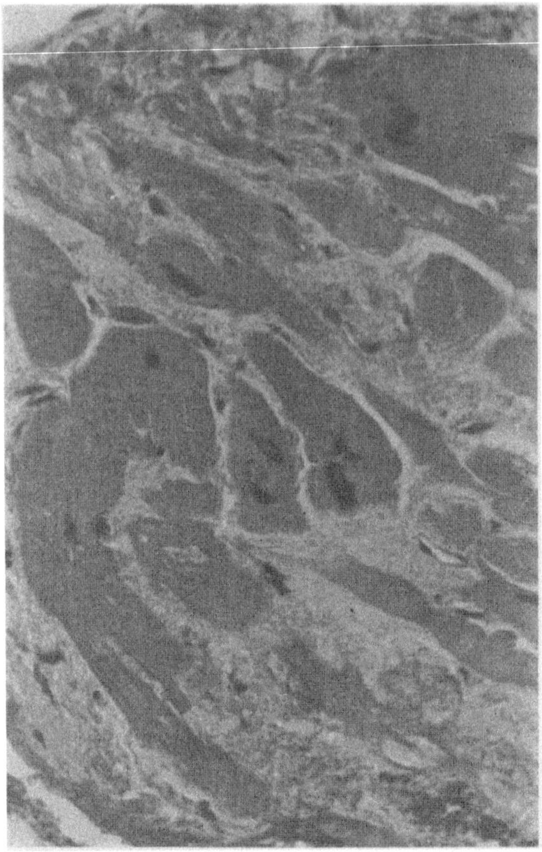

b

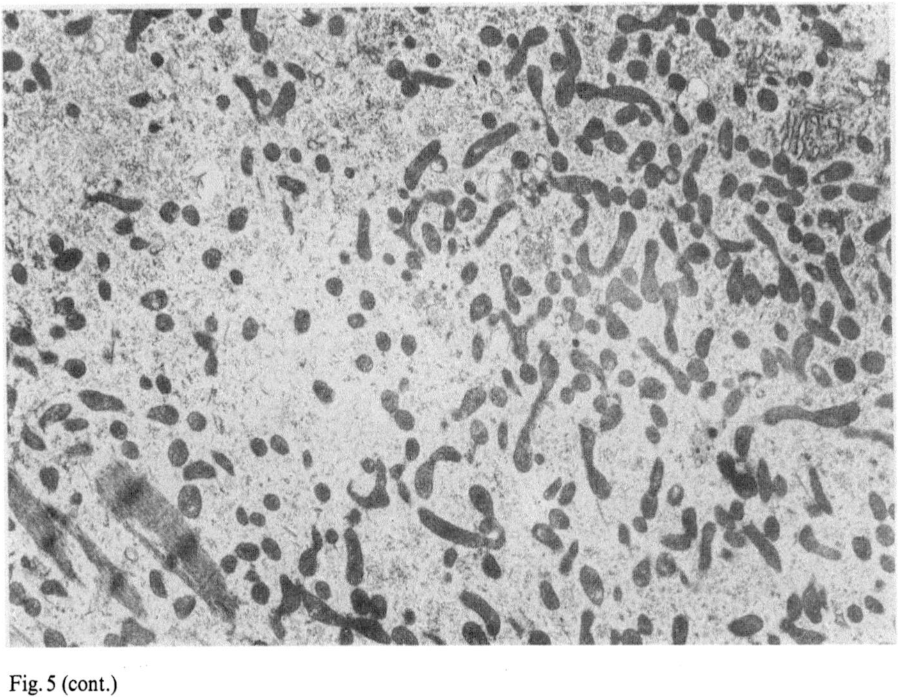

c

Fig. 5 (cont.)

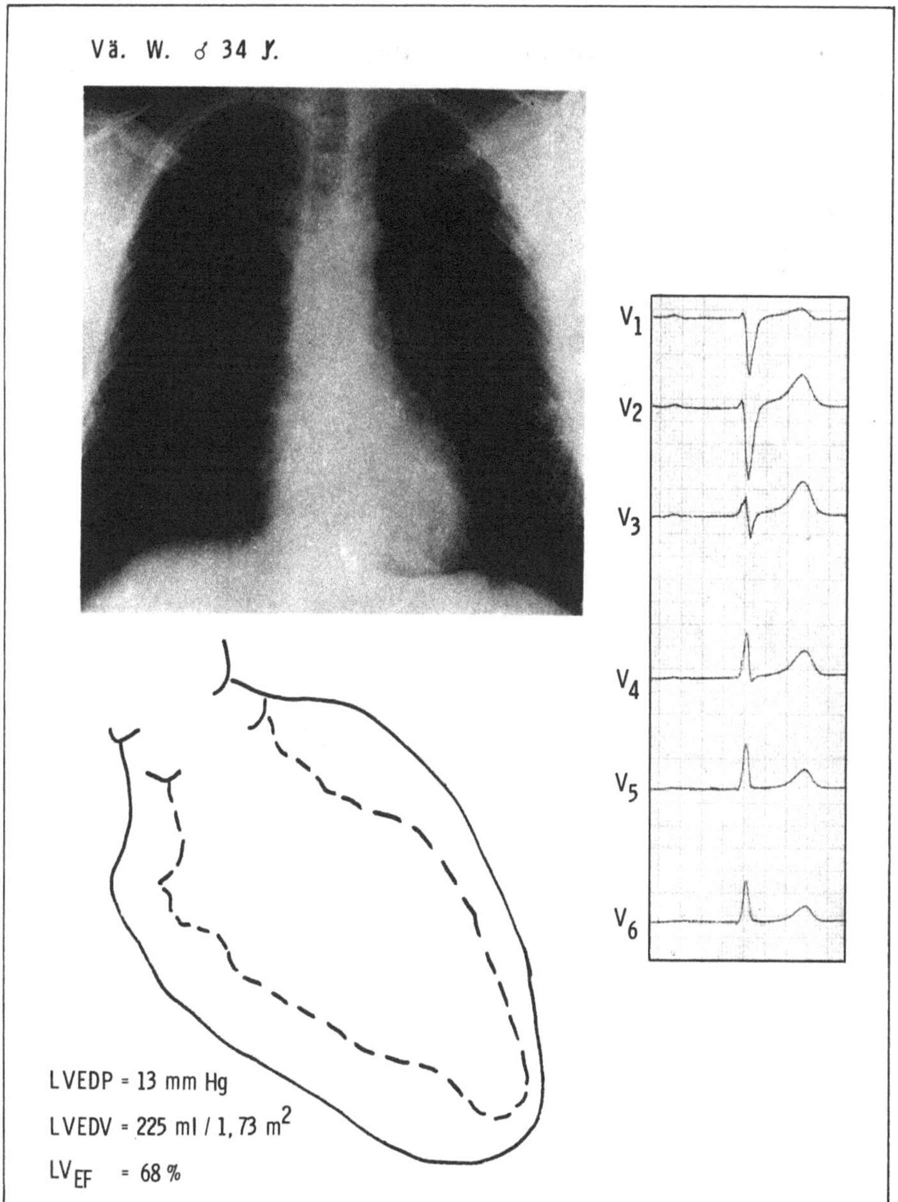

a

Fig. 6. Patient: Vä, W, male, 34y. (*a*) Clinical findings: no complaints. X-Ray: moderate cardiac enlargement. ECG: Av-block I. Sinusbradycardia. Heart catheterization: left ventricular enddiastolic pressure minimally increased. Left ventricular enddiastolic volume increased. Left ventricular ejection fraction within normal range. Course of disease: unchanged for 2 years. Myocardial biopsy: (*b*) Light microscopy: myocardial hypertrophy (mean fiber size 22.6 μ). (*c*) Electron microscopy: myocardial hypertrophy. Minor degenerative changes

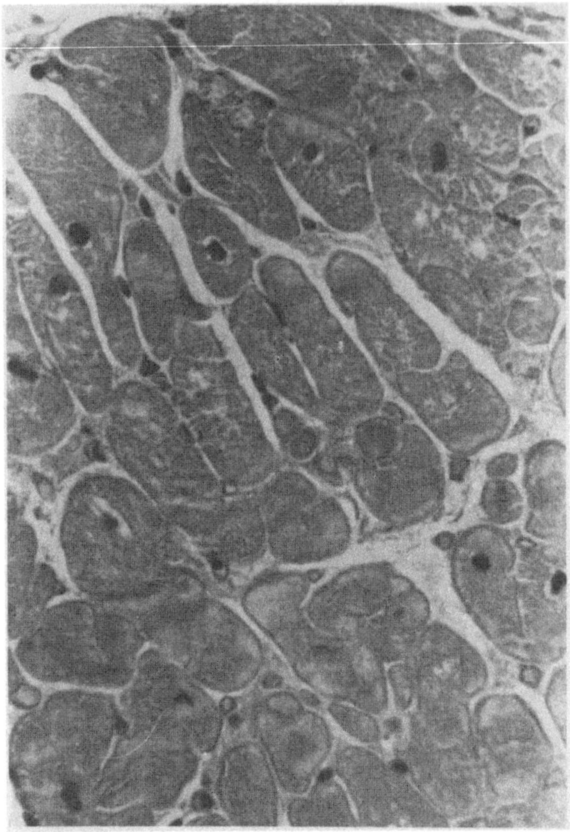

b

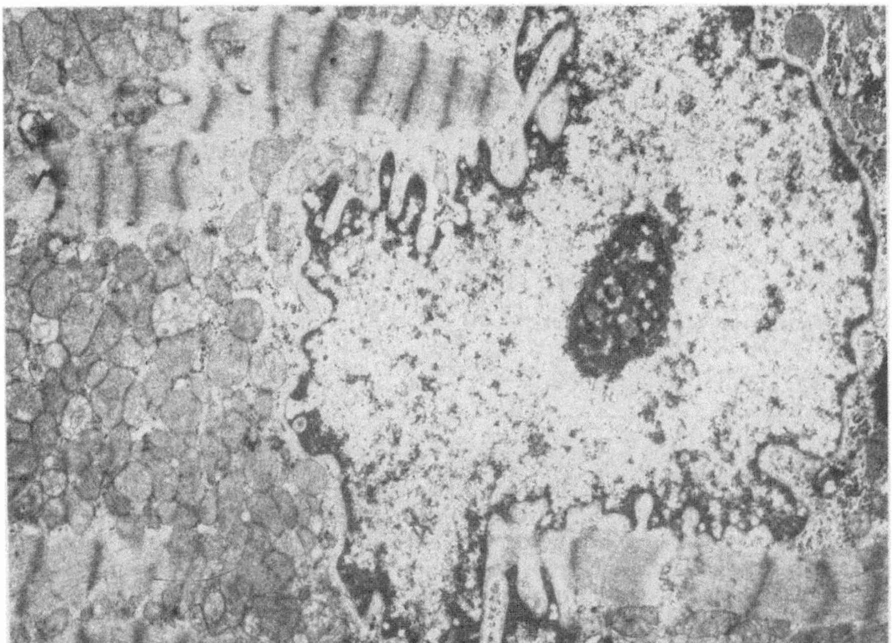

c

Fig. 6 (cont.)

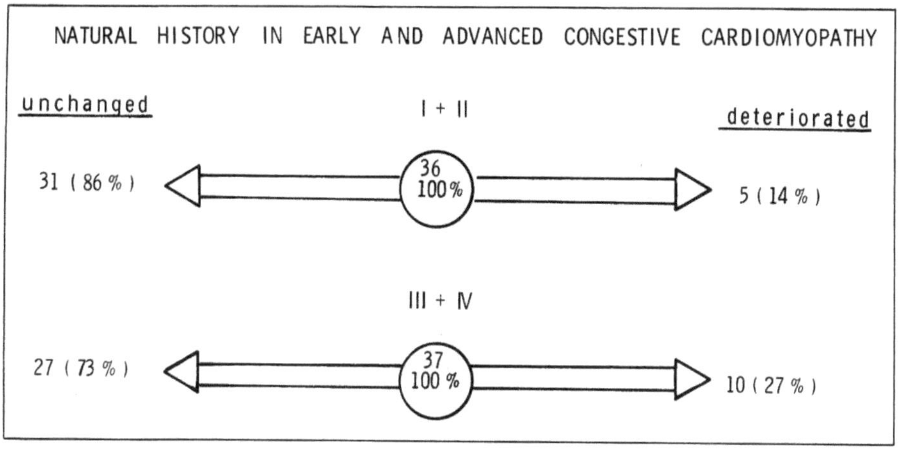

Fig. 7

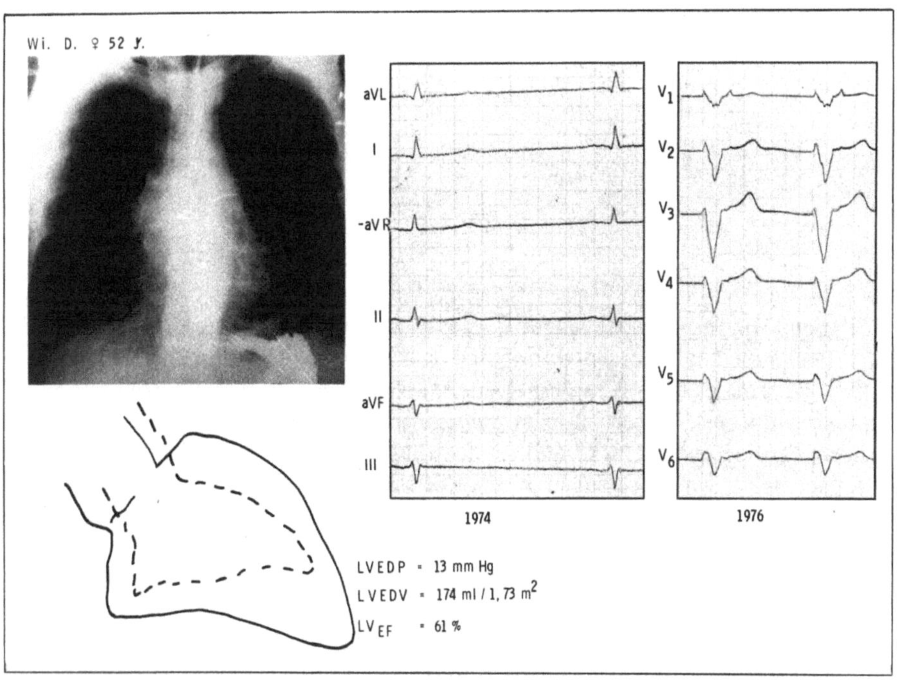

a

Fig. 8. Patient: Wi, female, 52 y. (*a*) Clinical findings: dizziness, chest pain. No signs of cardiac failure. X-Ray: moderate cardiac enlargement. ECG: Sinusbradycardia. SA-block. (1974) Heart catheterization: Left ventricular enddiastolic pressure: minimally increased. Left ventricular enddiastolic volume: minimaly increased. Ejection fraction: minimally decreased. Course of disease: cardiac failure after 2 years of observation. Pacemaker implantation, 1976. Myocardial biopsy: (*b*) Light microscopy: myocardial hypertrophy. Slight interstitial fibrosis (mean fiber size 27.5 μ). (*c*) Electron microscopy: severe myocardial hypertrophy with destruction of myofibrils and loss of mitochondria

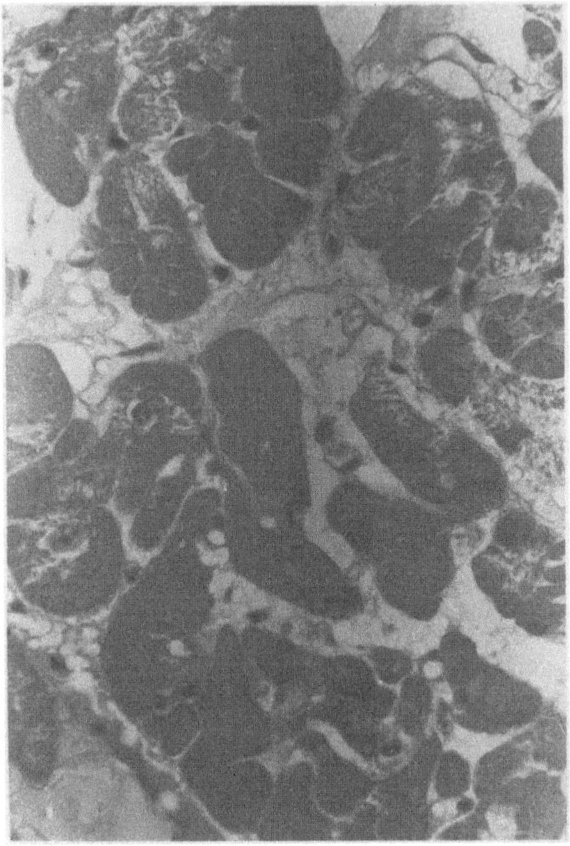

Fig. 8 b

Patients of the clinical stages I and II are of special interest. Of these 31 (86%) remained unchanged during the 1–3 years observation period, while 5 (14%)–2 females and 3 males, aged 23–52 years–developed progression of clinical symptoms. Three patients deteriorated in physical capacity, developed striking cardiac enlargement and myocardial failure. In one case, implantation of a pacemaker was necessary for relief of bradycardia.

The remaining two patients developed progressive cardiac enlargement and a decrease in cardiac efficiency. The ECG showed transition from temporary LBBB to permanent block in one case and aggravation of ventricular tachycardia in the other patient.

In all of these patients, left ventricular enddiastolic pressure and cardiac output at rest were normal. The ejection fractions were slightly decreased in two and were normal in three cases.

Light-microscopic examination revealed myocardial hypertrophy which was marked in three cases and mild in two. Electron microscopy showed signs of hypertrophy. Additionally all five patients exhibited marked degenerative changes. Three cases had destruction and loss of myofibrils and severe mitochondrial damage (Fig. 8). Two patients showed numerous myelin figures and

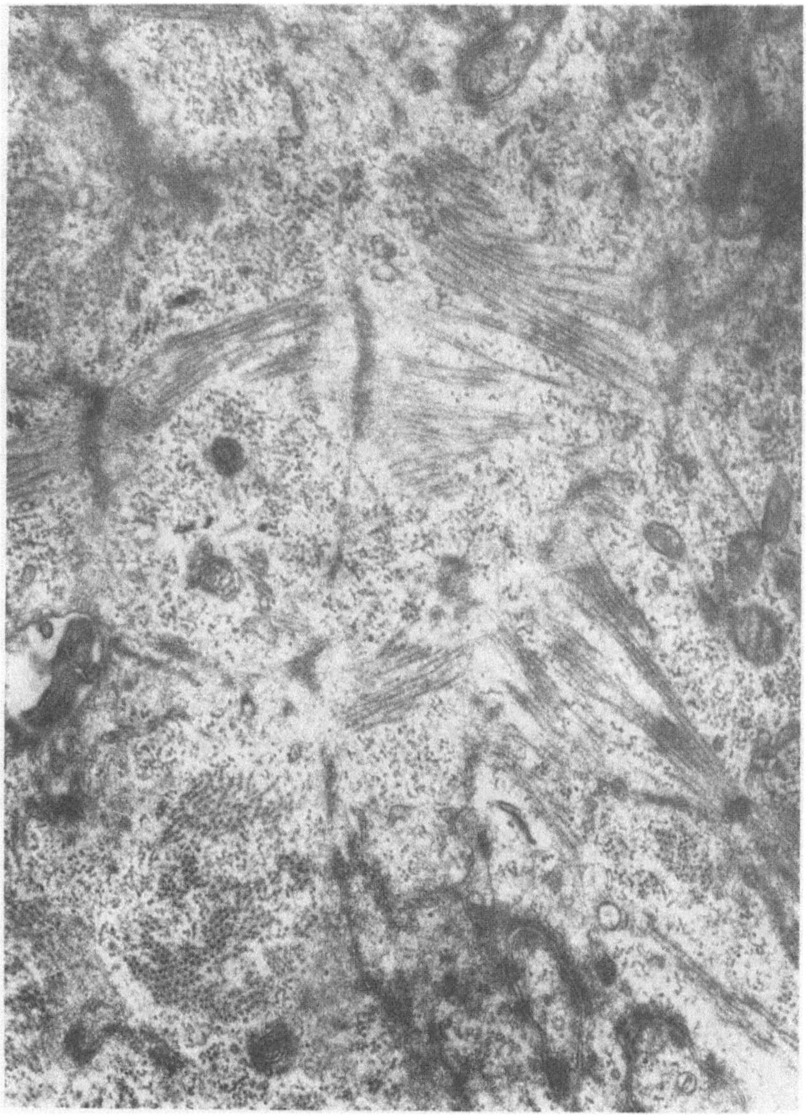

Fig. 8c

lipid droplets as well as dilatation of the sarcoplasmatic reticulum and small foci of myofibrillar disarray. In three cases the electron-microscopic score was considerably higher than was expected from the patients' ejection fraction. In two patients, scoring was in the upper range, as expected.

Discussion

Morphologic findings in myocardial biopsy normally correlated well with clinical and hemodynamic data obtained from patients with early and advanced COCM. Both cardiac hypertrophy and interstitial fibrosis increased with severity of clinical symptoms [1] and were mild to moderate in most cases during early stages and severe in advanced COCM. Existence of severe interstitial fibrosis extending to over more than 20% of the tissue specimen indicated advanced COCM. Conversely, absence of fibrosis did not allow the exclusion of advanced COCM entirely since marked variations within the same patient group were found.

An electron-microscopic score system developed for the study quantified cellular alterations due to hypertrophy and myocardial degeneration as well as interstitial changes. It was similar but more detailed than the scoring system used by Kuhn *et al.* [3]. Our score yielded a good correlability between clinical and morphologic findings. Variations among the same patient group were minimal. It is of interest that some patients with only mild clinical symptoms showed severe morphologic changes.

Among the hemodynamic data, the ejection fraction showed the best correlation with the electron-microscopic score.

In most patients onset of clinical symptoms occurred several years before final diagnosis of COCM was established by heart catheterization. One to three year follow-up after diagnosis revealed no progression of symptoms in 73% of the patients with advanced COCM. In contrast Kuhn *et al.* [3] described a rather rapid progression with high early mortality of the patients. The reasons for these differences are unknown.

Patients who died during follow-up (27%) exhibited extreme, severe morphologic changes equivalent to the terminal stage of the disease.

While clinical symptoms in most patients with early forms of CM remained unchanged during follow-up, five patients showed rapid progression of their disease. Myocardial biopsy was the only indicator of the degree of underlying CM. The present investigation thus demonstrates that in a series of patients the appearance of significant morphologic changes precedes manifest cardiac failure.

Summary

A combined clinical and morphologic study of early and advanced COCM showed good agreement between clinical and morphologic data. In some patients with early CM, ultrastructural changes of unusual degree were present. Five of 36 patients, stage I and II functional classification (NYHA), showed rapid clinical deterioration. In all five patients severe morphologic changes preceded the onset of clinical deterioration.

References

1. Ferrans, V.J., Massumi, R.A., Shugoll, A.N., Roberts, W.C.: Ultrastructural studies in myocardial biopsies in 45 patients with obstructive and congestive cardiomyopathy. In: Cardiomyopathies. Bajusz, E., Rona, G. (eds.). Munich: Urban & Schwarzenberg 1974
2. Jones, M., Ferrans, V.J., Marrow, A.G., Roberts, W.C.: Ultrastructure of crista supraventricularis muscle in patients with congenital heart diseases associated with right ventricular outflow tract obstruction. Circulation *51*, 39 (1975)

3. Kuhn, H., Breithardt, G., Knieriem, H.J., Loogen, F., Both, A., Schmidt, A.K., Strobandt, R., Gleichmann, U.: Die Bedeutung der endomyokardialen Katheterbiopsie für die Diagnostik und Beurteilung der Prognose der kongestiven Kardiomyopathie. Dtsch. med. Wschr. *100*, 717 (1975)
4. Maron, B.J., Ferrans, V.J., Roberts, W.C.: Myocardial ultrastructure in patients' chronic aortic valve disease. Amer. J. Cardiol. *35*, 725 (1975)
5. Roberts, W.C., Ferrans, V.J.: Pathologic anatomy of the cardiomyopathies. Hum. Path. *6*, 287 (1975)

Hypertrophic Obstructive Cardiomyopathy

24. Natural History of Hypertrophic Obstructive Cardiomyopathy and the Effect of Therapy

F. LOOGEN, H. KUHN, and W. KRELHAUS

Summary

In order to establish the usefulness of medical and surgical management of HOCM, 155 patients were followed for from 1 to 21 years (mean, 5.5 years). The patients were divided into three main groups:

1. Untreated group (47 patients)
2. Propranolol-treated group (77 patients)
3. Surgically treated group (31 patients)

The average follow-up period for group 1 was 6.7 years; it was for group 2 4.7 years, and for group 3 (postoperative) 5.0 years.

Medical treatment improved the symptoms in some cases. However, there was no significant difference between the clinical course of the untreated group and that of the propranolol group. Moreover, the difference between the mortality of the untreated group and that of the propranolol group was not significant ($P > 0.05$). The best clinical results were achieved in group 3 where 79% of the patients followed postoperatively showed an improvement of at least one clinical class (NYHA).

Hemodynamic control studies measured the outflow tract gradient and the left ventricular enddiastolic pressure. The average follow-up period for control catheterization in group 1 was 8.5 years (6 patients), and in group 2 it was 6.5 years (12 patients). These studies established that a) an increase of the pressure gradient was found only in patients whose condition had deteriorated, b) the enddiastolic pressure, however, had increased significantly independent of the clinical condition and propranolol therapy ($P < 0.005$). Recatheterizations were carried out in 21 patients of group 3 at an average of 20 months postoperatively. There was a significant reduction or abolition of the outflow tract gradient. Furthermore, a significant decrease of the enddiastolic pressure [(average pressure, preoperatively, 20.05 ± 8.45 mm Hg; postoperatively, 14.38 ± 5.11 mm Hg ($P < 0.005$)] was found. During an observation period up to 12 years after operation, a reobstruction was not observed. Two patients died in a follow-up period averaging 5 years postoperatively.

This study suggests that the clinical course and the prognosis was uninfluenced by propranolol in the majority of our patients with HOCM. Furthermore, the best clinical and hemodynamic results were obtained surgically, which also seems to improve the prognosis of HOCM.

In 1957 and 1958, the first anatomic and functional descriptions of hypertrophic obstructive cardiomyopathy (HOCM) were made by Brock and Teare [5, 26]. Although many communications dealing with different aspects of the disease have since been published, questions remain unanswered regarding etiology, diagnosis, prognosis and therapy.

The purpose of the present study is to elucidate the natural history of HOCM and the effect of therapy. Clinical and hemodynamic investigations were performed to help to answer the following questions:

1. Does the clinical course of untreated patients differ from that of treated patients?
2. Does the clinical course correspond with hemodynamic data?
3. What are the clinical and hemodynamic results of surgery?

Patient Profile and Methods

Out of a total of 210 patients suffering from HOCM, 155 patients were studied for a period ranging between 1 and 21 years (mean, 5.3 years). In 23 cases, the patients were followed for from 10 to 21 years. The entire series of 155 patients were functionally classified as:

a) 22 patients of functional class I
b) 64 patients of functional class II
c) 62 patients of functional class III
d) 7 patients of functional class IV

corresponding to the classification of the New York Heart Association (NYHA).

For the purpose of the study, patients were further classified into three groups:

1. Untreated group
2. Propranolol-treated group
3. Surgically treated group

The untreated group consisted of patients who received no medication because they either had no or only minimal complaints. There were in this group, however, also patients in whom propranolol treatment was started but discontinued after a short time for various reasons, most commonly because of adverse side-effects. Class I consisted of 17 patients, class II of 17 patients, class III of 12 patients, and class IV of 1 patient (NYHA). The follow-up time in this group was 6.7 years.

The propranolol group consisted of 6 patients of class I, 44 patients of class II, 23 patients of class III, and 4 patients of class IV. Their average follow-up period was 4.7 years. The dosage of propranolol depended on the clinical condition and on the heart rate (minimum 50–55 beats/min). The dosage of propranolol usually varied between 120 and 240 mg/day.

The surgically treated group consisted of 3 patients of class II, 25 patients of class III and 3 patients of class IV (NYHA). Twenty-eight patients were followed (the mean postoperative follow-up period was 5.0 years). Surgical intervention was undertaken in group III and IV patients when it became clear that conservative management was of no use. The three patients of class II showed a high pressure gradient (more than 100 mm Hg) and severe arrhythmias in one case. An additional 10 patients of our group who were operated on during the last 10 months were also included for the purpose of calculating the operation mortality, but the patients are not included in the follow-up study.

The surgical technique consisted in the last years of a transaortic myotomy and myectomy which was· performed in 23 cases. During the first years of surgical treatment different approaches were used. In three cases with severe mitral incompetence, an artificial mitral valve was implanted.

For statistical calculations, the Students t-test and the χ^2-test were used.

Results

Table 1 shows the functional class, the age at the time of diagnosis, and the age when the murmur was discovered. Of 155 patients, 23 were classified initially as functional class I, 64 as class II, 60 as class III, and 8 as class IV (NYHA). The mean age of the patients with the fewest complaints was 21.4 years, the average age of those patients with severe complaints (NAHA class IV) was 42.5 years. An increase of the functional class correlated with an increase of age, whereas detection of a heart murmur was independent of age (average, 18 years in all four groups).

Figure 1 shows a correlation between the functional class and the pressure gradient at rest. There was a good correlation between increasing functional class and increasing pressure gradient. The pressure gradient of patients of functional class III and IV was significantly higher ($P < 0.0005$) than that of patients of functional class II.

The natural history of untreated patients with HOCM is shown in Figure 2. Thirty-four patients (72%) were classified as functional class I or II. After a follow-up period of 6.7 years, the clinical condition remained unchanged in 28 cases (60%), 11 patients died, and 7 deteriorated.

The clinical course of the propranolol-treated patients with HOCM is summarized in Figure 3. Similar to the clinical course in the untreated group, the clinical condition was unchanged in 54 cases (70%) after 4.7 years follow-up. Definite deterioration was rarely observed (3 of 77 patients). Ten patients died. The numbers of patients who deteriorated and of those who died while receiving propranolol therapy are smaller than that of the untreated group. Bearing in mind, however, that the follow-up period of the propranolol group was only 4.7 years compared with 7.6 years in the untreated group, the difference between the two groups is insignificant.

Table 1. Functional class and age of 155 patients with HOCM.

NYHA class	No. of patients	Age at detection of heart murmur (years)	Age at the time of diagnosis (years)
I	23	17.9	21.4
II	64	18.7	32.9
III	60	17.0	33.2
IV	8	19.3	42.5

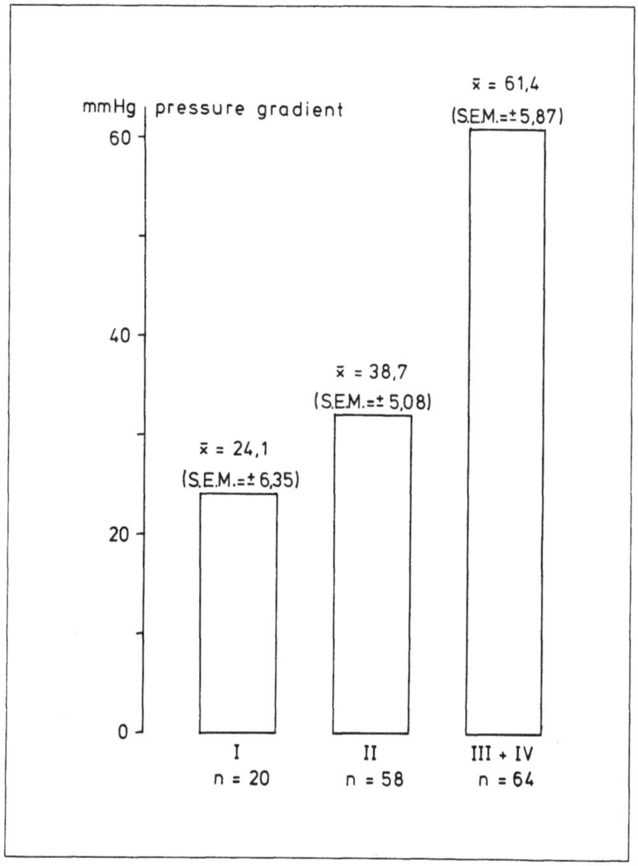

Fig. 1. Relation between functional class and pressure gradient at rest in HOCM. There was a significant difference between the mean pressure gradient of class II compared with class III and IV ($P < 0.0005$)

To determine whether there is a correlation between hemodynamic data and the clinical course, heart catheterizations were repeated after 8.5 years (on the average) in 6 untreated patients (Figs. 4 and 5) and in propranolol-treated patients after an average follow-up of 6.5 years (Figs. 6 and 7). In all cases which showed a deterioration of the functional class, an increase of the outflow tract obstruction and of the enddiastolic pressure was observed. Independent of the clinical condition, the enddiastolic pressure increased during the control period. [The enddiastolic pressure in the untreated group was 14.07 ± 1.97 mm Hg at the first examination and 22.08 ± 2.77 mm Hg at the second examination ($P < 0.025$). The enddiastolic pressure in the propranolol group increased from 14.60 ± 1.35 mm Hg to 18.36 ± 2.41 mm Hg ($P < 0.01$). For both groups, the increase was highly significant ($P < 0.0005$)].

The surgically treated group belonged mainly to functional class III (Fig. 8). The postoperative follow-up period averaged 5.0 years. Of 28 patients who were followed after surgery, 22 (79%) showed a distinct clinical improvement. There

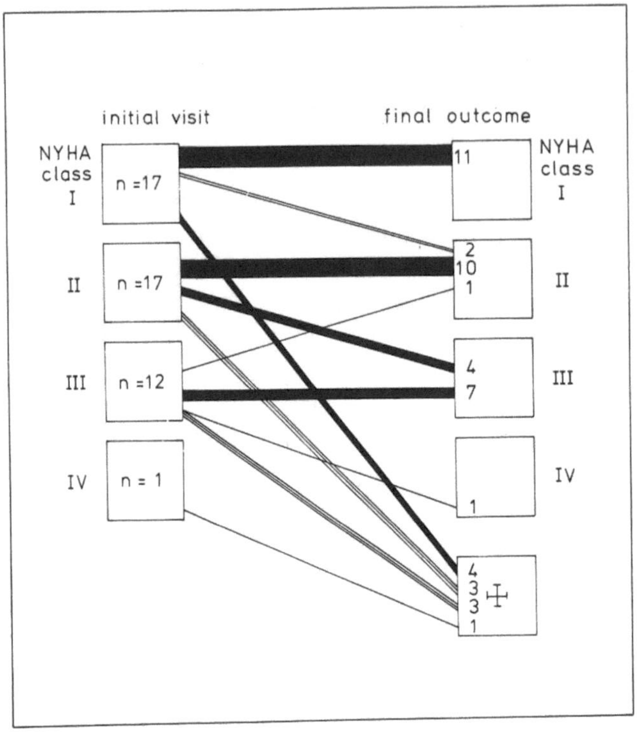

Fig. 2. Clinical course of untreated patients with HOCM ($\overline{x}$ = 6.7 years, n = 47)

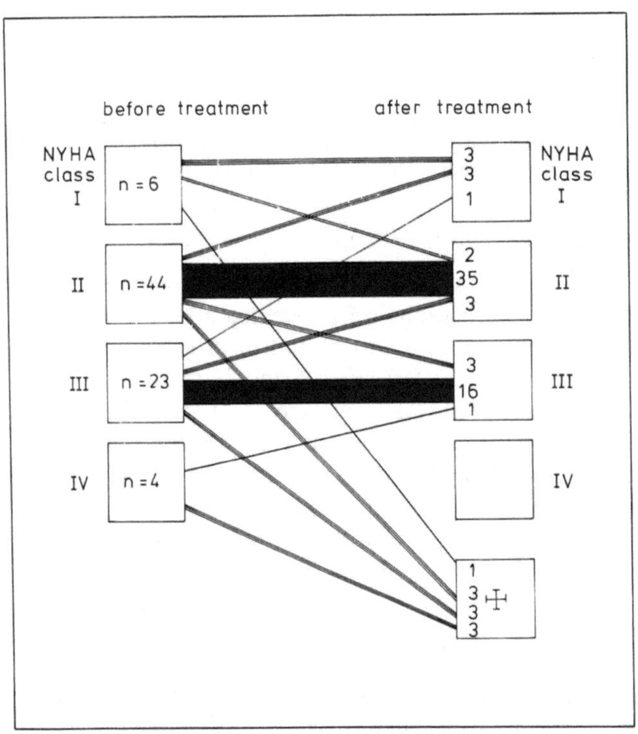

Fig. 3. Clinical course of propranolol-treated patients with HOCM ($\overline{x}$ = 4.7 years, n = 77). There was no significant difference between the number of propranolol treated and untreated patients of class II who deteriorated ($P > 0.05$ NS)

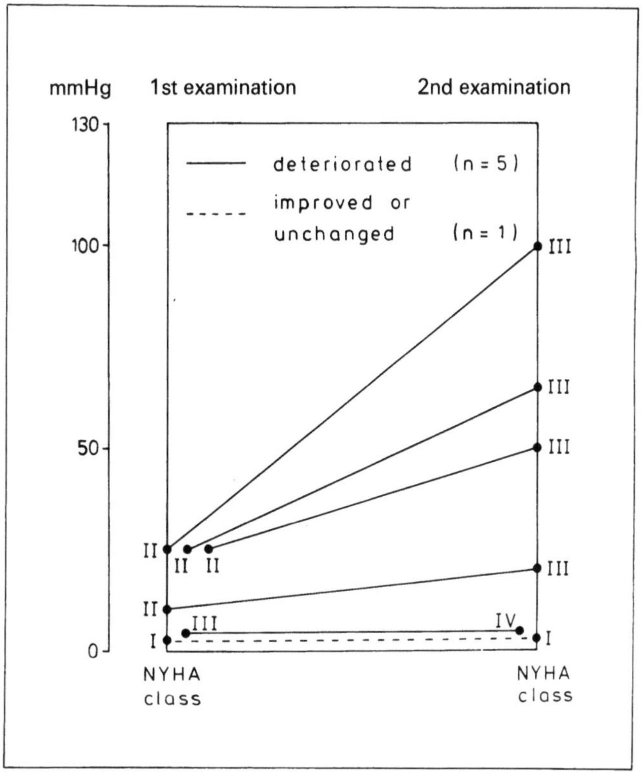

Fig. 4. Pressure gradient at rest in the course of untreated patients with HOCM ($\bar{x} = 8.5$ years, n = 6). With exception of one patient (*dashed line*), all patients had deteriorated

was no improvement in 4 cases, and it is noteworthy that 3 of these patients were children. Of 31 surgically treated patients, 5 died, 3 of them immediately after surgery. They were among our first patients who underwent operation for HOCM. One additional patient requiring an emergency operation due to shock died during operation, but is not included in this series. Two patients died 2–4 years after successful surgical treatment of unknown reasons despite clinical improvement.

To correlate preoperative hemodynamic data with postoperative results, recatheterizations were carried out in 21 surgically treated patients after an average of 20 months (Fig. 9). In 15 patients (72%), no pressure gradient was found at rest. In 5 patients, a pressure gradient between 15 and 30 mm Hg was still evident. One patient who did not improve postoperatively (a child) still had a pressure gradient at rest of 60 mm Hg.

Figure 10 shows the pre- and postoperative enddiastolic pressures. After operation, there was a significant decrease of the enddiastolic pressure [mean pressure preoperatively, 20.05 ± 8.45 mm Hg; postoperatively, 14.38 ± 5.11 mm Hg ($P < 0.0005$)].

The three patient groups are compared in Table 2. There was no great difference between the ages of the different groups. The follow-up period was

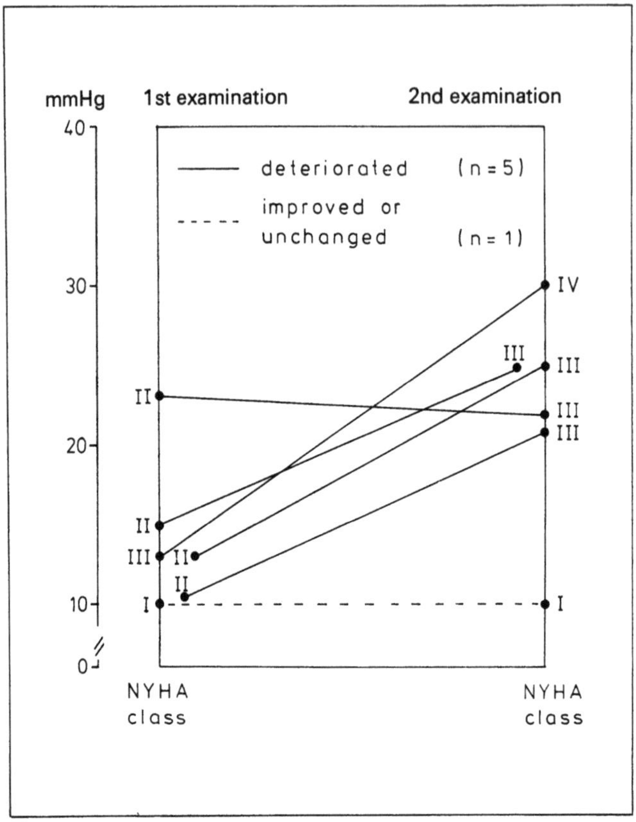

Fig. 5. Enddiastolic pressure in the course of HOCM [same patients as in Fig. 5 ($\bar{x}$ = 8.5 years, n = 6)]. There was a significant increase of the enddiastolic pressure at the second catheterization [from 14.07 ± 1.97 mm Hg at the first examination to 22.08 ± 2.77 mm Hg ($P < 0.025$)]. The *dashed line* indicates data for the one patient whose condition did not deteriorate

Table 2. Comparison of follow-up in three groups of patients with HOCM.

Group	Age (years)	Follow-up (years)	Clinical course (% of pts)			
			Stable	Improved	Deteriorated	Died
No treatment (n = 47)	33.1	6.7	60	2	15	23
Propranolol (n = 77)	39.0	4.7	70	10	7	13
Surgery (n = 28)	36.3	5.0	14	79	–	7

longest in the untreated group. Regarding the clinical course, the highest percentage of clinical improvement was seen in patients in the surgically treated group (79%). Two patients (7%) died postoperatively during the 5-year follow-up period – a relatively high incidence. Thirteen percent of the patients in the propranolol group died, and 23% of those in the untreated group died, but the follow-up period of the untreated group was considerably longer. Therefore, the difference is not significant ($P > 0.05$).

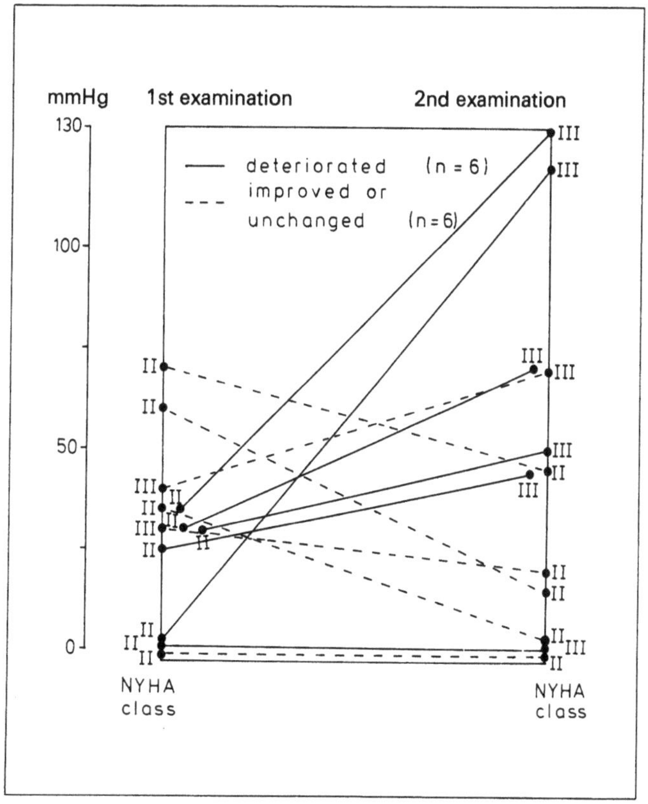

Fig. 6. Pressure gradient at rest in the course of HOCM, propranolol therapy ($\bar{x} = 6.5$ years, n = 12). Between the first and second examination, six patients had deteriorated (*unbroken lines*) and six patients had improved or were unchanged (*dashed lines*)

Since the groups under comparison belong to different functional classes, only the class III patients of each group were compared (Table 3). It can be seen that there is no marked difference when comparing the data of Table 2 with Table 3. This especially applies to the mortality rate. The rate of deterioration and "mortality" was lower in the propranolol group, although this difference was, however, not significant ($P > 0.05$).

The mortality in the surgically treated group is noteworthy. The overall operative mortality was 12% (Table 4). Of the first series when different operative techniques were used, 3 of the 13 patients died (23%). It must, however, be empha-

Table 3. Comparison of follow-up in three groups of patients with HOCM from functional class III.

Group	Age (years)	Follow-up (years)	Clinical course (% of pts)			
			Stable	Improved	Deteriorated	Died
No treatment (n = 12)	34.5	9.0	59	8	8	25
Propranolol (n = 23)	43.6	3.8	70	17	–	13
Surgery (n = 22)	34.2	5.2	13.5	82	–	4.5

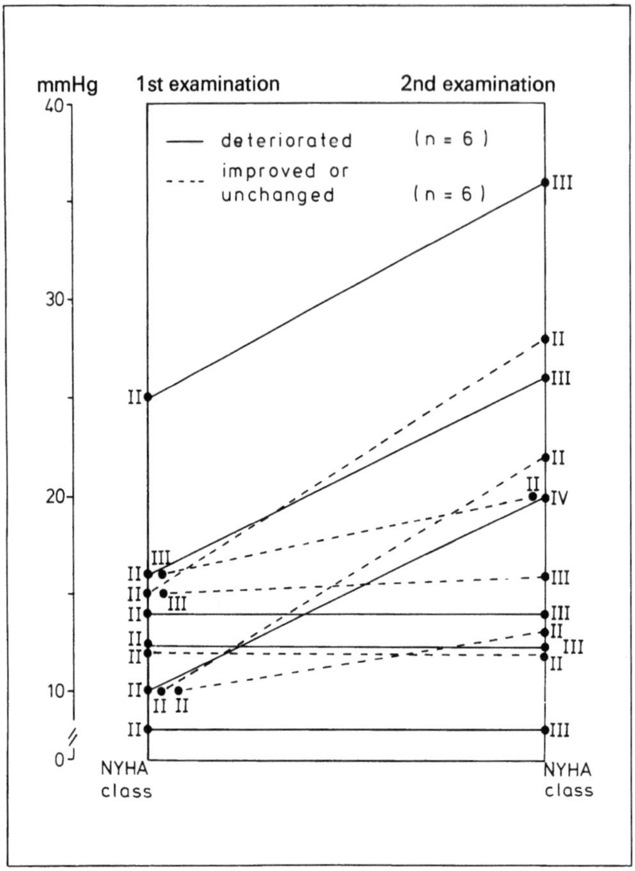

Fig. 7. Enddiastolic pressure in the course of HOCM, propranolol therapy [same patients as in Fig. 6 ($\bar{x} = 6.5$ xears, n = 12)]. There was a significant increase in the enddiastolic pressure from 14.60 ± 1.35 mm Hg at the first catheterization to 18.36 ± 2.41 mm Hg at the second catheterization ($P < 0.01$).

sized that the operative mortality was reduced considerably during the last 6 years [2 deaths out of 28 patients (7%)]. One of these patients suffered from a lentiginosis with cardiac manifestation and will be described elsewhere [17].

Under a "late mortality" (Table 4) 2 of the 28 patients also died of unknown causes 2–4 years postoperatively.

Discussion

It is well known that the natural history of HOCM is characterized by a slow progression. Our investigation supports this (Table 1), showing an increase of age and functional class. This indicates a progressive character of this myocardial disease.

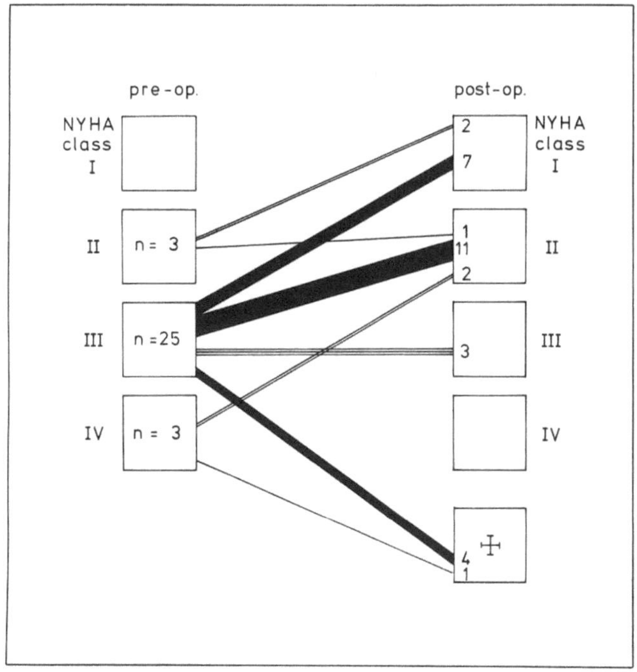

Fig. 8. Functional class pre- and postoperatively in HOCM ($\bar{x} = 5.0$ years, n = 31). The percentage of operated patients who improved was significantly higher than the percentage of propranolol treated patients who improved ($P < 0.01$)

Table 4. Mortality in surgically treated patients with HOCM.

Operation mortality						Late mortality [a]	
		1st period (1963–1969)		2nd period (1970–1976)		Follow-up study	
Pts. (n)	Overall Mortality (n)	Op. pts. (n)	Mortality (n)	Op. pts. (n)	Mortality (n)	Pts. (n)	Mortality (n)
41	5 (12.2%)	13	3 (23%)	28	2 (7%)	28	2 (7%)

[a] Late mortality in the series of follow-up patients is smaller (5.6%) than that in all surgically treated patients.

Hemodynamic investigation showed a good correlation between the functional class and the pressure gradient at rest in our patients (Fig. 1). This finding is not shared by all authors [11, 12] but was recently confirmed by others [7].

In many cases symptoms can be favorably influenced by medical treatment (Fig. 3). The percentage of improved patients is greater in the propranolol-treated group, than in the untreated group; this difference is, however, not statistically significant. Nor does propranolol influence the rate of sudden death [1, 9].

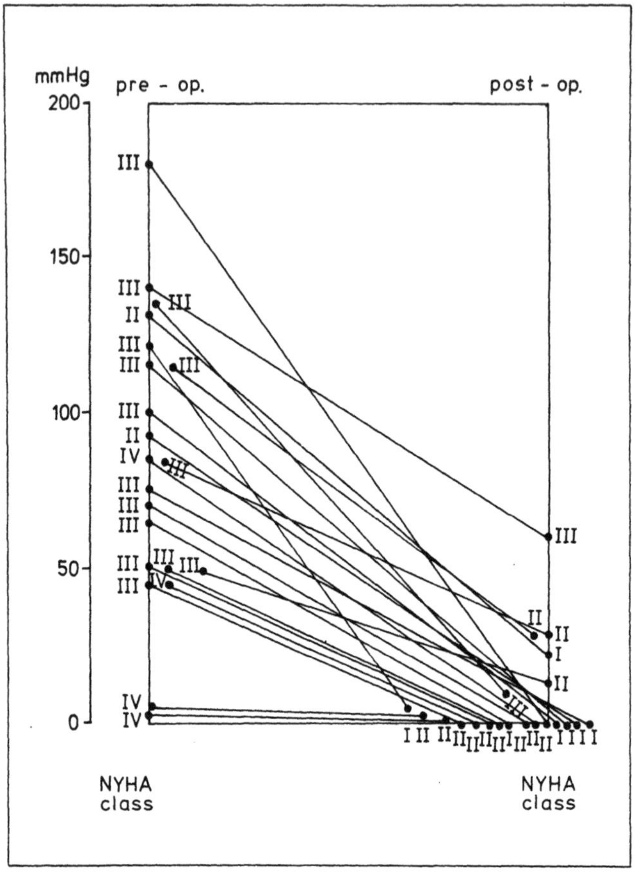

Fig. 9. Pressure gradient pre- and postoperatively ($\bar{x} = 20$ months, postoperatively, n = 21). In 15 patients, no pressure gradient was found at rest

In the majority of patients treated medically, clinical improvement corresponded with a decrease of the outflow tract obstruction but not with a decrease of the enddiastolic pressure (Figs. 4–7). Independent of the functional class, there was, however, a significant increase of enddiastolic pressure in the course of conservative management. This finding provides evidence that the hypertrophic process is progressive and accompanied by a decrease of myocardial distensibility. This also supports the suggestion that improvement in propranolol-treated patients is mainly due to a reduction of the outflow tract obstruction and agrees with the finding of a good correlation between outflow tract obstruction and clinical class.

Compared to medically treated patients, the definite clinical improvement in the great majority of surgically treated patients can be explained not only by the decrease of the outflow tract obstruction but also possibly by the decrease of the left ventricular enddiastolic pressure. We must, however, take into account that the period of hemodynamic control was much shorter ($\bar{x} = 20$ months) in

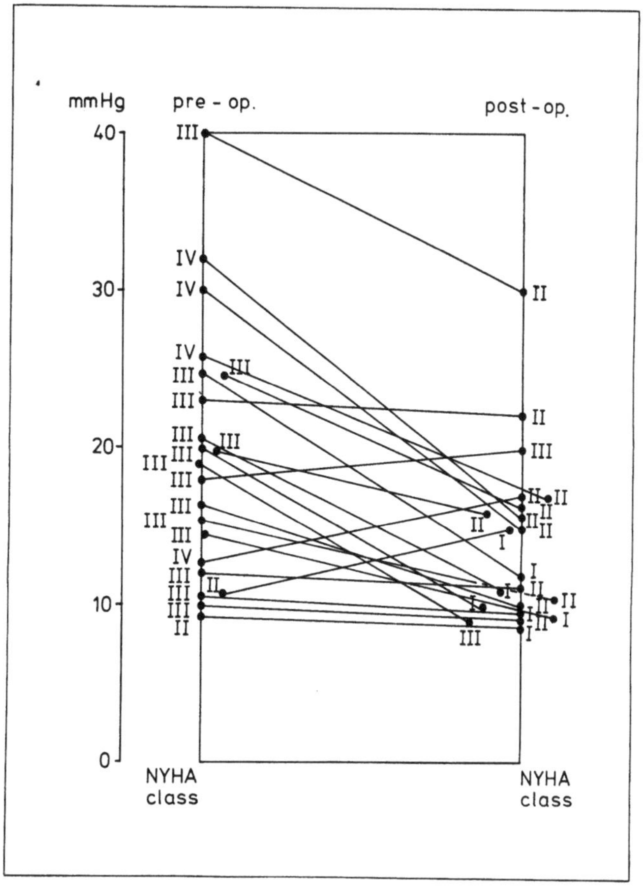

Fig. 10. Enddiastolic pressure pre- and postoperatively ($\bar{x} = 20$ months postoperatively, n = 21). There was a significant decrease of the enddiastolic pressure at the postoperative control ($P < 0.0005$)

this group than in the conservatively managed patients (untreated group, $\bar{x} =$ 8.5 years; propranolol group, $\bar{x} = 6.5$ years). It must be emphasized, however, that there was no reobstruction in a postoperative observation period of up to 12 years and that the clinical improvement in operated patients was long-lasting. These findings agree with the results of other authors [3, 4, 10, 15, 16, 20, 23, 24, 28].

Three of four surgically-treated patients who did not improve were children. The good results reported by Tajik *et al.* [27] show that good operative results in children with HOCM can be achieved.

It is well known that sudden death may occur at any stage of the disease [2, 9, 11, 18–21, 25]. Our study indicates that the rate of death is lower after surgery. Late mortality in patients following surgery was 7%, compared with 13% in the propranolol-treated group and 23% in the untreated group (Table 2).

Apart from the better clinical and hemodynamic results after surgery, there was a tendency toward fewer deaths in the late postoperative period, which has been confirmed by others [25]. These results support operative treatment of HOCM when propranolol treatment fails in patients of class III and IV and possibly also those patients in class II.

References

1. Adelman, A.G., Shah, P.M., Gramiak, R., Wigle, E.D.: Long-term propranolol therapy in muscular subaortic stenosis. Brit. Heart J. *32*, 804–811 (1970)
2. Adelman, A.G., Wigle, E.D., Ranganathan, N., Webb, G.D., Kidd, S.L., Bigelow, W.G., Silver, M.D.: The clinical course in muscular subaortic stenosis. A retrospective and prospective study of 60 hemodynamically proved cases. Ann. int. Med. *77*, 515 (1972)
3. Bigelow, W.G., Trimble, A.S., Wigle, E.D., Adelman, A.G., Felderhof, C.H.: The treatment of muscular subaortic stenosis. J. thorac. cardiovasc. Surg. *68*, 384 (1974)
4. Binet, J.P., Langlois, J., Conso, J.F., Planche, C.: Traitement chirurgical de 52 cardiomyopathies obstructives. Arch. Mal. Cœur *69*, 777 (1976)
5. Brock, R.: Functional obstruction of the left ventricle (acquired aortic subvalvular stenosis). Guy's Hosp. Rep. *108*, 126 (1959)
6. Cherian, G., Brockington, I.F., Shah, P.M., Oakley, C.M., Goodwin, J.F.: Beta-adrenergic blockade in hypertrophic obstructive cardiomyopathy. Brit. med. J. *1*, 895–898 (1966)
7. Emeriau, J.P., Fontan, F., Besse, P., Chauve, A., Coqueran, J.E., Bricaud, H.: Prognostic Value of Preoperative Left Ventricular Performance in Idiopathic Hypertrophic Subaortic Stenosis. 7th European Congress of Cardiology, Amsterdam, 1976
8. Flamm, M.D., Stenson, R.E.: Beta-adrenergic receptor blockade in hypertrophic subaortic stenosis. In: Circulatory Effects and Clinical Uses of Beta-Adrenergic Blocking Drugs, pp. 96–112, Amsterdam, Excerpta Medica 1971
9. Frank, S., Braunwald, E.: Idiopathic hypertrophic subaortic stenosis. Clinical analysis of 126 patients with emphasis on the natural history. Circulation *37*, 759 (1968)
10. Gerbaux, A., Hanania, G., Godefroid, Baragan, J., Maouad, J., Gay, J.: Resultats à long terme du traitement chirurgical de la myocardiopathie obstructive par intervention sur le septum interventriculaire. Arch. Mal. Cœur *69*, 791 (1976)
11. Goodwin, J.F.: Congestive and hypertrophic cardiomyopathies. *Lancet 1970* I, 731
12. Goodwin, J.F.: Prospects and predictions for the cardiomyopathies. Circulation *50*, 210 (1974)
13. Krelhaus, W., Kuhn, H., Loogen, F.: Todesfälle bei hypertrophischer obstruktiver Myocardiopathie. Verh. dtsch. Ges. inn. Med. *82*, 40 (1976)
14. Krelhaus, W., Kuhn, H., Körfer, R., Loogen, F.: Die hypertrophische obstruktive Myocardiopathie (HOCM) im Kindesalter – Krankheitsbild und Krankheitsverlauf. Verh. dtsch. Ges. paed. Kardiol. (Baden/Vienna) (1976)
15. Krelhaus, W., Kuhn, H., Loogen, F., Körfer, R., Schulte, H.D., Bircks, W.: Zur Operationsindikation bei hypertrophischer obstruktiver Myokardiopathie (HOCM). Z. Kardiol., Suppl. 3, 93 (1976)
16. Kuhn, H., Krelhaus, W., Loogen, F., Bircks, W.: Zur Operationsindikation der hypertrophischen obstruktiven Kardiomyopathie. Z. Kardiol. (in press)
17. Kuhn, H., Haensch, R., Lösse, B., Jehle, J.: Hypertrophische obstruktive Kardiomyopathie und Lentiginosis. Dtsch. med. Wschr. (in press)
18. Loogen, F., Gleichmann, U., Krelhaus, W.: Die obstruktive Myokardiopathie. Z. Kreisl.-Forsch. *60*, 1044 (1971)
19. Loogen, F., Krelhaus, W., Kübler, W.: Natural history of hypertrophic obstructive cardiomyopathy: Observation on 107 patients. In: Cardiomyopathies. Recent Advances in Cardiac Structure and Metabolism. Bajusz, E., Rona, G. (eds.), pp. 629–637. Baltimore: University Park Press 1973
20. Loogen, F., Krelhaus, W., Kuhn, H.: A Follow-up Study of Patients With Hypertrophic Obstructive Cardiomyopathy. 7th European Congress of Cardiology, Amsterdam, 1976
21. Loogen, F., Krelhaus, W., Kuhn, H.: Verlaufsbeobachtungen der hypertrophischen obstruktiven Myocardiopathie. Z. Kardiol. *65*, 511 (1976)

22. Loogen, F., Kuhn, H.: Classification and Natural History of Primary Cardiomyopathies. International Symposium on Myocardial Failure, Rottach-Egern, 1976 (in press)
23. Morrow, A.G., Reitz, B.A., Epstein, S.E., Henry, W.L., Concle, D.M., Itscoitz, S.B., Redwood, D.R.: Operative treatment in hypertrophic subaortic stenosis. Circulation *52*, 88–102 (1975)
24. Rothlin, M., Arbenz, U., Krayenbuhl, H.P., Turina, J., Senning, A.: Spätresultate nach Operationen bei muskulärer subvalvulärer Aortenstenose. Z. Kardiol. *65*, 501 (1976)
25. Shah, P.M., Adelman, A.G., Wigle, E.D., Gobel, F.L., Burchell, H.B., Hardarson, T., Curiel, R., De La Caldaza, C., Oakley, C.M., Goodwin, J.F.: The natural (and unnatural) history of hypertrophic obstructive cardiomyopathy. Circulat. Res. *34*, *35*, Suppl. II, 179 (1974)
26. Teare, D.: Asymmetrical hypertrophy of the heart in young adults. Brit. Heart J. *20*, 1 (1958)
27. Tajik, A.J., Giuliani, E.R., Weidman, W.H., McGoon, D.C., Brandenburg, R.O., Ritter, D.G.: Idiopathic hypertrophic subaortic stenosis in children. Circulation *47*, *48*, Suppl. IV, 222 (1973)
28. Tajik, A.J., Giuliani, E.R., Weidman, W.H., Brandenburg, R.O., McGoon, D.C.: Idiopathic hypertrophic subaortic stenosis. Long-term surgical follow-up. Amer. J. Cardiol. *34*, 815 (1974)

25. Analysis of Deaths in the Course of Hypertrophic Obstructive Cardiomyopathy

W. Krelhaus, H. Kuhn, and F. Loogen

Summary

Patients with HOCM die as often suddenly (13 cases) as after progressive deterioration (10 cases). Sudden deaths occurred especially in young patients – 10 of 13 patients who died suddenly were 20 years of age or younger. While the rate of sudden death decreases after age 20, the possibility of death from progressive deterioration in older patients increases with duration of the disease. These older patients who also had signs of heart failure, died on the average after 5 months, which suggests a poor prognosis if conservative management is continued.

Analyses of ECG-tracings of the patients who died showed that there is no obvious means of identifying patient groups at high risk of sudden death. Atrial fibrillation, however, may indicate an advanced stage of HOCM and may be a precursor of death after progressive deterioration.

A biventricular obstruction may also indicate special risk, both for sudden death and for death after progressive deterioration. A biventricular gradient at rest was found in 50% of the patients who subsequently died but only in 17% of those who lived ($P < 0.01$).

The results of interviews of relatives of the patients who died showed that sudden death occurred after heavy exercise in 8 of 10 cases.

By systematic ambulatory ECG monitoring in consecutive patients with HOCM, severe cardiac arrhythmias were detected in 20%, indicating a possible role of rhythm disorders for the final outcome of patients with HOCM. Rhythm control and eventually antiarrhythmic therapy seem to be necessary in patients with HOCM.

Follow-up studies of HOCM have shown that the course of the disease is characterized by a slow progression, which many studies have confirmed [1, 7–10, 12]. Sudden death in the course of the disease often occurs in spite of medical management. Several catamnestic studies, interviews of relatives of the deceased patients, and ambulatory ECG monitoring were performed to determine the incidence and cause of deaths and whether or not high risk groups of patients can be identified.

Patients Profile and Methods

Of 210 patients with HOCM, 26 died in the course of conservative management. Systematic inquiries were made of the relatives of the dead patients and of the family doctors to get information about the kind of death (sudden death or death after progressive deterioration) and the circumstances of death. The delay between the last ECG tracing and the incidence of death varied from a few days to 10 years ($\bar{x} = 2$ years and 1 month). The delay between the heart catheterization and the incidence of death varied from 6 months to 10 years ($\bar{x} = 2$ years and 10 months). Continuous ECG tracings were performed with a Siemens Meditape K recorder and analysed manually. The mean duration of registration was 6 h. For statistical calculation, the chi-square test was used.

Results and Discussion

Of 210 patients with HOCM, 13 died suddenly and 10 died after progressive deterioration in the course of conservative management. These findings show that complication in the course of HOCM is not exclusively sudden death. In 3 other cases, the circumstances of death could not be elucidated.

Table 1 shows the relation between the kind of death and the decades of life. Sudden death occurred especially up to age 20 and with decreasing frequency afterwards, while after age 20 death due to progressive deterioration, increased with age.

In an attempt to recognize clinical parameters which might indicate death after progressive deterioration, the clinical data about these patients is collected in Table 2. It can be seen that with exception of the infant, the presence of a heart murmur had been known for 19 years on the average. Symptoms were present for 16 years on the average. In all cases, there was for years dyspnea after mild exercise and half of the patients complained of angina. It seems to be important' that the time between the onset of heart failure and death varied from 1 week to 1 year, with an average of only 5 months. We may conclude that the prognosis is bad in patients with HOCM when heart failure is present if conservative management is continued. This finding is of importance for the indication of surgery which is discussed later in Chapter 26.

Table 3 analyses the clinical data of the patients who died suddenly. There was no relation to the functional class. Three patients had no complaints at all, and five patients had only minimal complaints. A history of syncopal attacks or of rhythm disorders was as rare in those who died as in the patients with HOCM who were living.

Table 4 compares the clinical data of the patients who died suddenly and of those who died after progressive deterioration. Sudden deaths occurred at a mean age of 19.5 years after a short duration of the disease (i.e., an average

Table 1. Death in HOCM in relation to age.

Age (years)	Sudden death (n = 13)	Death after progressive deterioration (n = 10)
1–20	n = 10	n = 1
21–40	n = 2	n = 3
>40	n = 1	n = 6

Table 2. Clinical data of patients with HOCM who died after progressive deterioration.

Patient	Age (years)				Duration of symptoms (years)[a]			
	Discovery of a heart murmur	Beginning of symptoms	Died	Sex	Dyspnea	Angina	Syncopal attacks	Tachy-cardias
E.H.	?	18	38	f	5	20	–	5
U.W.	?	15	32	f	9	17	–	1
J.P.	40	40	48	f	8	–	–	–
U.J.	?	?	71	m	+	–	+	–
H.P.	?	?	44	m	+	–	–	–
H.K.	22	?	51	m	+	+	+	+
H.R.	17	20	32	m	12	12	–	–
M.G.	19	22	47	f	25	–	–	+
S.W.	Birth	Birth	1	f				+
A.B.	36	36	47	f	11	11	+	–

[a] Pluses indicate that the symptom existed, but its duration was not known. Minuses indicate that the symptom did not exist

Table 3. Clinical data of patients with HOCM who died suddenly.

Patient	Age (years)					Duration of symptoms (years)[a]			
	Discovery of a heart murmur	Beginning of symptoms[a]	Died	Sex	NYHA class	Dyspnea	Angina	Syncopal attacks	Tachy-cardias
J.S.	7	8	10	m	III	2	–	–	2
M.D.	?	?	12	m	III	1	–	+	–
E.K.	14	14	16	m	II	+	–	–	–
A.H.	15	–	16	m	I	–	–	–	–
P.G.	?	?	12	m	III	+	–	–	–
D.S.	10	–	14	m	I	–	–	–	–
H.P.	?	–	18	m	I	–	–	–	–
J.S.	10	10	17	f	II	6	–	–	6
H.W.	?	?	42	m	II	+	13	–	–
A.M.	20	26	32	f	III	6	6	5	1
W.C.	31	32	34	m	II	2	–	–	–
A.Sch.	8	12	12	f	III	1	–	+	–
K.H.	12	12	19	f	II	7	–	–	–

[a] Pluses indicate that the symptom existed, but its duration was not known. Minuses indicate that the symptom did not exist

Table 4. NYHA class and age in HOCM patients who died.

	NYHA class	Discovery of a murmur (patients)	Mean age (years)	Duration of symptoms (years)
Sudden death	I–III	14	19.5	4
Death after progressive deterioration	IV	22	41	16

of 4.0 years between the beginning of the symptoms and death). Deaths after progressive deterioration occurred at a mean age of 41 years after an average duration of symptoms of 16 years. We may conclude that death after progressive deterioration occurred rather early and that the risk of a fatal outcome is high after a certain time of conservative management.

As already shown in Table 1, sudden deaths occurred mainly in young patients. Of 18 patients in whom the diagnosis was already made in childhood, nine died suddenly during an observation period which was 6.3 years in untreated patients and 4.2 years in propranolol-treated patients [5], as Table 5 shows. These poor results were confirmed by others [11, 13] who reported as poor results of conservative management of HOCM in childhood. Tajik reported about 5 deaths of 9 children after an observation period of 3.8 years, and Maron reported about 4 deaths out of 10 children after an average observation period of 8.0 years in an untreated patient group. Out of 11 propranolol-treated children, there were 4 deaths in the group of Maron *et al.* after an average observation period of 4.2 years. These findings show that the mortality in patients in which the diagnosis of HOCM was already made in childhood is high. Although the number of patients is too small to make definite conclusions, it seems that the prognosis of HOCM in childhood is not much influenced by propranolol therapy.

To determine whether there are electrocardiographic or hemodynamic data which may help to identify patients at a high risk of death, the data of the dead patients were compared to those of living patients. Table 6 shows that 3 of 10 patients (30%) who died after progressive deterioration suffered from atrial fibrillation, whereas atrial fibrillation occurred in only 5% of the living patients. Atrial fibrillation in HOCM is regarded as a sign of an advanced stage of HOCM, as reported by many investigators [1, 3, 4, 7]. Other ECG abnormalities, such as left or right axis deviation, left bundle branch block, or signs of biventricular hypertrophy, were seen more often in the group of patients who died, although the difference was insignificant ($P \ll 0.05$). Thus, although we have not seen any ECG abnormalities which could serve as an indicator of sudden death, atrial fibrillation may be a precursor of death after progressive deterioration.

Hemodynamic findings in both groups (dead and living) of patients with HOCM (Table 7) were compared in order to identify high risk groups. Findings show that there was no difference in the left ventricular outflow tract gradient and the left ventricular enddiastolic pressure of the patients who died and those who survived. It was striking, however, that a biventricular gradient at rest was

Table 5. Clinical course of HOCM in childhood (n = 22).

Therapy	Pts. (n)	NYHA class	Follow-up time (years)	Clinical course: Improvement	No change	Deterioration	Died
None	7	I–II	6.3	–	3	–	5
Propranolol	11	II	4.2	1	6	–	4
Operation	4	III	4.0	1	3	–	–

Table 6. ECG findings in HOCM patients who died (n = 26).

	Atrial fibrillation	Left or right axis deviation	LBBB	Left ventricular hypertrophy	Biventricular hypertrophy
Sudden Death (n = 13)	–	4	2	10	4
Death after progressive deterioration (n = 10)	3	4	3	7	2
Obscure (n = 3)	1	–	1	2	2
Total	4	8	6	19	8
ECG findings in patients who died	15%	31%	23%	73%	31%
ECG findings in living patients	5%	11%	10%	73%	18%

Table 7. Frequency of hemodynamic findings in HOCM patients who died (n = 26).

	Right ventricular resting gradient	Left ventricular resting gradient	Augmented LVEDP
Dead patients	50%	71%	75%
Living patients	17%	69%	70%

Table 8. Circumstances of sudden deaths in HOCM.

Heavy physical exercise (6)	Playing hockey	1
	Running upstairs	1
	Running for a bus	2
	Heavy physical exercise (lifting radiators, working at a building site)	2
Physical exercise probable (2)		
	In the schoolyard	1
	In a training camp	1
No physical exercise (2)		
Obscure (3)		

found in only 17% of patients who lived, but in 50% of those who died. This difference was significant ($P < 0.01$), indicating that a biventricular obstruction seems to mean an ominous prognosis.

In order to find some evidence for possible causes of sudden deaths, the relatives of the patients who died were interviewed. Table 8 shows the results of the inquiry: of six patients who died during or immediately after heavy exercise, one young patient died playing hockey; two children died after running for a school bus; and another child died after running upstairs. One patient died lifting radiators, and another patient died during heavy work at a building site. It seems obvious that physical exercise in patients with HOCM is associated with a high risk.

Although there is little conclusive information, the circumstances of death in our patients support strong arguments that the fatal events have been rhythm disorders. In one child who collapsed while playing in the school yard and died later, ventricular fibrillation could still be recorded in the hospital. Two additional patients were treated in other hospitals because of recurrent ventricular tachycardias.

Since incidence and type of rhythm disorders in patients with HOCM are important, ambulatory ECG monitoring was performed for 6 h on the average in 25 consecutive patients. Rhythm disorders were recorded in 11 patients (44%) (Fig. 1). Supraventricular premature beats were recorded in 32%, ventricular premature beats in 28%, in two cases as a repetitive ventricular ectopy. Atrial fibrillation was already known in three cases, a WPW syndrome in one. By continuous monitoring, another case of intermittant atrial fibrillation and another case of intermittant WPW syndrome were discovered. In four cases, supraventricular tachycardias have been recorded.

In 20% of the recordings, potential serious arrhythmias were found (ventricular premature beats > 10/100, repetitive ventricular rhythms, tachycardias).

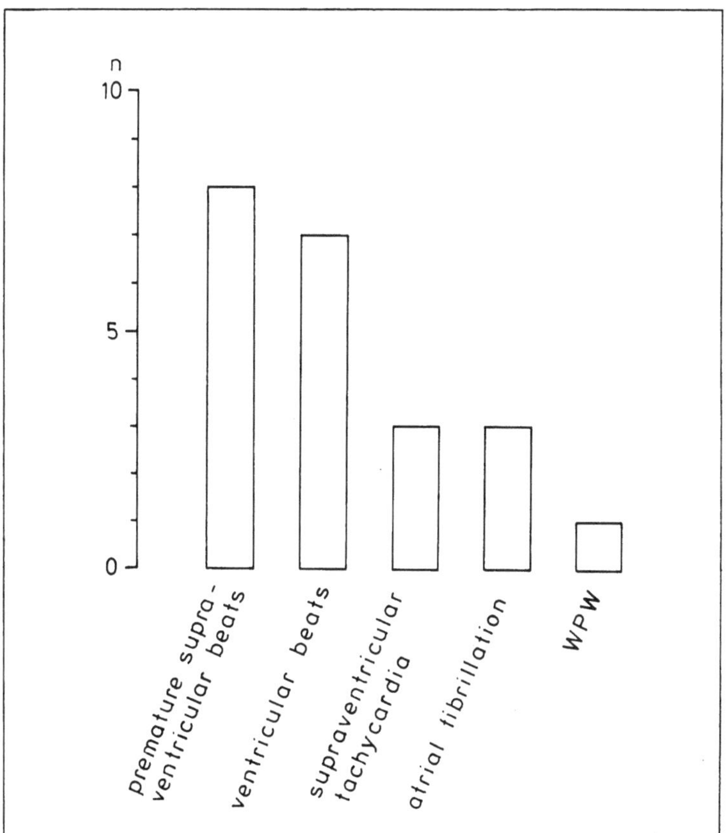

Fig. 1. Rhythm disorders in patients with HOCM (n = 25)

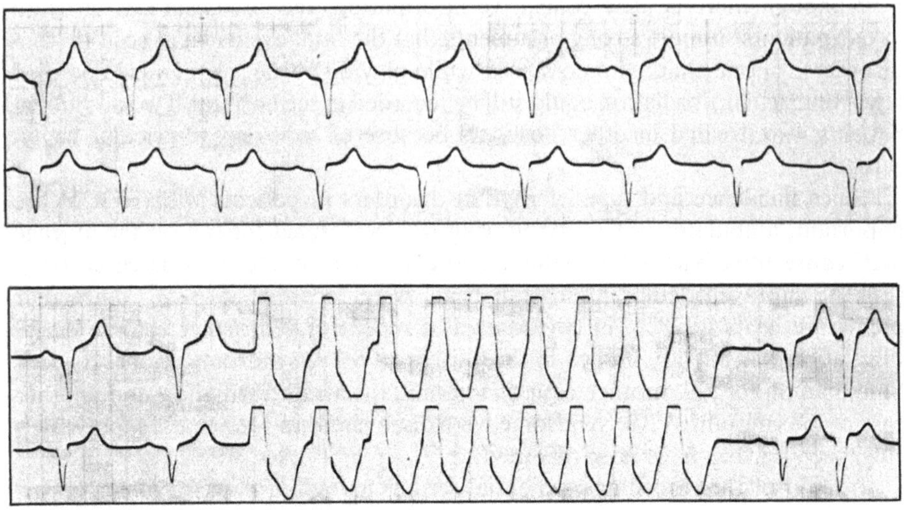

U. Stö. 35y. ♂ HOCM

Fig. 2. Repetitive ventricular ectopy in a patient with HOCM

Serious arrhythmias can probably be recorded in a much higher percentage if the periods of monitoring are longer. This is supported by the finding of repetitive ventricular rhythms (Fig. 2) in two patients. In one of these patients, the ventricular ectopy was seen after 10 hours of monitoring, whereas the ECG before was completely free of ectopic beats. In both patients, there were no complaints of dizziness, syncopal attacks or arrhythmias.

According to these observations, rhythm disorders in patients with HOCM are a frequent finding [2, 3, 6]. Rhythm controls and eventually an antiarrhythmic therapy seem to be necessary in patients with HOCM.

References

1. Frank, S., Braunwald, E.: Idiopathic hypertrophic subaortic stenosis. Clinical analysis of 126 patients with emphasis on the natural history. Circulation *37*, 759 (1968)
2. Ingham, R.E., Rossen, R.M., Goodman, D.J., Harrison, D.C.: Ambulatory electrocardiographic monitoring in idiopathic hypertrophic subaortic stenosis. Circulation *52*, Suppl. II, 93 (1975)
3. James, T.N., Marshall, T.H.: De subitaneis mortibus. Asymmetrical hypertrophy of the heart. Circulation *51*, 1149 (1975)
4. Krelhaus, W., Kuhn, H., Loogen, F.: Todesfälle bei hypertrophischer obstruktiver Myocardiopathie. Verh. dtsch. Ges. inn. Med. *82*, 40 (1976)
5. Krelhaus, W., Kuhn, H., Körfer, R., Loogen, F.: Die hypertrophische obstruktive Myocardiopathie (HOCM) im Kindesalter – Krankheitsbild und Krankheitsverlauf. Verh. dtsch. Ges. paed. Kardiol. (Baden/Wien) (1976)
6. Lever, H.M., Shah, P.M., Reeves, W.C., Nanda, N.C., Gramiak, R.: The relation of left ventricular outflow obstruction to ventricular arrhythmias in hypertrophic subaortic stenosis. Circulation *54*, Suppl. II, 105 (1976)

7. Loogen, F., Gleichmann, U., Krelhaus, W.: Die obstruktive Myokardiopathie. Z. Kreisl.-Forsch. *60*, 1044 (1971)
8. Loogen, F., Krelhaus, W., Kübler, W.: Natural history of hypertrophic obstructive cardiomyopathy: Observation on 107 patients. In: Cardiomyopathies. Recent Advances in Cardiac Structure and Metabolism. Bajusz, E., Rona, G. (eds.), pp. 629–637. Baltimore: University Park Press 1973
9. Loogen, F., Krelhaus, W., Kuhn, H.: A Follow-up Study of Patients With Hypertrophic Obstructive Cardiomyopathy. 7th European Congress of Cardiology, Amsterdam, 1976
10. Loogen, F., Krelhaus, W., Kuhn, H.: Verlaufsbeobachtungen der hypertrophischen obstruktiven Myocardiopathie. Z. Kardiol. *65*, 511 (1976)
11. Maron, B.J., Henry, W.L., Clark, C.E., Redwood, R., Roberts, W.C., Epstein, S.E.: Asymmetric septal hypertrophy in childhood. Circulation *53*, 9 (1976)
12. Shah, P.M., Adelman, A.G., Wigle, E.D., Gobel, F.L., Burchell, H.B., Hardarson, T., Curiel, R., Della Caldaza, C., Oakley, C.M., Goodwin, J.F.: The natural (and unnatural) history of hypertrophic obstructive cardiomyopathy. Circulat. Res. *34*, *35*, Suppl. II, 179 (1974)
13. Tajik, A.J., Giuliani, E.R., Weidman, W.H., McGoon, D.C., Brandenburg, R.O., Ritter, D.G.: Idiopathic hypertrophic subaortic stenosis in children. Circulation *47*, *48*, Suppl. IV, 222 (1973)

26. Indication for Surgical Treatment in Patients With Hypertrophic Obstructive Cardiomyopathy

H. KUHN, W. KRELHAUS, W. BIRCKS, H. D. SCHULTE, and F. LOOGEN

Clinical recognition of hypertrophic obstructive cardiomyopathy (HOCM) is generally attributed to Brock in 1957 [4]. Although since that time many pathologic-anatomic, clinical, hemodynamic, echocardiographic, and angiographic features of HOCM have been well established, the therapy of HOCM consisting mainly of administration of propranolol and/or surgery has remained controversial [11]. In part this situation might be caused by the fact that clinical experience today is based on relatively small numbers of patients and on relatively short comparative follow-up periods in patients with HOCM.

Long-term studies in patients with HOCM seen in our hospital up to December 1976 show that surgery for HOCM apparently gives the best clinical and hemodynamic results [8, 9, 16, and Ch. 24]. To investigate the usefulness and the indications of surgical treatment in larger numbers of patients with HOCM, our main results, which are reported in detail elsewhere [8, 9, and Ch. 24], will be compared with those of other authors, particularly comparative long-term studies in untreated, propranolol-treated, and surgically treated patients. Furthermore, the complications and the rate of early and late mortality in surgically treated patients will be considered.

Natural Course of HOCM

In Table 1 the clinical course of untreated patients is shown. Our results are compared with those of five other cardiology centers (the multicentric study of Shah *et al.* [17] includes the data of 4 centers), which show similar periods of observation. In the majority the patients belong to clinical class II. One can see that in most patients the clinical state was unchanged. The mortality rate was the same in the multicentric as in our study (23%). No patient died in the first group of Table 1 [11]. But one has to consider that this group consisted only of 11 patients and the follow-up period was the shortest (4.0 years compared to 6.6 years in our study).

Clinical Course of Propranolol Treated Patients

Table 2 lists results of studies on the long-term effect of propranolol. With regard to observation time, our results are only comparable with the multicentric study. The percentage of improved patients in the multicentric study of Shah *et al.* [17] was higher than that in our study. In the Shah study, the percent-

Table 1. Natural course of HOCM.

Author	Year	Pts. (n)	Follow-up period (years)	Clinical course (% of pts)			
				Improved	Unchanged	Deteriorated	Died
Parker *et al.*	1969	11	4.0	9	82	9	–
Shah *et al.* (multicentric study)	1974	30	5.2	3	71	3	23
Our results		47	6.7	2	60	15	23

Table 2. Clinical course of propranolol-treated patients with HOCM.

Author	Year	Pts. (n)	Follow-up period (years)	Clinical course (% of pts)			
				Improved	Unchanged	Deteriorated	Died
Stenson *et al.*	1973	13	1.4	62	23	15	–
Powell *et al.*	1973	29	1.3	42	34	17	7
Shah *et al.* (multicentric study)	1974	100	5.2	28	47	6	19
Our results		77	4.7	10	70	7	13

age of unchanged patients in the propranolol-treated group was lower than that of unchanged patients in the untreated group.

These findings are not in agreement with ours, which reveal a higher percentage of unchanged patients than did the multicentric study. This discrepancy might be due to the fact that our results were obtained in consecutive cases from one center, whereas the data from Shah *et al.* were summarized from four centers, i.e., a different selection and a different clinical classification of patients were possibly applied. Furthermore in the early years possibly the doses of propranolol administered to our patients were smaller. However in a preliminary report of a long-term study in England [5] in 1966, the doses were also very small, varying from 5–20 mg 3 times a day and yielding subjective improvement in 10 of 13 patients. Furthermore, it must be considered that the percentage of class III patients in the propranolol-treated group was higher than that in the untreated group (Table 3). Nevertheless, in both studies the percentage of unchanged patients is much higher than that of improved patients. Furthermore considering different follow-up periods of our patients, the percentage of deteriorated patients and patients who died was not improved by propranolol in either study.

Table 3. Clinical course of patients with HOCM.[a]

Therapy	Author	Pts. (n)	Follow-up period (Y)	Class (NYHA)	Improvement (%)	Deterioration (%)	Died: Follow-up (%)	Died: During surgery (%)
Untreated	Parker *et al.* 1969; Shah *et al.* 1974; Our results	81	5.7	II	3.1	11.0	21.2	–
Propranolol	Shah *et al.* 1974; Our results	168	5.2	II–(III)	20.5	6.5	16.5	–
Surgery	Tajik *et al.* 1974; Shah *et al.* 1974; Morrow *et al.* 1975; Gerbaux *et al.* 1976; Rothlin *et al.* 1976; Our results	304	5.6	III	79.0	1.0	8.0	3.1 (11.7)

[a] Data represents mean values calculated from previously published data. Operative mortality was 3.1% (11.7%). See Tables 7 and 8 for explanation.

Course of Surgically Treated Patients

Of 41 surgically treated patients, 75% preoperatively belonged to clinical class III (Table 4). Follow-up studies were performed on 28 patients who fulfilled the condition that the interval to the time of surgery was at least one year. Table 5 relates our clinical data to that on 28 patients (of 41 treated surgically before December 1976) in whom the interval to surgery was at least 1 year. The 7% of our patients who died (n = 2) was calculated from 28 patients of the follow-up study, but the 5.3% was calculated from the total of 36 patients who survived surgery. For the other studies, the percentage of patients who died was calculated only from the patients of the follow-up studies, as shown in the second column. Table 5 demonstrates, in agreement with our results, that improvement of clinical class can be observed in the great majority of patients, clinical class I often existing postoperatively [8–10]. Furthermore in contrast to hemodynamic controls in conservatively managed patients [8, 9, and Chapter 24, Loogen *et al.*], in most cases a reduction of left ventricular enddiastolic pressure and a complete abolition of left ventricular outflow tract gradient was consistently measured (Fig. 1). It has yet to be considered that the compatability

Table 4. Preoperative functional class (NYHA) of surgically treated patients with HOCM.

<table>
<tr><th rowspan="2">Author</th><th rowspan="2">Year</th><th rowspan="2">No. of operated pts.</th><th colspan="4">Functional class (%)</th></tr>
<tr><th>I</th><th>II</th><th>III</th><th>IV</th></tr>
<tr><td>Barratt-Boyes et al.</td><td>1971</td><td>30</td><td>3</td><td>44</td><td>30</td><td>23</td></tr>
<tr><td>Schmahl et al.</td><td>1974</td><td>11</td><td>–</td><td>–</td><td>23</td><td>73</td></tr>
<tr><td>Bigelow et al.</td><td>1974</td><td>39</td><td>5</td><td>8</td><td colspan="2">87</td></tr>
<tr><td>Tajik et al.</td><td>1974</td><td>43</td><td>7</td><td>21</td><td colspan="2">72</td></tr>
<tr><td>Morrow et al.</td><td>1975</td><td>83</td><td>–</td><td>1</td><td>70</td><td>29</td></tr>
<tr><td>Rothlin et al.</td><td>1976</td><td>35</td><td colspan="2">48</td><td colspan="2">52</td></tr>
<tr><td>Gerbaux et al.</td><td>1976</td><td>26</td><td>4</td><td>39</td><td>34</td><td>23</td></tr>
<tr><td>Our results</td><td></td><td>41</td><td>–</td><td>10</td><td>75</td><td>15</td></tr>
</table>

Table 5. Postoperative course of patients with HOCM.

Author	Year	Pts. (n)	Follow-up period (years)	Clinical course (% of reexamined pts) Improved	Unchanged	Deteriorated	Died
Barratt-Boyes *et al.*	1971	29	1.4	90	3	–	7
Tajik *et al.*	1974	35	7.0	72	17	–	11
Schmahl *et al.*	1974	10	1–7	90	10	–	–
Shah *et al.* (multicentric study)	1974	41	5.2	58	27	5	10
Morrow *et al.*	1975	61	5.7	97	–	–	3
Rothlin *et al.*	1976	32	5.0	78	16	–	6
Gerbaux *et al.*	1976	23	5.7	66	17	–	17
Our results		28	5.0	79	14	–	7

of these data is reduced by the fact that hemodynamic control periods varied greatly, i.e., from several months to several years, though in more comparable studies similar results were obtained [10].

Mortality in HOCM and Complications of Surgical Treatment

Severe complications of surgical treatment were ventricular septal defect, embolic events, mitral insufficiency, and aortic insufficiency. The percentage of 365 surgically treated patients summarized from the literature is small [i.e., 15 cases (4%), Table 6]. In addition, Tables 7 and 8 show the mortality of surgical treatment in HOCM, which without analysis of surgical techniques reaches an average of 11.7%. But mortality is much smaller (3.1%, Fig. 8) if different periods of surgical therapy are compared. Table 8 shows results obtained from reports in the literature which contained corresponding data.

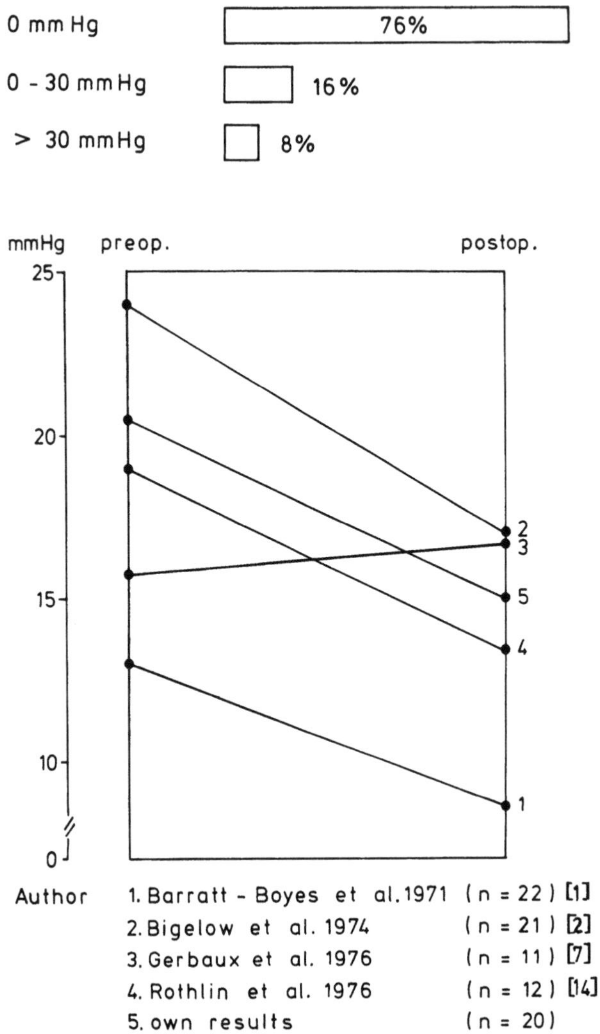

Fig. 1. Left ventricular enddiastolic pressure (a) (LVEDP) and mean postoperative outflow gradient of the left ventricle in HOCM [1, 2, 7, 10, 14, 15, 19]

In our earlier long-term studies the rate of patients who died tended to be smaller in surgically treated patients than in propranolol-treated patients [8, 9], i.e., out of 41 surgically treated patients, 36 survived surgery and only 2 of these 36 died during follow-up (5.6%), whereas out of 77 propranolol-treated patients 10 died (13%, Table 2). Similar observations were made by others [17, 7]. By comparing the mean mortality rate, calculated from data of different publications, this tendency seems to be confirmed (Table 3). The mortality rate appears to be twice as high in the propranolol group (16.5%) compared to the mortality rate in the surgically managed group (8.0%) during a fairly identical follow-up period (5.2 and 5.6 years, respectively).

Table 6. Complications of surgery in patients with HOCM.

Author	Year	n (pts.)	LBBB	AV-block III	VSD	Embol.	Mitral-I.	Aortic. I.
Barratt-Boyes *et al.*	1971	30	?	–	–	–	–	–
Cooley *et al.*	1971	54	?	1	3	–	1	1
Arbenz *et al.*	1974	30	25	3	–	–	–	–
Bigelow *et al.*	1974	39	?	3	–	–	–	1
Tajik *et al.*	1975	43	13	5	–	–	–	–
Morrow *et al.*	1975	102	?	3	5	?	?	?
Gerbaux *et al.*	1976	26	4	?	?	?	?	?
Our results		41	2	2	1	1	1	1

Table 7. Mortality of surgically treated patients with HOCM.

Author	Year	n (pts.)	Op.-mort. (% of pts)
Cooley *et al.*	1971	54	17
Barratt-Boyes *et al.*	1971	30	3
Shah *et al.* (multicentric study)	1974	58	26
Tajik *et al.*	1974	43	16
Morrow *et al.*	1975	102	6
Rothlin *et al.*	1976	35	3
Gerbaux *et al.*	1976	26	11.5
Binet *et al.*	1976	52	10
Our results		41	12
			$\bar{x} = 11.7$

Table 8. Mortality of surgically treated patients with HOCM as related to operative period.

Author	Year	Pats. (n)	Overall mortality (%)	1st period Op. period	(n)	Mortal. (%)	2nd period Op. period	(n)	Mortal. (%)
Bigelow *et al.*	1974	39	7.5	till 1965	9	33.3	1965–1973	30	0
Tajik *et al.*	1974	43	16.0	1958–1966	26	20.0	1966–1974	17	11.7
Morrow *et al.*	1975	102	6.0	1960–1970	48	12.5	1970–1975	52	0
Our results		41	12.0	1963–1969	13	23.0	1970–1976	28	7.1
			$\bar{x} = 9.4$			$\bar{x} = 18.0$			$\bar{x} = 3.1$

Conclusions and Comments

Many problems occur when data about treatment of HOCM from different publications is compared and if corresponding averages of the results are calculated. Problems include different doses of propranolol, different surgical techniques, different age distributions, different lengths of follow-up, different patients selection criteria, and modified definitions of clinical class, of early and late operative mortality, or of complications. Nevertheless, comparison of therapeutic results published in the literature seems to allow the following conclusions:

Surgical treatment of HOCM apparently yields the best clinical and hemodynamic results. The most frequent and effective technique today seems to be myotomy and myectomy of the ventricular septum, performed by transaortic approach [10]. Both the symptomatic and probably hemodynamic (reduction of LVEDP, reduction or complete relief of outflow tract obstruction) improvement seem to be long-lasting. Furthermore, today a relatively low complication and mortality rate at least in experienced centers can be assumed. A striking fact is that the late mortality rate of surgically treated patients tends to be distinctly smaller than that of propranolol-treated patients. This observation requires further studies.

The propranolol therapy of HOCM can also lead to long-lasting subjective improvement, but results from the literature, according to our former findings [8,9], seem to indicate no considerable difference between the natural life history and the course of propranolol-treated patients. New methods of conservative management of HOCM seem to be necessary. First results after applying verapamil in high doses have been reported (Kaltenbach *et al.*, Chapter 27).

The main reasons for advising surgical treatment of HOCM seem to be: 1. high probability of distinct subjective and hemodynamic improvement, 2. long-lasting effects, 3. distinct tendency of reduced late mortality rate. These results indicate that candidates for surgical approach should be primarily patients of clinical class III, in whom propranolol has proved ineffective. Furthermore, surgical treatment should be advised in all patients of clinical class IV, because long-lasting improvement in these patients by propranolol and other drugs (e.g. digitalis) cannot be expected [8] and because these patients show a very high mortality rate (Krelhaus *et al.*, Chapter 25), on the other hand the most impressive improvement by surgical repair is observed mainly in patients of clinical class IV [8,10]. Arguments for justifying surgical approach at least in patients with severe obstruction (i.e., obstruction to left ventricular outflow of more than 100 mm Hg present at rest) independently of clinical class and previous propranolol therapy are primarily: 1. high probability of complete, long-lasting relief of outflow tract gradient and reduction of LVEDP, 2. the possibly causative role of outflow tract gradient for the progression of the disease [8,9], and 3. the clear tendency of reduced late mortality rate independent of clinical class [8,9,15, Loogen *et al.*, Chapter 24).

References

1. Barratt-Boyes, B.G., O'Brien, K.P.: Surgical treatment of idiopathic hypertrophic subaortic stenosis using a combined left ventricular-aortic approach. In: Hypertrophic Obstructive Cardiomyopathy. Ciba Foundation Study Group, 37. Wolstenholme, G.E.W., O'Connor, M. (eds.), pp. 150–159. London: J. and A. Churchill Ltd. 1971
2. Bigelow, W., Trimble, A.S., Wigle, D., Adelman, A.G., Felderhof, C.: The treatment of muscular subaortic stenosis. J. Thorac. cardiovasc. Surg. *68*, 384 (1974)

3. Binet, J.P., Langlois, J., Conso, J.F., Planche, C.: Traitement chirurgical de 52 cardiomyopathies obstructives. Arch. Mal. Cœur *69*, 777 (1976)
4. Brock, R.: Functional obstruction of the left ventricle. Guy's Hosp. Rep. *106*, 221 (1957)
5. Cherian, G., Brockington, I.F., Shah, P.M., Oakley, C.M., Goodwin, J.F.: Beta adrenergic blockade in hypertrophic obstructive cardiomyopathy. Brit. med. J. *1*, 895 (1966)
6. Cooley, D.A., Leachman, R.D., Hallman, G.L.: Idiopathic hypertrophic subaortic stenosis: Surgical treatment including mitral valve replacement. Arch. Surg. (Chicago) *103*, 606 (1971)
7. Gerbaux, A., Hanania, G., Godefroid, A., Baragan, J., Maouad, J., Gay, J.: Résultats à long terme du traitement chirurgical de la myocardiopathie obstructive par intervention sur le septum interventriculaire. Arch. Mal. Cœur *69*, 791 (1975)
8. Loogen, F., Krelhaus, W., Kuhn, H.: Verlaufsbeobachtungen der hypertrophischen obstruktiven Myocardiopathie (HOCM). Z. Kardiol. *65*, 511 (1976)
9. Loogen, F., Kuhn, H.: Classification and natural history of primary cardiomyopathies. International Symposium on Myocardial Failure, Rottach-Egern, Juni 1976 (in press)
10. Morrow, A.G., Reitz, B.A., Epstein, S.E., Henry, W.L., Conkle, D.M., Itscoitz, S.B., Redwood, D.R.: Operative treatment in hypertrophic subaortic stenosis. Circulation *52*, 88 (1975)
11. Oakley, C.M.: Surgical correction of ASH. Circulation *19*, 951 (1975)
12. Parker, B.M.: The course in idiopathic hypertrophic subaortic stenosis. Ann. intern. Med. *70*, 903 (1969)
13. Powell, W.J., Whiting, R.B., Dinsmore, R.E., Sanders, C.A.: Symptomatic prognosis in patients with idiopathic hypertrophic subaortic stenosis (IHSS). Amer. J. Med. *55*, 15 (1973)
14. Rothlin, M., Arbenz, U., Krayenbühl, H.P., Turina, J., Senning, A.: Spätresultate nach Operationen bei muskulärer subvalvulärer Aortenstenose. Z. Kardiol. *65*, 501 (1976)
15. Schmahl, T.M., Flemma, R.J., Tector, A.J., Lepley, D.: Surgical management of idiopathic hypertrophic subaortic stenosis. Ann. thorac. Surg. *18*, 437 (1974)
16. Schulte, H.D., Bircks, W., Körfer, R.: Surgical results of idiopathic hypertrophic subaortic stenosis with special reference to the transaortic approach. 7th Congress of the Eur. Soc. Cardiol., Amsterdam, 20.–25. Juni 1976. Abstracts 1976: 221.
17. Shah, P.M., Adelman, A.G., Wigle, E.D., Gobel, F.L., Burchell, H.B., Hardarson, T., Curiel, R., Caldaza, C., Oakley, C.M., Goodwin, J.F.: The natural and unnatural history of hypertrophic obstructive cardiomyopathy. Circulat. Res. *34*, *35*, Suppl. II, 179 (1974)
18. Stenson, R.E., Flamm, M.D., Harrison, D.C., Hancock, E.W.: Hypertrophic subaortic stenosis. Amer. J. Cardiol. *31*, 763 (1973)
19. Tajik, A.J., Giuliani, E.R., Weidman, W.H., Brandenburg, R.O., McGoon, D.C.: Idiopathic hypertrophic subaortic stenosis, long term surgical follow up. Amer. J. Cardiol. *34*, 815 (1974)

27. Verapamil Treatment of Hypertrophic Obstructive Cardiomyopathy

M. Kaltenbach, R. Hopf, G. Kober, W.-D. Bussmann, M. Keller, and Y. Petersen

First described in the last century, HOCM is recognized today in a considerable number of patients. The severity of the disorder varies between severe disablement to a completely asymptomatic clinical picture.

Therapy must be adjusted to symptoms and prognosis. Today most patients are treated medically, while others require no therapy; surgery appears to offer the best treatment for a small group of patients [11,13].

Medical therapy with beta-blockers, especially propranolol, has now been in use for more than 10 years. Long-time follow-up reveals more scepticism than enthusiasm. It seems that the progression of the disease cannot be stopped, and that recurrence of symptoms is common [2,5,6,9,14,15].

Experimentally it has been shown that certain forms of CM can be prevented with calcium-inhibitive medication. This was shown for the hereditary CM of the Syrian hamster [10]. Recently similar findings were reported on experimentally Adriamycin-induced CM [1].

Although differences exist between the experimental animal CM and the disease in man, the final mechanism of myocardial damage may in all instances be attributed to a similar mechanism consisting of calcium overload of the myocardial cell [3,17].

As shown in preceding contributions, patients with HOCM may reveal remarkably high left ventricular contractility even in advanced stages of the disease. The high sensitivity to catecholamines and to digitalis is also well known. These properties could be related to an increased availability of intracellular calcium.

After a pilot study lasting 2 years a clinical trial with a calcium inhibitor, Verapamil, was initiated in a group of 22 patients, consisting of 18 males and 4 females, aged 19–44 years.

Methods

Subjective symptoms were evaluated from a questionnaire given to the patient. ECGs were taken every 3 months with special attention to accurate calibration. Phonograms and carotid pulse readings were repeatedly recorded. Echocardiograms were taken with the Picker System.

Heart volume was calculated from chest X-Rays in the supine position, and in addition conventional chest X-Rays in the standing position were taken. Right and left heart catheterization, selective coronary arteriography and cineangiography of the left ventricle in two planes were performed. Angiograms of the right ventricle were only taken if a systolic pressure gradient within the right ventricle was recorded.

Repeated catheter studies were done in 10 patients. In the follow-up study, after long-term treatment with Verapamil, right and left heart catheterization, selective coronary arteriography and ventriculography were repeated; in addition contractility of the left ventricle was studied by means of a Millar-double-tip catheter at rest and during exercise. Exercise was performed on a bicycle ergometer in supine position with a workload of 50–100 W for 6 min. After recovery from the first exercise test 10 mg Verapamil were injected within 10 min and a second test was performed with the same workload and the same duration of exercise. Pressure and contractility measurements (max dp/dt and dp/dt/p) were recorded through the double-tip catheter with one transducer in the apex and one in the outflow tract of the left ventricle.

Coronary artery diameters were measured in different locations from the cineangiograms using a TV camera mounted on a cineprojector for high magnification.

Left ventricular muscle mass was calculated from left ventricular free wall and left ventricular enddiastolic volume (LVEDV). LVEDV and left ventricular endsystolic volume (LVSV) were determined from outlines of the left ventricle in two planes (RAO and LAO). For calculations Simpson's rule by means of the computer system "Volumat" (Siemens) was applied.

Medication

Before the study most patients had been treated with beta-blockers, either propranolol 120–240 mg/day or Pindolol 7.5–15 mg/day, over several months or years. This and all other medication was stopped when treatment with Verapamil was started. After one week of treatment with 80 mg t.i.d., dosage was increased to 160 mg t.i.d., i.e., to 480 mg per day. In some patients the dose was further increased after several months to 120 mg 6 times daily (i.e., 720 mg/day). In long-term treatment the drug was always administered orally.

Results

Side Effects

One patient revealed a first-degree a-V block with an a-V interval of 0.3 s during administration of 480 mg Verapamil/day. After reduction of the dose to 240 mg, the pR interval became normal. In the remaining patients no change in pR interval could be measured.

Subjective Symptoms

Fifty percent of the patients reported lessening or complete relief of chest pain or breathlessness under effort. Twenty-two percent complained of dizziness, nausea, headache, or chest pain in the first weeks of treatment, but these symptoms disappeared under continued therapy. Twenty-eight percent of the patients had only minor subjective symptoms and noticed no essential change during therapy.

Heart Rate, Blood Pressure

The average heart rate decreased from 68 to 65 beats/min; the difference was statistically not significant. *Blood pressure* became normal in one patient with moderate hypertension; in the remaining patients no change was observed.

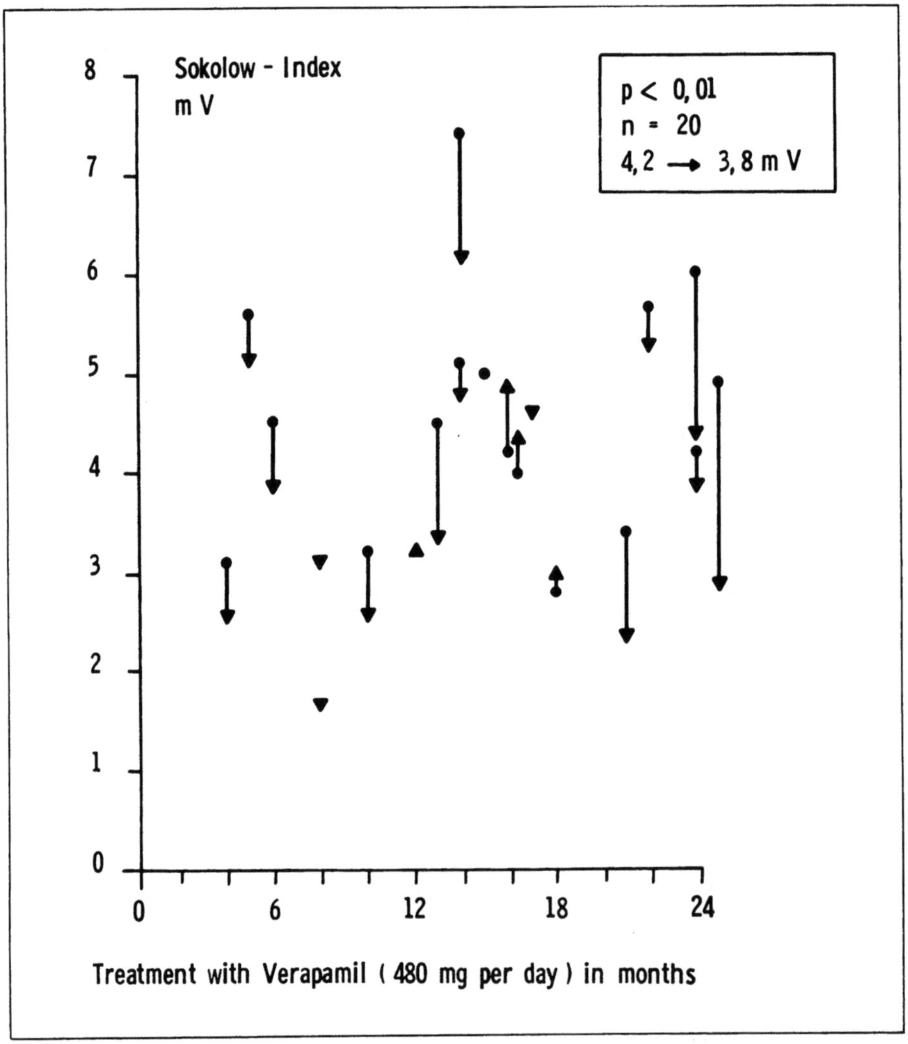

Fig. 1. Sokolow index (maximal S plus maximal R in $V_1 - V_6$) before and after treatment. Mean values show a significant reduction

Left Ventricular Hypertrophy in the ECG

Over 4–24 months (average 15 months) treatment a significant reduction in QRS amplitude occurred. The average Sokolow-index (maximal S + maximal R in Wilson V_1–V_6) decreased from 4.2–3.8 mV. Twelve patients showed a decrease of QRS amplitude, five patients were unchanged, and three showed an increase (Fig. 1). In patients with reduction of QRS amplitude a change of the ST-segment versus normalization could usually be observed (see Fig. 2). The changes in QRS amplitude during treatment with Verapamil were compared with the values obtained in the preceding period under beta-blockade (Fig. 3). During therapy with beta-blockers an unchanged or steadily increasing amplitude is usually observed, while a decrease under Verapamil occurs in most patients.

Phonocardiogram

The systolic murmur did not disappear during treatment; quantitative evaluations were not done. On auscultation, however, a decrease in loudness of the murmur was noticed in most patients. Carotid pulse traces revealed no significant changes.

Echocardiographic studies were carried out, but the results are inconclusive because the number of follow-up studies is too small. Further work is in progress.

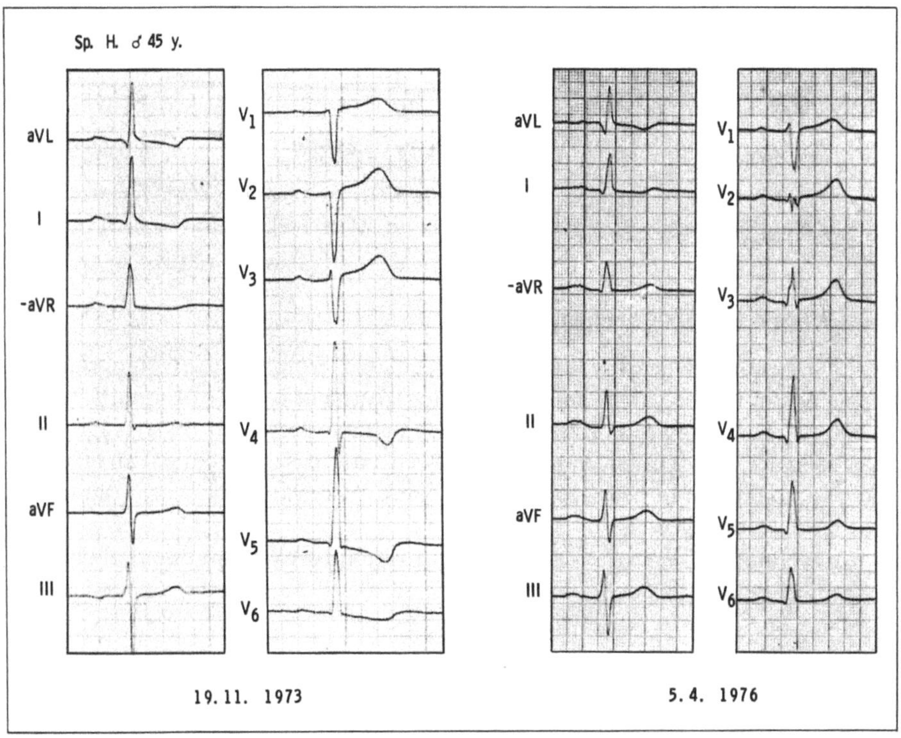

Fig. 2. Example of ECGs before and after treatment from a patient with HOCM

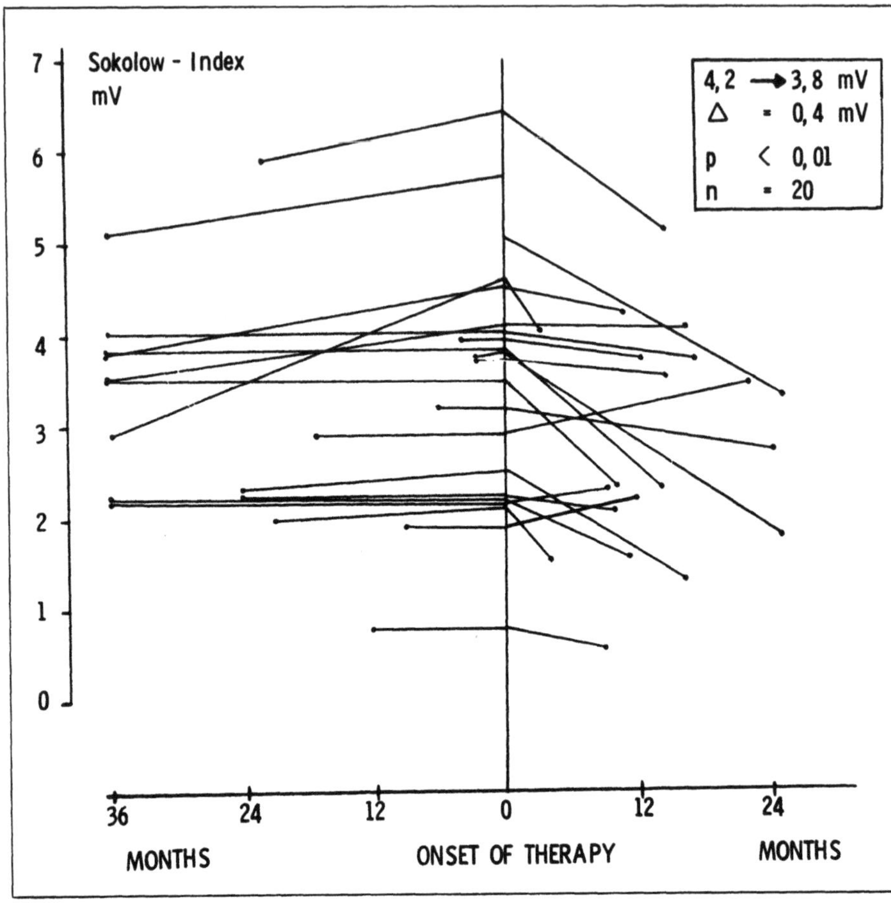

Fig. 3. Sokolow index in the precordial ECG during beta-blockers (left) and Verapamil treatment (right)

Chest X-Rays and Heart Volume

In 21 patients the heart volume was calculated from teleroentgenograms in supine position. The values before and after treatment over 2–24 months (mean 14 months) are shown in Figure 4. Heart volume decreased on average from 858–766 ml/1.73 m^2. Eighteen patients showed a decrease, one patient an increase, and two no change in heart volume. In Figure 5 the values of heart volume are shown on a time scale.

Conventional chest x-rays in standing position revealed no essential change; no signs of congestion were observed.

Heart Catheterization

Before the study all patients had undergone right and left heart catheterization, angiocardiography and selective coronary arteriography. Ten patients were recatheterized after 14–24 months of treatment (mean 19 months). The values

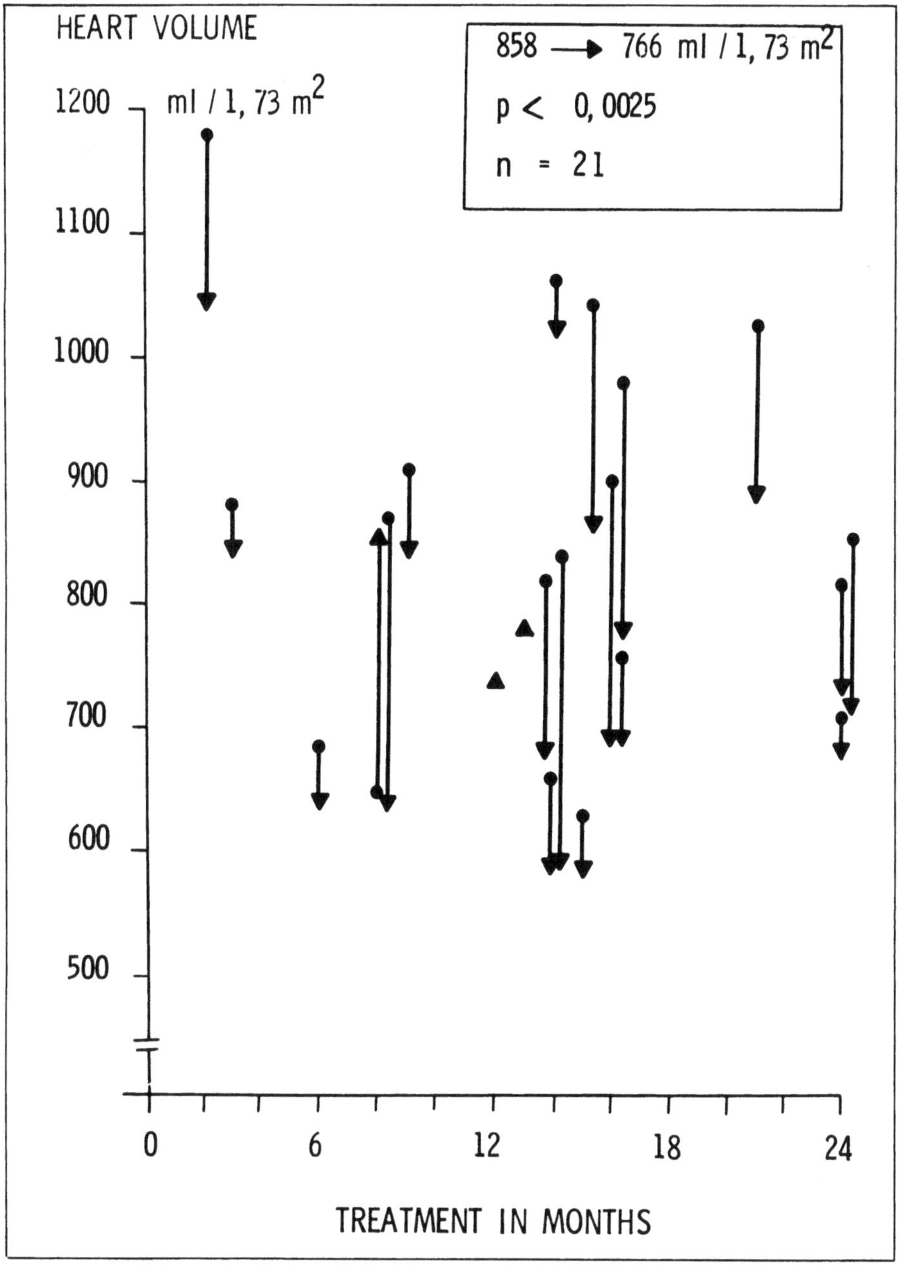

Fig. 4. Heart volume, calculated from two teleroentgenograms in supine position before and after treatment. Under Verapamil a significant reduction of the mean values occurred

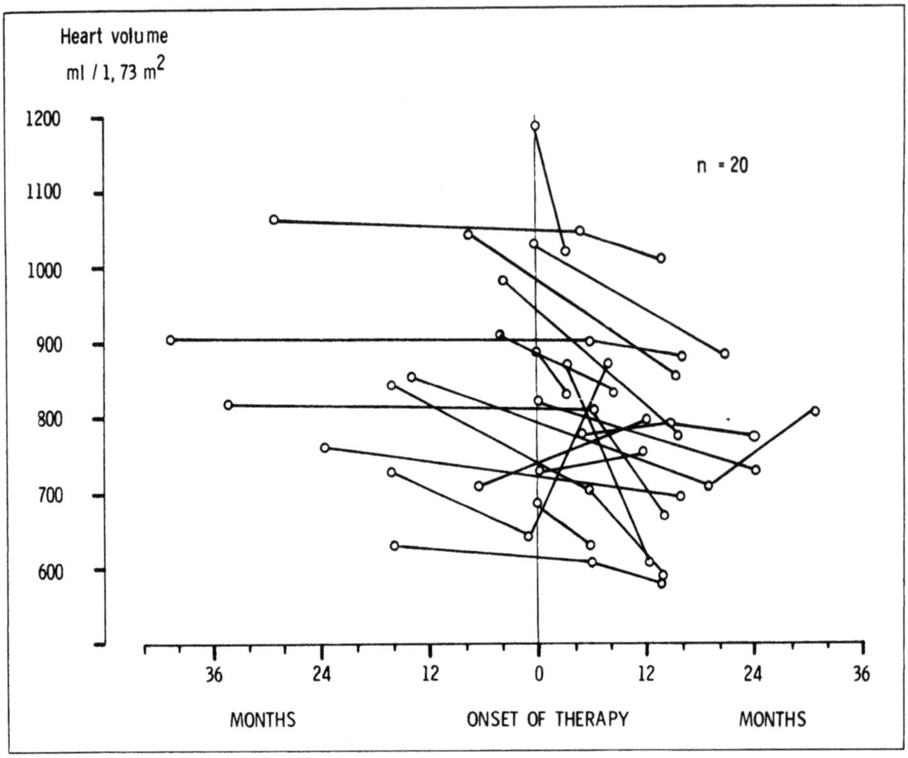

Fig. 5. Heart volume during beta-blocker (left) and Verapamil treatment (right). Note the decrease after the beginning of Verapamil treatment

obtained were compared with those of the first catheterization which was done prior to or at the time Verapamil treatment was started. In four patients the first catheterization was performed more than 1 year before the beginning of Verapamil treatment.

The intraventricular systolic pressure gradient in the left ventricle showed a reduction in five of eight patients; in one patient no gradient was present, and in one it could not be reevaluated. There were some differences among the resting gradient and the gradient during provocation (Fig. 6).

As Table 1 indicates LVEDP and ejection fraction (EF) showed no significant difference while left ventricular muscle mass (LVMM) decreased in seven and increased in three patients (Fig. 7). In the three patients with increased LVMM the first catheterization was performed 2–3 years prior to the beginning of the Verapamil treatment. After the first catheterization a further increase of LVMM may have occurred before Verapamil treatment was started.

Selective Coronary Arteriography

Two independent investigators measured coronary artery diameter at five different sites (Fig. 8). The investigators were not aware whether they were analysing

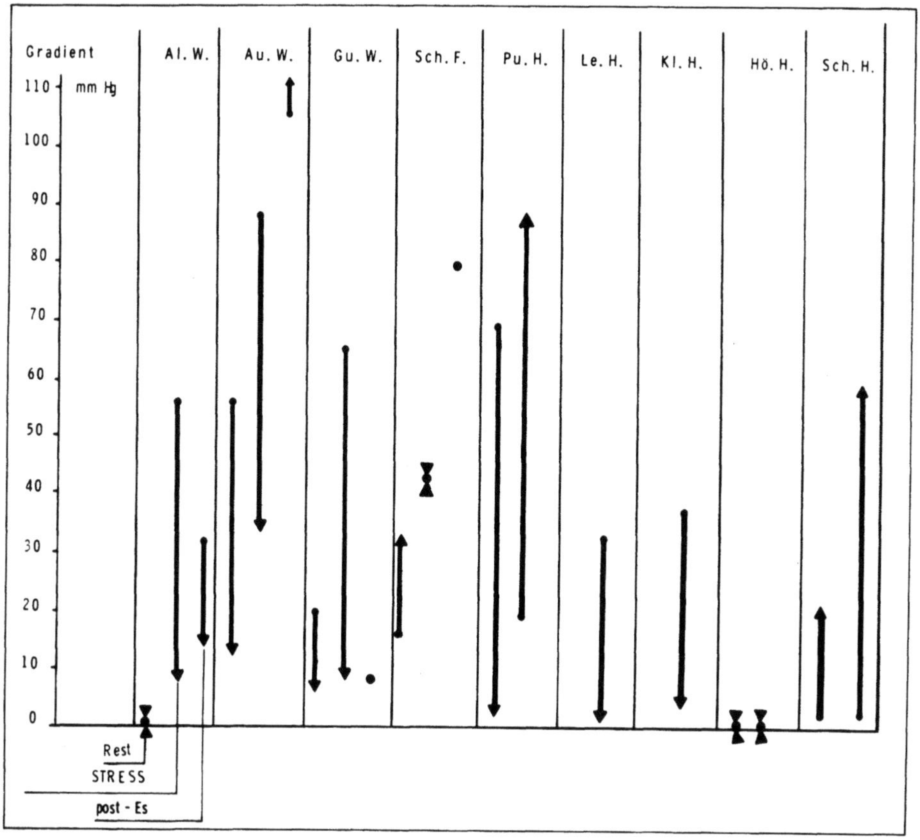

Fig. 6. Systolic pressure gradients within the left ventricle as measured at the time of the first and second catheterization

the first or the second angiogram of a given patient. The differences in X-ray magnification were corrected. Premedication was the same.

Seven patients showed a decrease, one an increase, and two unchanged coronary diameters (Fig. 8). On the average both coronary arteries were significantly reduced in diameter (8% RCA, 9% LCA) and in cross sectional area (15% RCA, 17% LCA) (see Fig. 9).

Table 2 summarizes the different values obtained. There is in general a good agreement among changes of different parameters such as interventricular gradient, left ventricular muscle mass, QRS amplitude, heart volume and coronary artery diameter.

Left Ventricular Contractility Under Acute Medication of Verapamil

Bearing in mind that the effect of Verapamil can be demonstrated by a change in contractility, i.e., a reduction of contractility at rest or during exercise, 11 patients with HOCM were studied by means of a Millar-double-tip catheter. Eight of them were treated with Verapamil prior to this investigation; three were not treated. After measurements under resting conditions an exercise test was per-

Table 1. Data of 10 patients with recatheterization. In the three patients with increased left ventricular muscle mass, the first catheterization was done 1–4 years prior to the beginning of Verapamil treatment.

PATIENT	Date of Catheterization	EDV ml/1,73 m²	EF %	Mm ml/1,73m²	Beginning of Verapamil treatment	Duration of treatment in months
Gu. W.	10.11. 1972 31. 8. 1976	105 142	63 63	148 101	6,75	14
Re. K.	7. 3. 1974 14. 9. 1976	85 89	78 76	122 110	4,75	15
Au. W.	11.12. 1974 7. 9. 1976	72 95	75 85	151 104	9,74	24
Sch. F.	19. 8. 1974 7. 9. 1976	149 146	88 93	154 112	9,74	24
Hö. H.	25. 6. 1973 27. 9. 1976	86 90	89 88	126 138	3,74	23
Sch. H.	26. 3. 1975 21. 9. 1976	201 109	80 71	417 318	7,75	16
Kl. H.	9. 3. 1972 23.11. 1976	109 131	85 86	349 296	4,75	19
Le. H.	29. 5. 1972 9.11. 1976	80 120	89 90	91 134	6,75	17
Pu. H.	29. 7. 1971 9. 11. 1976	117 179	90 91	232 301	5,75	18
Al. W.	11.12. 1974 14. 9. 1976	98 114	90 90	250 213	6,75	15
$\bar{x}$		110 121 p=0,20	82 83 p=0,35	204 182 p=0,1		

formed. After recovery, 10 mg Verapamil were given intravenously. A second exercise test was performed 10 min after injection.

Left ventricular systolic and enddiastolic pressure showed a decrease (LVSP 147 → 132; LVEDP 20 → 16 mm Hg). The pressure gradient was unchanged. The heart rate under exercise was significantly higher in the second test (Fig. 10). Contractility showed no essential difference before and after Verapamil injection, either at rest or under exercise. Figure 11 shows the values of max dp/dt. Figure 12 shows corresponding results before and after administration of a beta-blocker; in sharp contrast to Verapamil a marked reduction in resting contractility and complete abolition of contractility reserve can be demonstrated with identical methodology. Similar results were shown by Roskamm [12].

Discussion

The clinical impression during this study was that Verapamil offered a better therapeutic approach to HOCM as compared to the treatment with beta-blockers. Whenever a new drug is administered, a drug-free interval after some time of

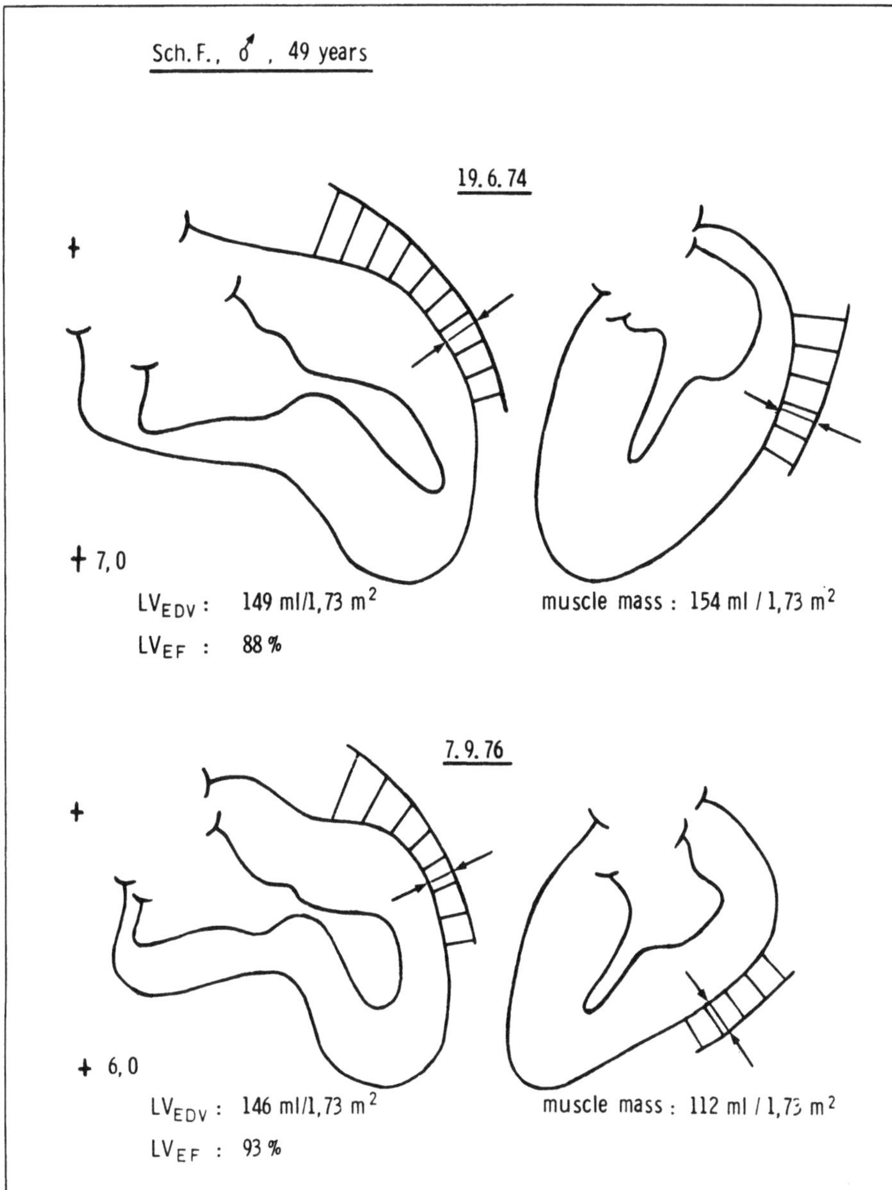

Fig. 7. Example of reduction in left ventricular muscle mass as calculated from free left ventricular wall in two planes and LVEDV determined from biplane angiograms using Simpsons' rule calculation

its application is desirable in order to assess the efficacy of the new medication. In the present investigation we did not, however, decide to interrupt the treatment.

The subjective and objective changes of symptoms must be interpreted in the light of the changes that were present during pretreatment with beta-blockers.

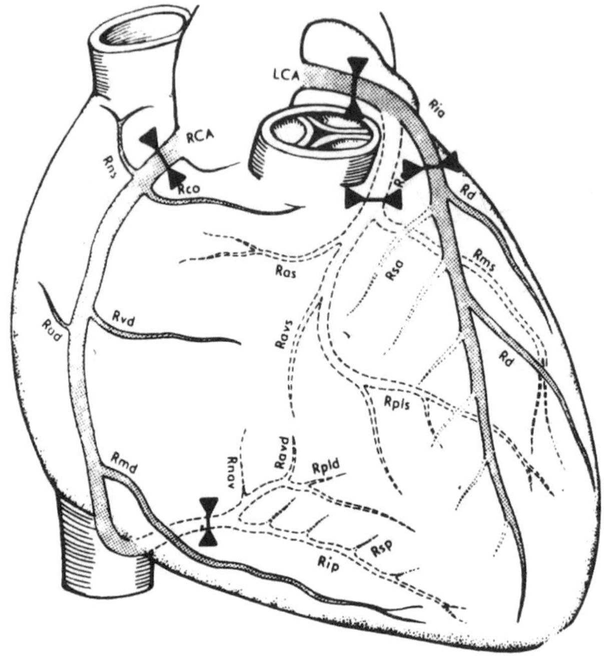

Diameter ⌀					
LCA	4.40 →	4.03 mm²	- 9 %	p < o, ol
RCA	2,72 →	2,50 mm²	- 8 %	p < o, ol
		Cross section area⊖		
LCA	15,19 →	12,58 mm²	-17 %	p < o, ol
RCA	5,81 →	4,91 mm²	-15 %	p < o, ol
	before	after	n=10	
	treatment			

Fig. 8. Measurement of coronary artery diameter in five different locations. The reduction in diameter and cross sectional area after Verapamil treatment is calculated from mean values for the right (RCA) and left (LCA) coronary artery

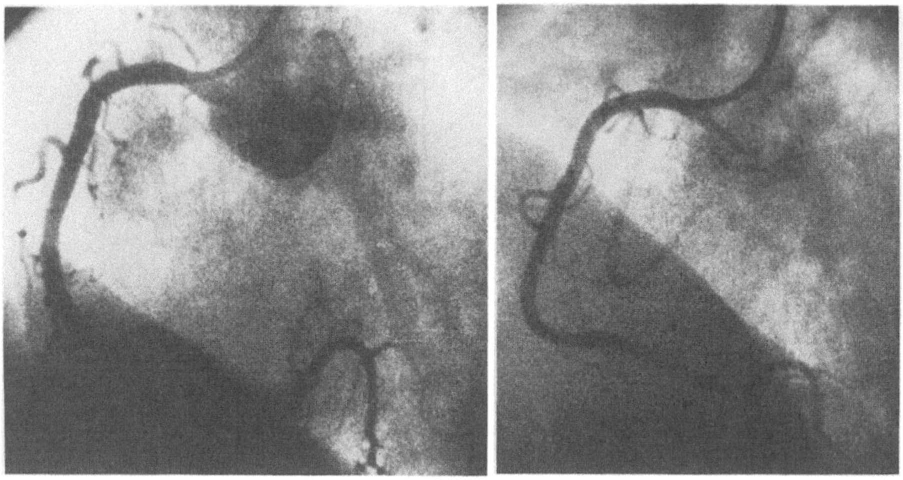

before treatment after treatment

Au. W. ♂ 48 Y

Fig. 9. Example of reduction in coronary artery diameter

Table 2. Changes in data of heart catheterization, ECG, heart volume, and coronary artery diameter in 10 patients.

PATIENT	GRADIENT	LV muscle mass		SOKOLOW-INDEX		Heart volume		Cor. art. diam.	
	mm Hg	ml/1.73m^2	%	mV	%	ml	%	mm	%
Gu. W.	20 65 ↓ 4 6	148 101	-32	5,3 4,7	-11	817 669	-18	5,9 4,9	-17
Re. K.	28 52	122 110	-10	3,5 2,3	-34	763 694	- 9	4,9 4,2	-14
Al. W.	0 56 ↓ 0 4	250 213	-15	1,7 2,1		633 581	- 8	4,1 3,6	-12
Au. W.	56 89 ↓ 9 24	151 104	-31	6,0 4,0	-33	820 731	-11	3,8 3,6	- 5
Sch. F.	15 43 =↑ 32 43	154 112	-27	4,2 4,2	0	711 657	- 8	3,9 3,9	0
Hö. H.	0 0 0 0	126 138	+ 9	2,9 3,1	+65	853 810	- 5	4,2 3,1	-26
Sch. H	0 60 ↑ 21	417 318	-24	>5 5	-x	1045· 856	-18	6.0 5,8	- 3
Kl. H	40 ↓ 4	349 296	-15	3,2 2,5	-22	645 872	+26	3,4 3,4	0
Le. H.	35 ↓ 1	91 134	+32	5,5 5,2	- 5	901 880	- 2	5.0 4,5	-10
Pu. H.	75 20 ⇕ 4 93	232 301	+23	3,6 4,9	+27	960		2,9 ,3,4	+15

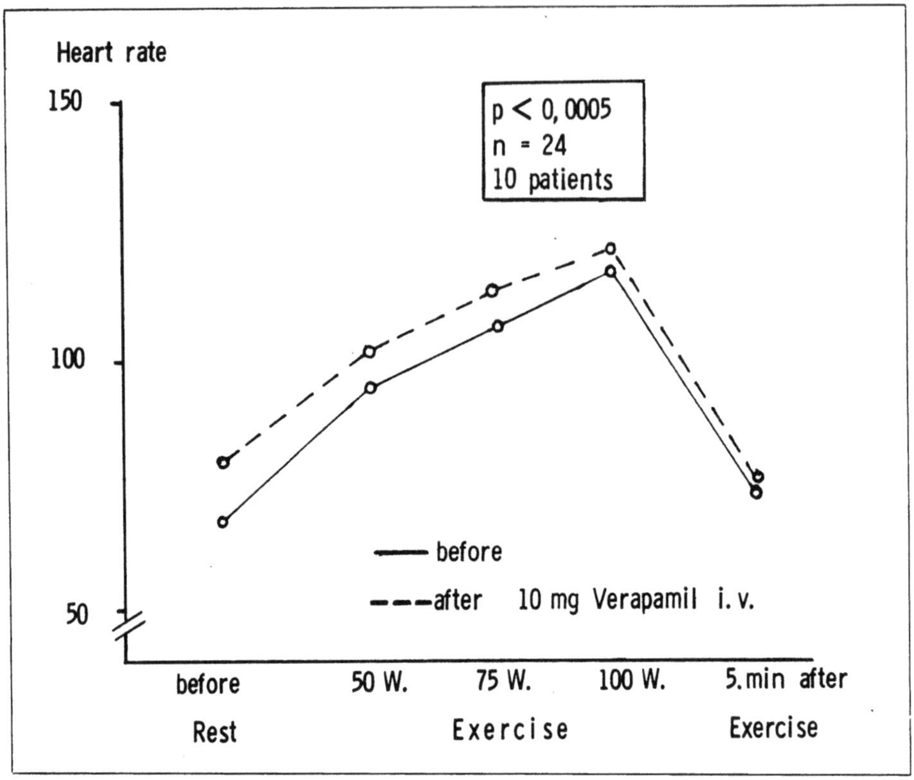
Heart rate
150
100
50
p < 0,0005
n = 24
10 patients
before
after 10 mg Verapamil i.v.
before
Rest
50 W.
75 W.
100 W.
Exercise
5.min after
Exercise

10

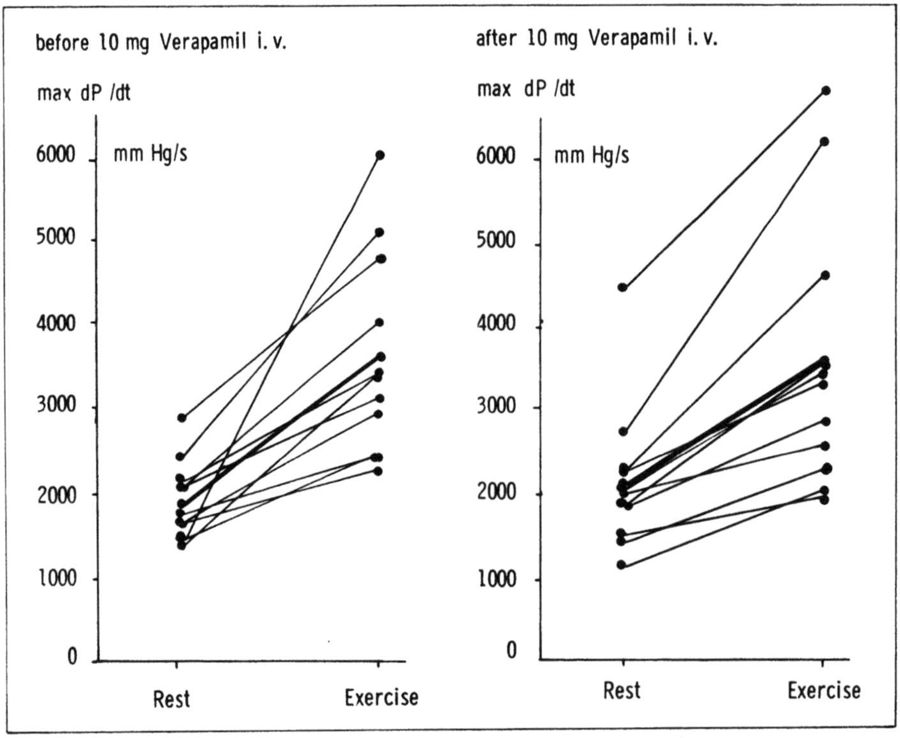
before 10 mg Verapamil i.v.
max dP /dt
mm Hg/s
6000
5000
4000
3000
2000
1000
0
Rest
Exercise
after 10 mg Verapamil i.v.
max dP /dt
mm Hg/s
6000
5000
4000
3000
2000
1000
0
Rest
Exercise

11

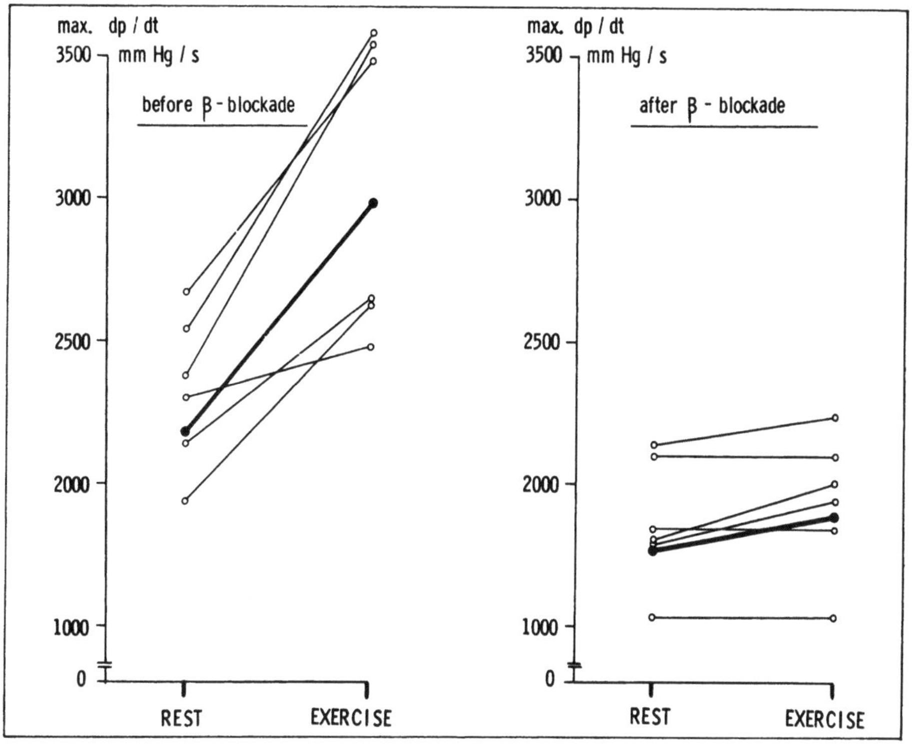

Fig. 12. Reduction in contractility and abolishment of contractility reserve after beta-blockade

It might be argued that the dose of 240 mg Propranolol daily was not as high as some authors favor. This dose, however, was not exceeded because testing of antianginal activity of beta-blockers by our own group had clearly shown that larger doses were hardly more effective. Therefore, no attempt to use increased doses was made. The question remains open whether high doses could have achieved better results. It is also possible that high doses of Propranolol reveal some nonspecific calcium-inhibitive effects.

Chest X-Rays and Heart Volume

It is known that heart volume changes can be induced by different drugs, e.g. acute administration of a beta-blocker leads to an approximately 10% increase in heart volume. We have no knowledge of any influence on heart size by acute administration of Verapamil. In this study only long-term changes were observed; influences of acute drug administration or withdrawal were avoided. The di-

◁ Fig. 10. Heart rate in the exercise tests during left heart catheterization. After 10 mg Verapamil i.v. heart rate is increased

Fig. 11. Unchanged contractility and contractility reserve after Verapamil as measured with a Millar-double-tip catheter

minished heart volume after Verapamil differs from the increase after chronic beta-blockade. It also seems important that during Verapamil no signs of cardiac failure were observed.

Heart Catheterization

The comparison of pre- and posttreatment data shows improvement in 7 out of 10 patients; in 3 it was difficult because the first cardiac catheterization was done a considerable time prior to the beginning of Verapamil treatment. From the data available it is likely that the patients under continued treatment with beta-blockers had deteriorated and the improvement achieved by Verapamil was masked by this deterioration.

Selective Coronary Arteriography

By selective coronary arteriography it is well established that vasodilators, such as nitroglycerin, increase coronary diameter [4]. A quantitative evaluation is therefore only possible if the influence of an acutely administered drug can be ruled out. Also any difference in X-ray magnifications of two studies must be taken into account when comparing coronary artery dimensions. The approximately 16% reduction in coronary artery cross sectional area seen in this study is considered real because all precautions mentioned above have been carefully observed. In an earlier study [8] a relationship between left ventricular muscle mass and coronary artery cross sectional area has been shown (Fig. 13). Accord-

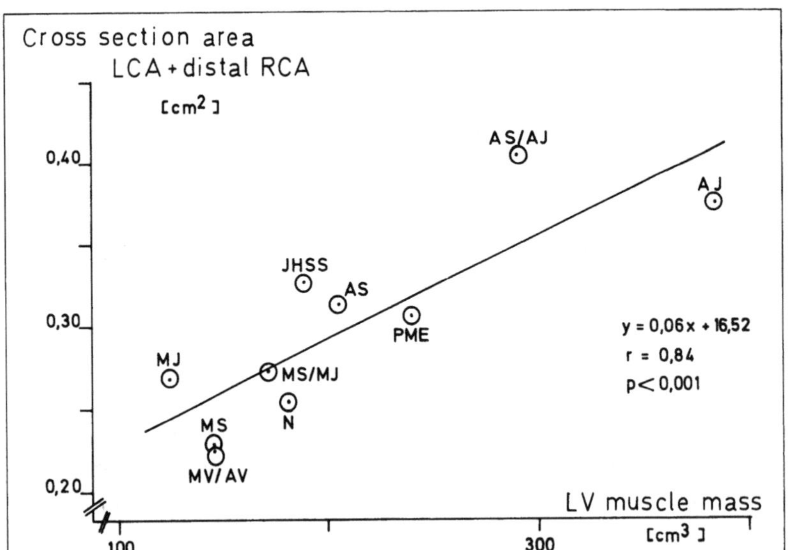

Fig. 13. Relationship of coronary artery cross section area and left ventricular muscle mass in different groups of patients (from Kober et al. [8] (1973). *MI*, Mitral insufficiency; *MS*, Mitral stenosis; *MV/AV*, Mitral and aortic valvular disease; *n*, normal; *JHSS*, HOCM; *AS*, Aortic stenosis; *PME*, Cardiomyopathies; *AJ*, Aortic insufficiency

ing to these findings it can be assumed that the observed reduction in coronary artery dimension is the consequence of a decreased ventricular muscle mass. In the context of this study the finding seems of particular interest because it reflects reduction of left ventricular hypertrophy by a factual assessment obtained by a method which is completely independent of all other measurements.

It is *concluded* from clinical data, the patients' subjective symptoms and a variety of objective measurements, that the treatment of HOCM with Verapamil has yielded encouraging results. Compared to beta-blocker therapy the superiority of this treatment appears to be clearly established.

References

1. Daniels, J.R., Billingham, M.E., Gelbart, A., Bristow, M.R.: Effect of Verapamil and Propranolol on Adriamycin-Induced Cardiomyopathy in Rabbits. 49. Sess. Am. H. Assoc., 1976, Abstr. 70
2. Edwards, R.H.T., Kristinsson, A., Warrell, D.A., Goodwin, J.F.: Effects of propranolol on response to exercise in hypertrophic obstructive cardiomyopathy. Br. Heart J. *32*, 219 (1970)
3. Fleckenstein, A.: Myokardstoffwechsel und Nekrose. In: Herzinfarkt und Schock. Heilmeyer, L., Holtmeier, H.J. (eds.). Stuttgart: Georg Thieme 1969
4. Gensini, G.G.: Coronary Arteriography. New York: Futura Publishing 1975
5. Goodwin, J.F.: Congestive and hypertrophic cardiomyopathies. A decade of study. Lancet *1970/I*, 731
6. Hubner, P.J.B., Ziady, G.M., Lane, G.K., Hardason, T., Scales, B., Oakley, C.M., Goodwin, J.F.: Double-blind trial of propranolol and practol in hypertrophic cardiomyopathy. Br. Heart J. *35*, 1116 (1973)
7. Kaltenbach, M., Hopf, R., Keller, M.: Calciumantagonistische Therapie bei hypertroph-obstruktiver Kardiomyopathie. Dtsch. med. Wschr. *101*, 1284–1287 (1976)
8. Kober, G., Spahn, G., Becker, H.-J., Kaltenbach, M.: Weite und Querschnittsfläche der großen, epikardialen Koronararterien bei Herzmuskelhypertrophie. Z. Kardiol. *63*, 297–310 (1973)
9. Loogen, F., Krelhaus, W., Kuhn, H.: Verlaufsbeobachtungen der hypertrophischen obstruktiven Myokardiopathie (HOCM). Z. Kardiol. *65*, 511–521 (1976)
10. Lossnitzer, K.: Genetic induction of cardiomyopathy. In: Handbuch der experimentellen Pharmakologie. Born, G.V.R., Eichler, O., Farah, A., Herken, H., Welche, A.D. (eds.). Berlin-Heidelberg-New York: Springer-Verlag 1975, Vol. XVI, p. 309
11. Morrow, A.G.: Operative treatment in hypertrophic subaortic techniques, and the results of pre- and postoperative assessments in 83 patients. Circul. *52*, 88–102 (1975)
12. Roskamm, H.: Die Kontraktilitätsreserve des gesunden linken Ventrikels bei körperlicher Belastung nach Beta-Rezeptorenblockade. Z. Kreisl.-Forsch. *61*, 802 (1972)
13. Rothlin, M., Arbenz, U., Krayenbühl, H.P., Turina, J., Senning, A.: Spätresultate nach Operationen bei muskulärer subvalvulärer Aortenstenose. Z. Kardiol. *65*, 501–510 (1976)
14. Stenson, R.E., Flamm, Jr., Harrison, D.C., Hancock, E.W.: Hypertrophic subaortic stenosis. Clinical and hemodynamic effects of long-term propranolol therapy. Am. J. Cardiol. *31* (1973), p. 763–773
15. Sowton, E.: Beta-Rezeptorenblocker bei hypertropher Cardiomyopathie. In: Die Beta-Blocker – Gegenwart und Zukunft. Schweizer, W. (ed.). Bern: Huber 1976, p. 239
16. Witzke, D.J., Kaye, M.P.: Hypertrophic Cardiomyopathy Induced by Administration of Nerve Growth Factor. 49. Sess. Am. Assoc. 1976, Abstr. 344
17. Wrogemann, K., Pena, S.D.J.: Mitochondrial calcium overload. A general mechanism for cell-necrosis in muscle diseases. Lancet *1976/I*, 672

Conclusions

It has become evident that CM is a rather frequent diagnosis. Although the nature of the disease is basically unknown, considerable progress in diagnosis and therapy has important clinical and therapeutic consequences.

The diagnosis of congestive CM on clinical and noninvasive findings alone is uncertain. Coronary arterial disease can be ruled out by selective coronary arteriography. In these cases myocardial biopsy has proved to be of great value, especially in identifying other forms of CM, such as sarcoidosis or amyloidosis, which may be clinically indistinguishable from congestive CM.

Distinguishing congestive CM from myocarditis can be difficult, though it has been achieved in some instances. Diffuse myocarditis is rare, and often small foci of inflammatory cells are found in the myocardium obtained at biopsy; however, a diagnosis of myocarditis in these instances cannot be justified.

In the majority of patients suspected of having congestive CM, only changes of a hypertrophied, dilated heart are found. Despite this, biopsy in these patients is justifiable because unexpected diagnoses may be made. Furthermore, myocardial biopsy offers information about the natural history and prognosis of congestive, dilated CM which cannot be obtained by clinical, noninvasive, hemodynamic or angiographic data. There is persuasive evidence that a poor prognosis of the disease can be anticipated in some instances only by myocardial biopsy. In other patients, however, despite severe clinical, hemodynamic and angiographic findings with severe impairment of left ventricular contraction, a remarkably stable course and an unchanged clinical condition may be observed over many years. The clinical value and importance of myocardial biopsy must be considered perhaps with respect more to prognosis than to a specific diagnosis.

By contrast, HOCM is well defined, and diagnosis can be made clinically and by noninvasive techniques with a high degree of accuracy. Myocardial biopsy has confirmed the characteristic changes of the disease previously defined by postmortem examination or by material obtained at surgery. The characteristic appearances of HOCM are disarray of myocardial fibers and fibrils on histologic and electron-microscopic examination. Although these appearances are not unique, quantitative changes rather than qualitative changes permit a pathologic diagnosis in many cases and furthermore help to define the degree and localization of this disorder. Hypertrophy changes, small vessel involvement and various degenerative changes of subcellular structures are less helpful findings.

In most of the patients suspected of having CM, biopsy has not so far thrown any light on the nature of the underlying disease process or processes.

Further valuable information can be anticipated. It seems likely that immunologic and biochemical studies may increase our understanding of the underlying disease or diseases.

Although myocardial biopsies have been clearly established to be of great value from both scientific and practical points of view, general application of the method is not justified. The use of this technique should be limited to centers where high standards of invasive techniques exist.

Therapy for CM remains, in most instances, symptomatic. Considerable clinical improvement can be achieved in HOCM, which may present in a wide clinical spectrum. Treatment sometimes includes surgery. In drug therapy, the concept of calcium inhibitors offers a new therapeutic approach, while beta-blocker therapy is today regarded with scepticism by several authorities.

Subject Index

MIX
Papier aus verantwortungsvollen Quellen
Paper from responsible sources
FSC® C105338

If you have any concerns about our products,
you can contact us on
ProductSafety@springernature.com

In case Publisher is established outside the EU,
the EU authorized representative is:
Springer Nature Customer Service Center GmbH
Europaplatz 3, 69115 Heidelberg, Germany

Printed by Libri Plureos GmbH
in Hamburg, Germany